Management of Facial, Head and Neck Pain

BARRY C. COOPER, D.D.S.
Associate Professor of Clinical Otolaryngology
New York Medical College
Director of Myofacial Pain Center
Department of Otolaryngology — Head and Neck Surgery
New York Eye and Ear Infirmary
New York, New York

FRANK E. LUCENTE, M.D.
Professor and Chairman
Department of Otolaryngology
New York Medical College
Chairman, Department of Otolaryngology —
 Head and Neck Surgery
New York Eye and Ear Infirmary
New York, New York

1989
W.B. SAUNDERS COMPANY
Harcourt Brace Jovanovich, Inc.
Philadelphia   London   Toronto   Montreal   Sydney   Tokyo

W. B. SAUNDERS COMPANY
Harcourt Brace Jovanovich, Inc.

The Curtis Center
Independence Square West
Philadelphia, PA 19106

Library of Congress Cataloging-in-Publication Data

Management of facial, head, and neck pain [edited by]
Barry C. Cooper, Frank E. Lucente
p. cm.

1. Headache. 2. Neck pain. 3. Facial pain.
4. Orofacial pain. I. Cooper, Barry C. II. Lucente,
Frank E. [DNLM: 1. Facial Pain—therapy. 2. Headache—
therapy. 3. Neck. 4. Pain—therapy. WE 705 M267]

RC936.M32 1989 617'.51—dc19

DNLM/DLC

ISBN 0–7216–2841–9   88-39758

Editor: W. B. Saunders Staff
Designer: Liz Schweber
Production Manager: Bill Preston
Manuscript Editor: Ruth Low
Illustration Coordinator: Brett MacNaughton
Indexer: Diana Witt

Management of Facial, Head and Neck Pain   ISBN 0–7216–2841–9

© 1989 by W. B. Saunders Company. Copyright under the Uniform Copyright Convention. Simultaneously published in Canada. All rights reserved. This book is protected by copyright. No part of it may be reproduced, stored in a retrieval system, or transmitted in any form or by any means, electronic, mechanical, photocopying, recording, or otherwise, without written permission from the publisher. Made in the United States of America. Library of Congress catalog card number 88–39758.

Last digit is the print number: 9   8   7   6   5   4   3   2   1

*This book is dedicated
To Gayle, David, and Sheree
To Bernice, Frank, and Stephen
and, most especially,
To patients who are in pain
and
To the doctors who seek to cure them*

*Wherever the art of medicine is loved,
there is also love of humanity.*

Hippocrates

Contributors

YOUNG B. CHOO, M.D.
Professor of Clinical Otolaryngology, New York Medical College, Valhalla, New York; Director, Otology, New York Eye and Ear Infirmary, New York, New York
Otalgia

DAVID L. COOPER, M.D.
Department of Surgery, State University of New York Health Science Center at Syracuse, Syracuse, New York
Perspectives in Head and Neck Pain

MONICA DWECK, M.D.
Department of Ophthalmology, New York Eye and Ear Infirmary, New York, New York
Head Pain Associated With the Eye

SHELDON GOLDSTEIN, M.D.
Clinical Instructor in Anesthesiology, State University of New York, Brooklyn, New York; State University of New York Health Science Center at Brooklyn, Brooklyn, New York
Management of Chronic Pain of the Head and Neck: An Anesthesiologist's Perspective

KEVIN C. GREENIDGE, M.D., M.P.H., F.A.C.S.
Associate Professor of Clinical Ophthalmology, New York Medical College, Valhalla, New York; Chief, Department of Ophthalmology, Director of Glaucoma Services, Metropolitan Hospital Center, New York, New York; Attending Surgeon, New York Eye and Ear Infirmary, New York, New York
Head Pain Associated With the Eye

JEFFREY T. KESSLER, M.D.
Clinical Associate Professor of Neurology, Cornell University Medical College, New York, New York; Attending Neurologist, North Shore Uni-

versity Hospital, Manhasset, New York; Assistant Attending in Medicine (Neurology), St. Francis Hospital, Roslyn, New York
Neurological Causes of Head and Face Pain

CHARLES P. KIMMELMAN, M.D.
Associate Professor of Otolaryngology, New York Medical College, Valhalla, New York; Director of Resident Training, Department of Otolaryngology, New York Eye and Ear Infirmary—New York Medical College, New York, New York
Rhinologic Causes of Facial Pain

ALLEN LEBOVITS, Ph.D.
Clinical Associate Professor of Anesthesiology and Psychiatry, State University of New York, Brooklyn, New York; State University of New York Health Science Center at Brooklyn, Kings County Medical Center, Brooklyn, New York
Management of Chronic Pain of the Head and Neck: An Anesthesiologist's Perspective

MATHEW LEFKOWITZ, M.D.
Director, Pain Management Service, Assistant Professor of Anesthesiology, State University of New York, Brooklyn, New York; State University of New York Health Science Center at Brooklyn, Kings County Medical Center, and Long Island College Hospital, Brooklyn, New York
Management of Chronic Pain of the Head and Neck: An Anesthesiologist's Perspective

KENNETH F. MATTUCCI, M.D., F.A.C.S.
Professor of Clinical Otolaryngology–Head and Neck Surgery, New York Medical College, Valhalla, New York; Chief, Division of Otolaryngology–Head and Neck Surgery, North Shore University Hospital, Manhasset, New York; Chief, Division of Otolaryngology, St. Francis Hospital, Roslyn, New York; Surgeon Director, Department of Otolaryngology–Head and Neck Surgery, New York Eye and Ear Infirmary, New York, New York
Otalgia

ROBERT L. PINCUS, M.D.
Assistant Professor of Otolaryngology, New York Medical College, Valhalla, New York; Director, Department of Otolaryngology–Head and Neck Surgery, Lincoln Hospital, Bronx, New York
Oropharyngeal, Laryngeal, and Neck Pain

THIRUMOORTHI V. SESHAN, M.D.
Assistant Professor of Rehabilitation Medicine, New York Medical College, Valhalla, New York; Attending Staff, Westchester County Medical Center, Valhalla, New York, Lincoln Hospital Center, Bronx, New York, and Metropolitan Hospital Center, New York, New York
Rehabilitation Management of Neck Pain

Contributors

DAVID A. SHAPIRO, M.D.
Associate Clinical Professor of Psychiatry, Cornell University Medical College, New York, New York; Faculty, Columbia University Psychoanalytic Center for Training and Research, New York, New York; Associate Attending Psychiatrist, The New York Hospital, New York, New York
The Psychiatric Aspects of Head, Neck, and Facial Pain

Preface

Facial, head, and neck pain provide a challenge to the clinician. The management of these types of pain may involve diagnosis and treatment by specialists from fields as diverse as ophthalmology and dentistry, otorhinolaryngology and neurology, and anesthesiology and radiology.

What makes these pain disorders so difficult to diagnose is that often a single thorough history and physical examination are not enough. Any one clinician may be unable to pinpoint an etiology or an illness that explains the patient's symptoms but may be able to rule out abnormalities that can be treated. In the end, the patient is referred to another specialist in the hope that he or she can make the correct diagnosis. However, the problem for the clinician often is deciding to whom to refer the patient.

We hope that through reading this book the clinician will develop an understanding of this complex subject and of the frequent need for involvement of a variety of specialists in providing optimum patient care.

The approach to facial, head, and neck pain discussed in this text is multidisciplinary. It involves a team of specialists, each with a knowledge and appreciation of their colleagues' fields and the broad range of diseases involved. This knowledge enables each specialist to make appropriate referrals to the correct specialists. Team members may include internists, dental specialists, neurologists, otolaryngologists, ophthalmologists, anesthesiologists, psychiatrists, physiatrists, and radiologists.

Perhaps just as important, the informed doctor is able to assure patients that they do indeed have a problem and that they will be directed to another physician or dentist for definitive diagnosis and treatment. The value of this service to the patient and the tremendous gratitude and respect it will engender should not be underestimated.

This book arose out of a series of symposia on "New Dimensions in the Management of Facial, Head and Neck Pain" that have been held during the past several years in the New York Eye and Ear Infirmary, sponsored by the Department of Otolaryngology of The New York Medical College. The material presented in those symposia, as in this book, was organized by specialty and covered the diagnosis, etiology, and treatment of facial, head, and neck pain syndromes that fall under the scope of each specialist.

It is the hope of all the contributors to this book that it will enlighten readers, help them develop a better understanding of the subject of facial, head, and neck pain, and motivate them to assemble their own team of specialists. With the dynamic interaction of the members of such a multidisciplinary group, effective, comprehensive patient care can be delivered.

BARRY C. COOPER, D.D.S.
FRANK E. LUCENTE, M.D.

Acknowledgments

The editors gratefully acknowledge the assistance of the many persons whose efforts contributed to the production of this book:

Mary Slisz, Administrator of the Department of Otolaryngology, New York Medical College, New York Eye and Ear Infirmary, who coordinated the entire project;

Donna B. Adkins and Rita Dowland, our dedicated typists;

Lisa McAllister, Ruth Low, Liz Schweber, and Bill Preston from W. B. Saunders Company, who nurtured the book through the publication process.

Contents

Chapter 1 **Perspectives in Head and Neck Pain** 1
   Frank E. Lucente and David L. Cooper

Chapter 2 **Neurological Causes of Head and Face Pain**............... 23
   Jeffrey T. Kessler

Chapter 3 **Otalgia** 53
   Kenneth F. Mattucci and Young B. Choo

Chapter 4 **Head Pain Associated With the Eye**........................ 77
   Kevin C. Greenidge and Monica Dweck

Chapter 5 **Rhinologic Causes of Facial Pain** 99
   Charles P. Kimmelman

Chapter 6 **Intraoral Pain**.. 115
   Barry C. Cooper

Chapter 7 **Oropharyngeal, Laryngeal, and Neck Pain** 131
   Robert L. Pincus

Chapter 8 **Craniomandibular Disorders**............................... 153
   Barry C. Cooper

Chapter 9 **Rehabilitation Management of Neck Pain**................ 255
   Thirumoorthi V. Seshan

Chapter 10 **The Psychiatric Aspects of Head, Neck, and Facial Pain**... 287
   David A. Shapiro

Chapter 11 **Management of Chronic Pain of the Head and Neck: An Anesthesiologist's Perspective**.......................... 299
Mathew Lefkowitz, Sheldon Goldstein, and Allen Lebovits

Index... 331

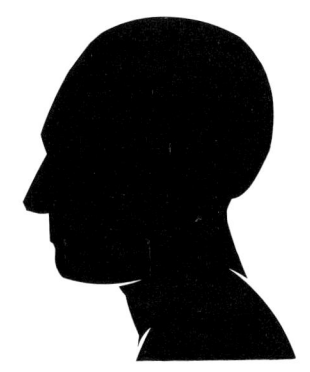

PAIN IS A MORE TERRIBLE LORD OF MANKIND THAN EVEN DEATH HIMSELF.
— Albert Schweitzer

Chapter 1
Perspectives in Head and Neck Pain

Frank E. Lucente and David L. Cooper

Pain in the head and neck is ubiquitous and serves as a continuous source of aggravation to millions of patients as well as a constant diagnostic and therapeutic challenge to physicians and other health care workers in many specialties. Approximately 45 million Americans annually have headaches that are sufficiently severe or frequent to prompt them to seek medical attention. Half of those who seek help consider the pain to be a major disruptive force in their daily lives. Headaches have an enormous economic impact on the country, accounting for approximately 132 million lost work days and resulting in an estimated $8 billion of lost productivity and expenditures for health care and medicines.

For the individual patient, the impact of pain in the head and neck varies from a minor annoyance to an incapacitating disability. The experience of pain itself as an unpleasant sensation is accompanied by the psychological distress of knowing that this sensation is occurring in a region of many important structures whose functions include communication, cognitive perception, and maintenance of physical appearance or beauty. This dual physical and psychological impact of head and neck pain makes the need for prompt diagnosis and efficient treatment even more pressing.

Perhaps the most difficult part of understanding pain is trying to comprehend the dual nature of the experience of pain. The perception of pain results from activation of the nociceptive afferent sensory system and transmission of impulses along known neuroanatomic pathways. The analysis and processing of these "painful" impulses, likewise, can be anatomically localized in the brain and understood without much difficulty.

For most persons, the mental state or emotion that is truly the basis for the experience of pain is elusive. Why does the same stimulus in two individuals, or in the same individual on different occasions, produce such different emotional responses? Science is still far from understanding the complex neurophysiological changes that affect this difference.

In this introductory consideration of the perception of pain, we might appropriately examine it from a number of different perspectives. We propose to examine the historical perspectives of pain in the context of medicine in past civilizations. We will review both the neuroanatomic pathways and structures that are responsible for the sensory input to the pain system and the neurophysiology and neuroendocrinology of the processing, interpretation, and modulation of pain. In considering the clinical aspects of pain, we stress the importance of a multidisciplinary approach to pain by many medical specialists in order to formulate the correct diagnosis. We will also examine the economic perspective and present data about the financial impact of pain on both the individual and on society as a whole. From the pharmacologic perspective we shall focus on the use of pharmaceutical agents in the management of pain as well as on some of the problems encountered in employing these medications. Finally, from the perspective of psychobiology we consider the impact of acute and chronic pain on the individual person as well as some of the problems related to management of head and neck pain.

Historical Perspectives of Pain

Pain has been a genuine and immediate concern to humans throughout history. However, as noted by Todd, "Man's attitudes and beliefs have been shaped by magical, demonological, theological, philosophical, and practical influences in varying degrees and with shifting emphasis."[1] Therefore, the meaning of pain in today's society may be more appropriately considered in the light of its role in previous years.

Ancient Civilizations

The perception of pain and its causes has varied throughout history in relation to the status of medicine in general and the perception of disease in particular. In *primitive and early societies* the source of pain was thought to be external, such as the Babylonian concept of disease as the result of an intrusion of a magical force or insidious evil spirit into the body. Disease resulted from sin or witchcraft, and cures were sought in spells and incantations. Pain was viewed as a punishment for such sin.

In this same land between the Tigris and Euphrates, one can also see the beginnings of the practice of medicine. Competing with the exorcist-priests were early physicians who attempted to study diseases by rational means. Lists survive of diseases, their symptoms, and effective drugs. In addition, one cannot forget the Code of Hammurabi, which delineated practical guidelines for surgical treatment of disease and the responsibility of the surgeon.

> If a surgeon has opened an eye infection with a bronze instrument and so saved the man's eye, he shall take ten shekels. If a surgeon has opened an eye infection with a bronze instrument and thereby destroyed the man's eye, they shall cut off his hand.[2]

In the face of such admonitions, it is not surprising that medicine became a descriptive art. Pain was viewed as a punishment for sin, and religious forces dominated the medical field.[1]

The first advances in elevating disease above the mystical level can be found in *ancient Egypt*. Evidence of this advance is seen in the rational empiricism of the Edwin Smith papyrus, a document copied by scribes of the sixteenth century B.C. from earlier medical writings ascribed to the era of Imhotep of the Third Egyptian Dynasty. Imhotep was a physician, architect, astronomer, and builder of pyramids. The Smith papyrus describes dozens of clinical situations for which the author gives a diagnosis and suggests a treatment. Diseases are classified as "an ailment that I will treat," "an ailment with which I will contend," or "an ailment not to be treated," reflecting an empirical knowledge of the prognosis of such diseases. This document also represents the first rational approach to treatment above mere folk remedies.

The Egyptian civilizations did not prohibit human dissection, and extensive studies were performed on mummies. Perhaps as a result of these studies, the knowledge of the anatomy of the human body increased, and the concept arose that disease was related to particular organs. However, the Egyptians felt that there was a separate god ruling over each organ and limb and that one must appeal to that deity to drive out the demons of the organ and restore health. It was through the left nostril that the evil spirits entered the body. It is interesting to note that the role of the brain was virtually ignored, and the heart was endowed with great importance. The heart and its vessels were the seat of sensory and motor activity. The Egyptians apparently had no knowledge of a peripheral or central nervous system.

In *India*, as far back as 4000 B.C., there were records of hundreds of remedies for pain derived from mineral, plant, and animal sources. Around 500 B.C., Indian physicians had well-organized concepts of disease as originating in anatomic loci, and they interpreted disease as representing a disturbance in physiology. However, religion again intruded—namely, in the birth of Buddhism during the fifth century B.C., and scientific discovery once again fell under a pall, with spiritualism prevailing.

The ancient *Chinese* interpreted the human situation as representative of the harmonious universe. Harmony was the result of a balance being achieved between yin and yang, the terms used to designate the two primitive forces. Yang and yin were essentially opposites, with yang representing the strong, aggressive force also associated with heat and light.

Yin denoted the cold, passive, dark, and weak force. The five organs thought to be important in the body were the heart, liver, lungs, spleen, and kidneys. The brain had no vital function but was thought to be simply a soft substance in the skull. Similarly, there was no particular brain center. Pain was thought to result from disturbances of the balance between yin and yang, such as might occur in emotional extremes. The Chinese divided the body into many parts, each having a specific focal representation that was of great significance to the acupuncturists. Pain was thought to have many foci, and the skill of the acupuncturist was used to identify the specific point at which the insertion of the needles would relieve pain in the afflicted part of the body.

The Greco-Roman World

During the period in which the development of civilization centered in *Hellenic Greece,* there was great effort in the vital intellectual community to study a world operating in an orderly manner in accordance with rational natural laws that could be ascertained by appropriate study.

Numerous philosophers expounded various theories about the meaning of observed phenomena. Alcmaeon, a student of Pythagoras (566–497 B.C.), was perhaps the first great medical figure of this period. Alcmaeon performed numerous animal dissections and on the basis of these studies elaborated a theory that posited the brain as the center of sensory appreciation. Unfortunately, his theories were ignored by those who felt that intellectual exercises were more important than anatomic studies in discerning the explanation of sensory perceptions.

However, shortly thereafter, the medical principles of Hippocrates of Cos (c. 460–360 B.C.) took hold and laid the basis for much of modern medicine. There is much evidence that Hippocrates and those who studied with him were greatly concerned with the causes and relief of pain. They focused on pain as a manifestation originating within the body, whether from an imbalance of the purported primal elements (hot, cold, moist, dry) or from other imbalances, and studied many medications in attempting to relieve pain. Among these substances were opium, hemlock, and mandrake.

Despite the theories of disease, a consideration of the humors and a scant choice of treatments did not permit the physician to do much. One of the best things he could expect to do was to predict the outcome of disease, a skill that results from experience with a large number of cases. Hippocrates devoted a volume, *Epidemics,* to such studies.

> Philistes in Thasos had for a long time pain in the head, and at last fell into a state of stupor and took to his bed. Heavy drinking having caused continuous fevers the pain grew worse. At night he grew hot at the first.
> First day. Vomited bilious matters, scanty, at first yello, afterwards increasing and of the colour of verdigris; solid motions from the bowels; and uncomfortable night.

Second day. Deafness; acute fever' tension of the right hypochondrium, which fell inwards. Urine thin, transparent, with a small quantity of substance, like semen, floating in it. About mid-day became raving.
Third day. Uncomfortable.
Fourth day. Convulsions; exacerbation.
Fifth day. Died early in the morning.

Some astonishing physiological inaccuracies appeared even in the writings of the most revered intellectuals of this time. Plato (427–322 B.C.), for instance, for whom the heart was the center of sensory experience, felt that control of sensitivity to pain was a function of the cardiovascular system.

In *Alexandria*, the extensive anatomic dissections of Herophilus (315–280 B.C.) facilitated the identification of the brain as the seat of motor and sensory function. His dissections focused on distinguishing between arteries and nerves and on tracing the course of the latter to and from the spinal cord and brain. Erasistratus of Cheor later distinguished between the cerebral and cerebellar cortices. Both attempted to locate the seat of the soul somewhere within the brain, with Herophilus placing it in the fourth ventricle and Erasistratus placing it within the cerebellum. Although their conclusions have been disproved, the quality of their work has led to recognition of Herophilus as the father of human anatomy and Erasistratus as the founder of experimental physiology.[3]

The importance of their pioneering work in stressing the role of anatomy in the understanding of pain led the Roman Celsus (first century A.D.) to write in *De Re Medicina*:

Moreover, as pain and also various kinds of disease arise in the internal parts, they hold that no one can apply remedies for these who are ignorant of the parts themselves: hence, it becomes necessary to lay open bodies of the dead to scrutinize their viscera and intestines . . . for when pain occurs internally, it is not possible for one to learn what hurts the patient unless he has acquainted himself with the portion of each organ or intestine; nor can a diseased portion of the body be treated by one who does not know what that part is.[4]

Turning to *Rome*, we see an evolution of the view of pain in earlier work, characterized by stoic indifference and an interest in studying the causes of pain. Although many of the early theorists could not produce scientific studies to substantiate their speculations, the Greek physician Galen (131–201 A.D.), who served as physician to the aristocracy and surgeon to the gladiators, began animal dissections that revealed new information about sensory and motor innervation. He "concluded that pain was the lowest form of conscious sensation, caused by either dissolution of continuity in tissues (cuts, burns, overdistention of hollow viscera, etc.) or by sudden violent commotion in the humors (pressure and tensions)."[1] Unfortunately, Galen attempted to determine why physiologic phenomena occurred rather than how, and his writing acquired an etiologic aspect that reduced its scientific value but endowed it with a veneer of which the church fathers approved. Interestingly, Galen did understand that illnesses presented with symptoms and that more information was needed to make a diagnosis.

> What is more manifold, more complicated, and more varied than disease? Or how does one discover that a disease is the same as another disease in all its characteristics? Is it by the number of the symptoms or by their strength and power? . . . [I]f one were to be satisfied with mere observation of the number of symptoms by themselves without requiring to consider also their order, and which is first and second and third, some advantage might probably be derived therefrom. Now, however, it is found that by changing the order of some of the symptoms and by removing them from their places, or acting similarly in the case of some diseases, this disease is not only different from the foregoing one, but is frequently its reverse, because the similarity and consistency are void and perverted.[5]

Fortunately, the encyclopedic records that he maintained have endured as a testament to his fine anatomic descriptions and as evidence of the scientific activity in Rome during his lifetime. With his death, scientific productivity in this region waned.

The Dark Ages and the Rebirth

During the subsequent Dark Ages, the weight of church dogma and mystical attitudes toward pain promoted martyrdom and gave voluntary suffering an exalted aura of spiritual beauty, thereby forestalling further scientific exploration into the physical causes of pain. However, even during the Dark Ages, a school of medicine arose in *Persia,* where native Persian influences merged with influences of Syrian, Jewish, Hindu, and Chinese scholars. A school of medicine was founded by the Nestorians in Jundishapur. Perhaps the most prominent physician of this time was Avicenna (980–1063), whose medical textbook, *Canon,* influenced medical practice for ensuing centuries. He was obviously familiar with the writings of Hippocrates, Aristotle, Galen, and other Europeans and drew his notions of pain from them, including an attempt to discern a central pain force within the cerebral hemispheres. The Arab literature already contained an extensive list of drugs used for relief of pain. From that list he focused on three groups of analgesics: those that treated the cause of pain, those that had anesthetic properties, and those of a more supportive nature. In the years after Avicenna's death the site of medical progress shifted back to Europe, particularly to the Iberian peninsula, where the moorish influences introduced by Jewish scholars who had flourished under Islam were already being felt.

The Renaissance brought intellectual and scientific activity back to *western Europe.* The fortuitous interest of the legal profession in autopsies brought about a resurgence of interest in human dissection, but the oppressive role of the church at this time made it necessary for much dissection to be performed in secrecy. Among the leaders in this field was Leonardo da Vinci, who demonstrated great proficiency in mapping out the anatomic intricacies of the brain, spinal cord, and peripheral nerves. He reportedly regarded pain as an intense manifestation of the sense of touch. He was able to map out the sensory distribution of cutaneous nerves by cutting the nerves and noting the region of deficit.

Due to the pressure of the church, which viewed pain as an act of God that was to be endured rather than suppressed, little attention was apparently paid to the development of anesthetic medications. However, records indicate that physicians were aware of the narcotic effects of opium. Also, Ambrose Paré used carotid compression for anesthesia, and other practitioners of medicine used belladonna, atropine, and other substances to treat pain.

At the same time as this re-exploration of anatomy was taking place, the science of physiology was reborn. Perhaps the ultimate achievement in anatomic and physiologic research was the animal studies of William Harvey, summarized by his statement in 1628 that "it must therefore be concluded that the blood in the animal body moves around in a circle continuously, and that the action or function of the heart is to accomplish this by pumping. This is the only reason for the motion and beat of the heart."

The eighteenth and nineteenth centuries saw the birth of the germ theory of disease and the cell theory. By the 1870s, when Claude Bernard concluded his "Cours de physiologie," he acknowledged that "the most complex organism is a vast mechanism which results from the assemblage of secondary mechanisms. The most perfect animal possesses a circulatory system, a respiratory system, and a nervous system. . . . They exist not for themselves but from the cells, for the innumerable anatomic elements which form the organic edifice."[7] Neuroanatomy was established, and the concepts of cell theory set the stage for the science of neurophysiology to follow.

The centuries of the Renaissance saw few advances in the understanding and management of pain. The next milestone occurred in the 1800s, when C. Bell and E. Magendie defined the roles of the anterior and posterior nerve roots, allowing the understanding of the physiology of pain to advance many steps beyond that of the ancient Alexandrians. In the 188 years since then, numerous further advances have been made. The mechanism for nerve conduction of painful stimuli along various neural pathways, the sensory receptor apparatus, the neurochemical basis of impulse transmission, and many more aspects have been elucidated.

As we ponder these new discoveries, it may be useful to recall the evolution of this knowledge during the preceding several thousand years and to interpret the questions that we continue to pose within the context of the intellectual atmosphere of each of the preceding ages.

The Neurologic Perspective

Current concepts of the neuroanatomy and neurophysiology of pain have evolved through centuries as a result of planned research and serendipitous discoveries, some of which have been described in the previous section. The anatomic basis of many painful sensations in the head and neck is now understood as a stimulus originating at a peripheral nociceptive site and being conducted along nerve fibers and across synapses to areas where recognition and interpretation occur.

Afferent Pain Pathways

Traditionally, two theories were proposed to explain pain sensation. Von Frey's "specific" theory postulated that pain, touch, warmth, and cold each have distinctive end-organs in the skin, and each has discrete neuroanatomic pathways to the brain. In contrast, Goldscheider's "intensive" theory held that any sensory stimulus, if intense, could produce pain. Pain resulted from the summation of sensory impulses, and there were no specific "pain" receptors. Modern theories have reconciled these two disparate views.

Two types of afferent fibers exist, each carrying different types of sensation. They are the fine, slow unmyelinated C fibers (0.4 to 1.1 microns [μ] in diameter) conducting at 0.5 to 2 meters per second, and the thinly myelinated fast A-delta fibers (1.0 to 5.0 μ in diameter) conducting at 5 to 15 meters per second, which originate at free nerve endings in the skin and visceral organs. Free nerve endings are branching nerve fibers covered by Schwann's cells but not laminated by myelin. These fibers respond to both noxious and innocuous stimuli. There are also several special sensory receptors, including the Ruffini end-organs for warmth, the bulb of Krause for cold, and the corpuscles of Meissner and Pacini for perception of touch.

In a simplified discussion, these afferent fibers pass through the dorsal root into the dorsal horn of the spinal cord, where they occupy the lateral part of the root entry zone and form the tract of Lissauer, along with proprioceptive fibers. The fibers from special sensory organs pass through the more medial portions of the dorsal root. Nociceptive afferents synapse in the superficial layers with secondary neurons, then cross in the anterior spinal commissure to ascend in the anterolateral fasciculus to the brainstem and thalamus. A second, faster spinoreticulothalamic pathway also exists. These nociceptive fibers end in the nucleus ventralis posterolateralis (VPL) of the thalamus.

At the thalamic level, the fibers involved in the perception of pain are not organized in a discrete locus separate from other sensory afferents. As one continues to ascend from the thalamus to the cortex and limb system, the response of particular fiber tracts to nociceptive input becomes less clear. The nuclei of VPL send axons to the postcentral cortex and the upper bank of the sylvian fissure, areas that are concerned with reception of tactile stimuli and proprioception and with discriminative sensation. The face is represented in the area immediately superior to the sylvian fissure. These nerve fibers are activated by noxious stimuli, not by thermal or proprioceptive input. However, stimulation of any area of the cortex itself does not produce the sensation of pain.

The Neurophysiology of Pain

The stimulus causing pain in a particular type of tissue is unique to that tissue. Skeletal pain is caused by ischemia (such as angina), injuries to connective tissue sheaths, necrosis, hemorrhage, and injection of irritating solutions. An aching pain occurs with prolonged contraction. Gastrointestinal pain is caused by engorgement or inflammation of the mucosa or by smooth muscle distention or spasm. Migraine headaches are thought to be caused by excessive pulsation and distention of skeletal muscles. Proteolytic enzymes are released when tissue is damaged and act on gamma globulins to liberate nociceptor-stimulating substances. These substances may include bradykinins, histamine, prostaglandins, serotonin, and potassium.

In order to explain the differences in perception of pain with minor and more significant stimuli, Melzack and Wall proposed the "gate-control theory" of pain. According to their work in 1965 and Wall's further refinement in 1980, both the large A-delta fibers and the small C fibers synapse with a transmitting neuron and an interposed inhibitory neuron. With mild pain, large fiber activity predominates, and there is an inhibitory influence on the transmitting neuron. No pain is perceived. However, with significant stimuli, small C-fiber activity predominates, blocking the inhibitory neuron. The impulses pass to the transmitting neuron, and the patient experiences severe pain.

Modern theories of neurophysiology try to reconcile the gate theory with the specific and pattern-intensive theories. The gate theory was the first effort to explain the central summation of impulses and the spinal and supraspinal pain-modulating systems.

Clinical Types of Pain

Pain in different regions is characterized differently. Pain can be localized because the nerve fibers are segmentally organized into dermatomes. The facial structures and anterior cranium lie in the field of the trigeminal nerves; the back of the head is innervated by the second cervical nerve; the neck is innervated by the third cervical; the epaulet area, by the fourth cervical; and the deltoid area, by the fifth cervical. Deeper structures have segmentally organized afferent nerve fibers as well, although they do not directly correlate with the skin dermatomes. This is important in understanding the concept of referred pain.

Pain in the skin progresses in two stages—first a pricking pain evoked by penetration of the skin, and then a stinging or burning pain several seconds later. Nerve ischemia blocks the pricking first pain transmitted by the large A-delta fibers. Deep pain from visceral organs or the skeletomuscular system is aching in character but may be knifelike if intense. The pain is felt to be deep to the body surface and is poorly localized and diffuse, perhaps due to the paucity of nerve endings in the viscera.

Deep pain from visceral organs may be referred to the skin. In this case, the pain is felt in the skin dermatome corresponding to the same spinal nerve level that innervates that visceral organ. Visceral organs are often innervated by several spinal nerve levels, accounting for the diffuse nature of referred pain. This referred pain relates to the fact that ascending spinal pain fibers are more frequently activated by the greater abundance of skin afferents. For example, the complex innervation of the laryngopharynx and the external auditory canal by vagal afferents does much to explain how a patient with carcinoma of the piriform sinus may present with otalgia.

The pool of neurons in adjacent segments of the spinal cord can be altered, for example, by chronic activation in a segment and may result in poor localization of pain, called *aberrant reference*. Cervical arthritis or gallbladder disease results in constant activation and can shift cardiac pain either caudad or cephalad from its usual locale.

Patients may also have altered thresholds (*hyperalgesia*) or increased sensitivity (*hyperesthesia*) to painful stimuli. *Hyperpathia* denotes an excessive reaction to pain, usually with a raised threshold. In cases of chronic pain there is both a defect in pain perception and an increased sensitivity to typically non-noxious stimuli. Chronic pain is thus diffuse and is modified by fatigue and emotion. Chronic stimulation of central structures, such as the thalamus, may result in autonomous overactivity, which remains after peripheral pathways are no longer activated, as in *phantom pain*.

Neuroendocrinology

In a classic study, Beecher found that wounded soldiers required far less narcotic for pain relief than did civilians undergoing elective surgery, despite the fact that the soldiers sustained greater injuries.[7] This fact prompted neuroscientists to search for a reason for such changes in the thresholds for pain or endogenous analgesia. What has come back from this work is the discovery of a system of endogenous analgesia, very similar in action to the administration of opiates. In fact, administration of an opioid antagonist, naloxone, reverses this endogenous analgesia.[8]

In 1969, Reynolds showed that electrical stimulation of the ventrolateral periaqueductal gray matter in the rat induced profound analgesia.[9] Likewise, stimulation of the medical and caudal regions of the diencephalon and the rostral bulbar nuclei produced sufficient analgesia to permit surgery. Neurophysiologists have shown that the action of this endogenous analgesic system as well as that of opioid administration occurs in laminae I and V of the dorsal root of the spinal cord. There is evidence that opioid compounds bind to presynaptic areas of the primary sensory neurons and inhibit release of their transmitter, substance P. It is also thought that endogenous opioid compounds, such as enkephalin, are released by spinal interneurons synapsing with the presynaptic regions of the afferent neurons.

This endogenous pain-modulating system acts both centrally, at the level of the midbrain and limbic system, and peripherally, at the level of the spinal cord. Deficiencies in brain endorphin levels may account for persistent pain and may also explain opioid addiction. Endorphins reduce pain and eliminate symptoms of withdrawal.

Hughes was one of the first to discover specific naturally occurring peptides, the *endorphins*, which means "the morphine within." The two most widely studied compounds are beta-endorphin and enkephalin. Beta-endorphin, a fragment of the pituitary hormone beta-lipotropin, is found predominantly in the midbrain regions mentioned above. In contrast, enkephalins are found predominantly in the spinal cord interneuron systems that modulate pain sensation. There are at least six subtypes of opiate receptor sites identified to date. The differences among them may explain the various pharmacologic effects of different endorphins and narcotics.

Kelly and associates have studied both analgesia and hyperalgesia induced by experimental stress.[10] They noted that the analgesia was naloxone-sensitive and that the hyperalgesia was not. Removal of the pituitary gland enhanced both effects. However, removal of the adrenal gland eliminated the hyperalgesia and enhanced the analgesia.[9] Beecher noted that soldiers experienced analgesia to primary wounds but complained markedly of pain caused by inept venipuncture.[6] The animal studies of Kelly and others now give evidence that suggests that there are different neuroendocrine systems for mediation of stress-induced differences in responsivity to nociceptive stimuli.[9]

Interestingly, endorphins may explain the "placebo effect," and the efficacy of acupuncture. It has been shown that the opiate antagonist naloxone interferes not only with the pain suppression of narcotics but also with the pain relief of placebos. It is possible that placebos shut off pain through activation of an endogenous system causing the release of endorphins.

Modulation of pain transmission most likely also involves descending pain control systems containing serotoninergic as well as endorphin links. This is important in understanding the use of certain serotonin-agonists in patients with chronic pain.

The neuroendocrine events that transpire during the production and transmission of painful phenomena continue to be a focus for much research. It is hoped that future work will facilitate greater understanding of these phenomena because efficient pain control will be enhanced by this information.

The Clinical Perspective

The diagnosis and treatment of patients suffering from facial, head, and neck pain present a challenge to any clinician faced with a given patient. This is largely due to the broad range of causes of facial and head pain, each falling seemingly within the purview of a different specialist. Often, a clinician may be able to obtain a good history and perform a physical examination that directly suggests a specific cause of the pain. However, all too often, patients relate rather vague clinical histories and have nonspecific physical findings. With these patients, the diagnosis is far from clear. The general practitioner or specialist to whom the patient initially presents may be able to rule out abnormalities that he or she can treat but may be unsure where to refer the patient next.

This book will demonstrate that facial, head, and neck pain is a complex field involving many specialists in a variety of fields. The importance of a multidisciplinary approach to head and neck pain should not stop when the clinician has established a group of specialists to use as sources of referral. The multidisciplinary approach to this type of pain requires that each clinician involved have a general knowledge of the entire spectrum of etiologies possible so as to be able to make appropriate referrals to the correct specialists. In addition, the well-informed member of the multidisciplinary team should have a good conception of the optimal workup and the likely diagnostic possibilities.

Pain is unquestionably a physical phenomenon, and formulating the diagnosis requires attention to both the physical setting in which it occurs and the physical characteristics of the phenomenon itself. In approaching the patient with pain, it is a good idea to determine all clinical parameters including location, intensity, duration, and periodicity, circumstances of onset, exacerbating and ameliorating factors, concurrent symptoms, and previous response to therapy. One should also record pertinent life habits such as alcohol ingestion, smoking, dietary patterns, caffeine use, and sleeping patterns. Among the other pertinent aspects of the history are menstrual and hormonal history, past medical illnesses and surgery, use of prescription and nonprescription drugs, and environmental aspects of the home and work setting.

Although it is impossible to review the history-taking and diagnostic workup for each cause of facial, head, and neck pain in this introduction, it is important to consider the application of this multidisciplinary approach to the problem of headaches. In the diagnosis of headache, the most important clues to the etiology of the headache can be gleaned from a detailed and relevant history. The importance of the headache history is emphasized by the number of patients who present with no physical or neurologic signs of their ailment. However, the goal of history-taking should not be to identify immediately a particular headache syndrome because patients often have many types of headaches, and the new onset of a particular type of headache or change in headache pattern may be of great significance. Some physicians advocate charting of daily headaches by the patient to assess patterns.

The *onset* of headaches and the length of time the patient has suffered from them offer important clues to etiology. Vascular headaches often start in childhood and adolescence and in the second and third decades of life. Patients may present with a 20-year or more history of these migraine or cluster headaches. Onset of migraine headaches is frequently preceded by a prodrome consisting mainly of ocular symptoms. Headaches of middle age or following a specific stressful incident or emotional trauma may imply an etiology related to stress and emotional factors. Headaches can occur following head trauma and may persist for years. The sudden onset of severe headache with neurologic signs may also provide a clue to emergent neurologic conditions. Morning headaches that worsen during the day are typically seen with sinus conditions.

The *location* of headaches is often of great help in diagnosis. Bandlike headaches are most often due to tension or are muscular in origin. Unilateral headaches may be vascular or related to focal intracranial abnormalities. Generalized headaches may indicate altered intracranial pressure or may be associated with psychogenic disease. Ocular headaches may signify ocular disease or may be cluster headaches.

Frequency, duration, and *severity* of headaches may also help in revealing a typical pattern. Migraine headaches may vary in association with the menstrual cycle, whereas cluster headaches are more frequent in spring and fall and occur in bouts for several weeks or months. Although migraines may last hours to days and are described as throbbing or pulsating in nature, cluster headaches usually last less than 4 hours and are felt as a deep, boring, and severe pain. Muscle tension headaches are typically of long duration, occur persistently over years to decades, and are described as an aching, dull, nagging pain. Headaches of worsening severity during a short period of time may indicate an expanding intracranial lesion.

When a patient presents with a headache, it is important to identify the cause of the headache as fully as possible. During the patient's initial presentation, a full medical and surgical history should be taken. This should include a history of head or neck trauma, recent medical or dental procedures, seizures, syncopal episodes, neck stiffness, cerebrovascular disease, previous surgery on the head and neck, and previous surgery to remove tumors elsewhere that may have metastasized to the brain. The history should include a survey of systemic diseases that may involve the head and neck and may present with headache, as well as diseases of the eyes, ears, nose, and throat.

A detailed family history of headaches and other neurologic diseases should be taken. Migraines are known to show a hereditary linkage. A menstrual and obstetric history should be taken and correlated with changes in the headache history. The patient should be questioned about previous therapies and diagnostic studies that have been performed. A history of past and present medications and their effectiveness may also be helpful in making the differential diagnosis. The examining physician should also evaluate the mental status of the patient to assess mood, range of affect, memory, intelligence, and orientation. In this way, insight can be gained into the patient's level of anxiety, agitation, and coping mechanisms.

Physical examination should be thorough and should include not only the entire head and neck region but other pertinent regions as well. The selection and performance of laboratory tests and other examinations will be guided by clinical impressions. It is frequently necessary to perform a physical examination on several occasions and to elicit additional historical information before the correct diagnosis can be made. It is often particularly helpful to examine the patient during an acute or typical episode of pain.

The general appearance of the patient is often very revealing. Patients with migraine headaches often are well dressed and meticulous and come with a detailed list of symptoms, medications, and charts of headache frequency. A patient presenting with telangiectases, facial flushing, accentuated glabellar creases, and coarse cheek skin may have cluster headaches. Neurofibromatosis with café-au-lait spots may indicate an increased predilection for intracranial neuromas or meningiomas. Examination may also reveal signs of a disease that may include headaches as a manifestation, including hypertension, cervical spinal abnormalities, hypothyroidism, and syndromes associated with hypersecretion of pituitary hormones (such as hyperprolactinemia and Cushing's disease). Simply noting a patient's gait as he or she enters the office may reveal signs of cerebellar disease.

Examination of the head may reveal muscle pain on palpation, sounds heard in the temporomandibular joints with movement, hardened temporal arteries, evidence of inflammation or infection, or tenderness over the sinuses. The neck and cervical spine should be examined for tenderness, muscle spasm, and decreased range of motion.

Neurologic examination should begin with a complete evaluation of cranial nerve function. Dysfunction in any of these nerves may provide telling evidence about both central nervous system and peripheral abnormalities that might manifest as headaches. The olfactory nerve (cranial nerve I) can be tested with some aromatic substance. Loss of the sense of smell may be associated with headaches in sinus conditions. A careful evaluation of the eyes must be performed. Gross examination of the visual fields can be performed by confrontation to assess field cuts from occipital lobe lesions or pressure on the optic nerve (cranial nerve II). Extraocular movements to the positions of cardinal gaze and pupillary light reflexes may reveal signs of compression in the oculomotor (cranial nerve III), trochlear (cranial nerve IV), and abducens (cranial nerve VI) nerves. Funduscopic examination may reveal signs of optic atrophy, papilledema, hemorrhages, organic brain disease, systemic hypertension, and diabetes. When headaches or head pain are associated with trigeminal neuralgia, examination may reveal trigger points or dysfunction in the trigeminal nerve (cranial nerve V). Examination of facial movements may provide clues to lesions involving the facial nerve (cranial nerve VII), either peripherally or centrally. Because headaches are often associated with tinnitus, vertigo, and deafness, examination of the auditory-vestibular nerve (cranial nerve VIII) should be performed as well to rule out ear or posterior fossa lesions. Abnormalities of the remaining cranial nerves are not typically associated with headaches.

Neurologic examination of the motor and sensory systems should be performed and deep tendon and pathologic reflexes should be elicited to search for localizing signs of central nervous system disease that may manifest as headaches. Such abnormalities may involve ischemic brain insults, traumatic damage, or hemorrhage.

Although most headaches are not manifestations of serious organic disease, some diagnostic workup is indicated when patients are seen for the first time. An initial evaluation generally includes skull films and computed tomographic and electroencephalographic studies when indicated. Since in many patients with headaches the symptoms are aggravated by angiography, spinal punctures, and other tests, these tests should be ordered cautiously.

Although sometimes overused or dismissed as unnecessary and without value, *plain skull films* can be very important. Lateral and anteroposterior films must be properly aligned to be of any clinical use. Skull films may reveal fractures, splitting of sutures, increased vascular markings, abnormal size of the sella turcica or erosion of the sella, metastatic disease, and shifts of the pineal gland signifying displacement secondary to contralateral mass lesions. *Electroencephalograms (EEG)* should be performed in some instances to rule out organic brain disease. Lesions may be revealed by focal EEG abnormalities or general dysrhythmias.

Lumbar puncture, or spinal tap, is indicated if infection is suspected. Signs of meningeal infection include occipital headache, fever, and neck rigidity. Cerebrospinal fluid (CSF) can be collected for culture, cell counts, and composition analysis. However, caution must be used in performing lumbar punctures because patients with brain tumors and associated increased intracranial pressure may undergo brainstem herniation when fluid is removed quickly. When patients have headaches due to raised intracranial pressure in the absence of a mass lesion, the diagnosis of benign intracranial hypertension (pseudotumor cerebri) must be considered; this is confirmed by spinal puncture with evidence of very high CSF opening pressure.

The diagnosis of intracranial disease, whether it be tumor, abscess, hemorrhage, or other process, has been revolutionized by the advent of *computed tomography (CT)* and *magnetic resonance imaging (MRI)*. The common use of CT scanning has replaced invasive techniques of pneumoencephalography, angiography, ventriculography, and radioisotope scanning. CT scans, with and without contrast, enable physicians to noninvasively differentiate hemorrhage from tumor, monitor the progression of mass lesions, accurately diagnose supratentorial abscesses, and follow patients' progress postoperatively. In studying headache, CT is valuable in excluding brain tumors, chronic subdural hematomas, hydrocephalus, and benign intracranial hypertension. It can also spot cerebral edema in the immediate period of migraine headaches.

Magnetic resonance imaging is one of the newest diagnostic tools in neurology. In the study of headache, MRI can detect even more occult organic etiologies. Scanning can be performed in frontal, sagittal, or axial projections with greater clarity of soft tissues than is possible with CT. In addition, MRI provides better images of the posterior fossa (CT is encumbered by bony artifact) and thus is more sensitive for detecting posterior fossa lesions that may be associated with headache.

Various techniques have been developed for studying the cerebral circulation. *Cerebral angiography* and the newer *digital subtraction angiography* make possible the visualization of the cerebral circulation. The diagnosis and localization of aneurysms and arteriovenous malformations can now be made more easily preoperatively. Rupture of a berry aneurysm is a major cause of subarachnoid hemorrhage and presents as an explosive severe headache.

Positron emission tomography (PET) allows study of the function and physiology of the brain. Using positron-emitting radioisotopes tagged to compounds, scientists can study the functioning brain in vivo. PET scanning is still a research tool owing to its cost and the necessity for a cyclotron to generate the isotopes, but it may yield some insight into the changes that take place in brain physiology during headache.

The multidisciplinary approach to the diagnosis and management of facial, head, and neck pain involves a dynamic interaction among a coordinated team of physicians whose primary goal is to deliver better, more comprehensive patient care. It involves not only cooperation but also knowledge. The team of physicians and dentists treating the patient must have a complete understanding not only of their specialty field, but also of the broad range of diseases involved.

Approaching facial, head, and neck pain as part of a multidisciplinary team takes time, effort, and a willingness to learn continually. In turn, the physician provides a valuable service to the patient by being more informed about all aspects of head and neck pain and thus being able to suggest referrals with clear ideas as to other possible diagnoses to be ruled out. Perhaps more important, the physician is able to assure the patient that he or she does indeed have a problem and will be directed to another physician who will be able to diagnose and treat the illness more definitively.

The Pharmacologic Perspective

For centuries the management of pain has focused on the use of pharmacologic agents. As noted above, some remedies described in the Edwin Smith papyrus of the sixteenth century B.C. are still employed today. Some pharmacologic agents currently employed have been formulated through careful experimental studies, whereas others have been discovered serendipitously. The efficient use of pharmacologic agents is predicated on the recognition that pain is an emotion resulting from activation of the nociceptive afferent system and thus has both physical and psychological components.

Foley notes that pain involves both a sensory perception and an affective response.[11] Pain may also be characterized as acute or chronic. Chronic pain patients can be further divided into (1) patients with chronic medical illnesses for whom narcotic and non-narcotic analgesics are generally used; (2) patients with chronic pain associated with a specific pain diagnosis, such as low back pain; and (3) patients with chronic pain and no specific diagnosis.

In discussing the clinical management of pain, Foley notes that drug therapy is the basis of therapy for most patients with pain.[11] Treatment usually begins with the use of the nonopioid analgesics. In general, nonopioids alleviate headaches, myalgias, arthralgias, and integumental pain. Compounds such as the nonsteroidal anti-inflammatory agents (NSAIDs) act peripherally to inhibit the acute inflammatory response associated with tissue injury and are potent prostaglandin synthetase inhibitors.[12] The newer nonsteroidal drugs such as diflunisal (Dolobid), a salicylate derivative, are as potent (500 mg bid) as codeine (25 mg qid) or pentazocine (50 mg qid) and have a far easier dosing interval and produce no tolerance or physical dependence as do these narcotics.

Narcotic analgesics can be divided into three groups: natural opium alkaloids and derivatives, synthetic narcotics, and mixed agonist-antagonists. The opioids each act at different receptor subtypes and consequently have varied actions, potencies, and pharmacokinetics. The mixed agonists-antagonists have agonist activity at certain opioid receptors and antagonist properties at others. It should be noted that nearly all narcotic medications have some potential for abuse and that tolerance and physical dependence occur with chronic administration. In prescribing these medications one should understand not only the pharmacologic action of the drugs used but also the duration of the analgesic effect and the consequences of withdrawal of the medication. In addition, it is important to know the difference between the duration of pain relief and the duration of other effects, such as central nervous system excitability, mood changes, sedation, and respiratory depression from each drug.

A third group of analgesic drugs is referred to as the adjuvant analgesics. These produce or potentiate analgesia by mechanisms other than those mediated by the opiate receptor system. These drugs include the anticonvulsants, phenothiazines, steroids, antihistamines, and amphetamines. Within this category also, one must consider the antidepressant amitriptyline (Elavil), which is used commonly at low doses in the treatment of chronic pain due to neurologic or neoplastic disease. The use of these medications will be discussed in more detail in a later chapter in this text.

In the management of acute pain, the physician and patient are both frequently concerned with the possibility of addiction, especially if narcotics are used. However, such concern with addiction should not cause physicians to purposely undermedicate patients. Studies have shown that patients receiving narcotics for short periods for real pain do not develop any long-term psychological dependence despite the development of minor tolerance. It is far better to use adequate pain relievers including narcotics and monitor the patient for signs of physical and psychological dependence. If physical dependence occurs, tapering can be done in a supportive environment.

The Economic Perspective

Although it is difficult to obtain accurate statistics about the number of patients afflicted with head and neck pain during any period of time and the economic cost in insurance payments and lost work days, it is safe to estimate that the economic impact of such pain on the country is enormous. Some recent surveys have indicated that the cost of treating either acute or chronic pain at all sites is approximately $90,000,000,000 annually.[13]

In 1980 Ng and Bonica estimated that 36 million persons suffer from migraine headaches, and an additional 60 million have other types of headache.[14] They estimated that 124 million work days were lost per year, with a resultant cost of $6.2 billion annually. They also estimated that the health care cost for management of pain in this group was $1.2 billion, for a total cost to the country of $7.4 billion. Figures on other chronic pain states such as orofacial pain, neuralgic pain, and vascular pain were less readily available, but Ng and Bonica estimated that the total cost for these was an additional $4 billion annually.

Regardless of individual variations in estimates of the costs of pain diagnosis and therapy, the economic impact of these diseases is tremendous, and the number of people suffering from pain is enormous. We pay a high price for pain in the form of morbidity and physical suffering.

The Psychobiologic Perspective

The final perspective in which pain might be understood is the psychobiologic perspective, a term used to emphasize the mind-body interaction that is central to the pain experience. There are many aspects to this perspective that are relevant to understanding the patient with head and neck pain and to designing a plan for therapy.

In view of the complex biologic and psychological factors involved in the causation and perception of pain, it is reasonable to suggest that formulations for therapy must include attention to both factors. Physical pain is appropriately treated by identifying and eradicating the source, whether that be inflammatory, infectious, neoplastic, degenerative, or other. The psychological components require similarly intensive investigation and determination of appropriate therapy, which may involve psychiatric or psychological counseling, pharmacologic therapy, environmental adjustment, and other factors. It is well recognized that failure to determine the psychological components of the experience of pain, to treat them effectively, and to provide the same extensive follow-up and support that are part of the management of physical pain may cause any proposed program of therapy to be unsuccessful.

Numerous psychiatric and psychological factors are involved in the management of the patient with pain. Kornfeld points out that the word *pain* is derived from Latin and Greek roots meaning punishment.[15] The manner in which pain and punishment are linked during childhood can later affect the adult's response to pain.

It is important to realize that the physician may have developed attitudes to pain during his or her formative years, and those attitudes may influence his or her response to patients' complaints of pain. For example, the physician who was raised to tolerate pain may encourage such practices from patients and may be intolerant of patients who complain openly of pain.

In diagnosing and treating the patient with pain in the head and neck, it is necessary to keep in mind the strong psychological investment of most people in structures in this region, since they often endow the pain with a special significance. For example, pain involving the organs of speech (larynx) and hearing (ear) may be interpreted by the patient as posing a threat to the ability to communicate. At the other extreme, a patient may present with laryngitis or throat pain as a conversion symptom that reflects a psychological conflict concerning communication.

Patients with facial, head, and neck pain may exhibit profound denial of their illness or the potential etiologies of their symptoms. For example, it is not uncommon for a patient with an ear infection to place much more emphasis on the attendant hearing loss than on the possibility of extension or dissemination of the infection to intracranial and other vital structures, even when assured that the hearing loss is likely to be temporary. Similarly, the patient with hoarseness, throat pain, and a neck mass may focus more attention on the loss of vocal ability than on the possibility that this constellation of symptoms strongly suggests the presence of cancer.

The clinician must determine what the patient is experiencing as pain, and how he or she interprets that pain. It is important to understand what the patient expects from therapy. Relief of pain without restoration of a lost and important function may not result in a satisfied patient. For example, the patient with pain on swallowing may regret the loss of the pleasant sensations involved with the ingestion of food but may otherwise pay little attention to the medical importance of this symptom. Also, patients with impairments of smell and taste may focus more on lost pleasure than on physical impairment. Treatment must focus on eliminating the pain and restoring the lost sense of smell or taste as well as on addressing the patient's psychological response to loss and recovery.

Psychological Pain

Emotional factors undoubtedly play a direct role in the production of pain. Kornfeld observes that pain that is truly psychogenic in origin should be treated as such. Therapy may include the use of a mild analgesic and perhaps a minor tranquilizer such as diazepam (Valium) or oxazepam (Seras). It is particularly important for the physician to be available for frank and open discussions about the origin of pain in these instances.

Hackett has developed a 7-point scale called the Madison scale that is used to help evaluate the relative significance of psychogenic factors in a patient's complaint of pain.[16] In the Madison scale each characteristic is rated on a scale from 0 to 4; a score above 15 suggests the need for further psychiatric intervention. The scale factors are as follows:

M	Multiplicity	Pain occurs in more than one place or in more than one variety
A	Authenticity	Patient very much wants the physician to believe the pain is real
D	Denial	Patient denies the presence of any emotional problems
I	Interpersonal relationships	Patient shows evidence of disturbance at the mention of the name of someone who may have something directly, indirectly, or symbolically to do with the patient
S	Singularity	Patient stresses that he has a singular and unusual pain that distinguishes him from all other patients
O	"Only You"	The patient emphasizes that "only you can help me, doctor"
N	Nothing helps	The patient stresses that nothing has worked in his previous therapy

When those characteristics are noted and the patient is complaining of severe pain, it is prudent to obtain psychiatric consultation. Other forms of pain that call attention to the need for psychiatric assistance are those associated with a conversion reaction, severe depression, or a compensable injury.[15]

Patients with depression often report pain as a predominant symptom, and most patients with chronic pain are depressed. Although depression may be either primary or secondary to the pain, treatment with antidepressants may be of therapeutic value. Trials with amitriptyline have shown excellent results.

Patients with chronic hysteria and compensation neurosis may present with intractable pain. Compensation neurosis is often associated with persistent headaches, neck pain (whiplash injuries), low back pain, and so on. Frequently, patients with these disorders are so persistent in their complaints that they undergo unnecessary surgery. The clinical presentation often involves insomnia, weakness, fatigue, depression, and anxiety. Hysterical women may present with scarred abdomens from repetitive surgery to the appendix, ovaries, fallopian tubes, uterus, and gallbladder.

Conclusion

Pain is a part of our daily practices. We can choose to treat pain simply as part of the illnesses we treat or as a reflection and product of the psychological state of the individual in pain. In fact, as we have shown, pain can be approached in various ways, ranging from the most scientific neuroanatomic and neurophysiologic bases to the clinical perspective, and from the historical approaches to pain to its current economic impact.

Pain often provides a challenge to clinicians. It may seem to relate clearly to a specific cause, or it may exist without any objective evidence of a disease process. Pain may be a primary response to activation of the nociceptive afferent system. Conversely, pain may present as a chronic complaint for purposes of secondary gain, whether for economic compensation or social purposes.

Our approach to facial, head, and neck pain should be multidisciplinary, involving the participation of a team of specialists in a variety of fields. Each physician brings to the group a knowledge of the complex intricacies of his or her own field, but each must also learn enough about the other specialties to be able to appreciate the types of therapy performed and to refer patients properly for diagnosis and treatment. It is left to the remainder of this text to provide an understanding of the ways in which different specialists approach pain in the face, head, and neck in terms of diagnosis, etiology, treatment, and prognosis.

References

1. Todd, E. M. Pain: Historical perspectives. In Aronoff, G. M. (ed.). Evaluations and Treatment of Chronic Pain. Baltimore, Urban and Schwarzenberg, 1985, pp. 1–16.
2. Hamurabi Code, Babylonia, cited in Todd, E. M. Pain: Historical perspectives. In Aronoff, G. M. (ed.). Evaluations and Treatment of Chronic Pain. Baltimore, Urban and Schwarzenberg, 1985, pp. 1–16.
3. Seeman, B. Man Against Pain. New York, Chilton, 1962.
4. Keele, K. D. Anatomies of Pain. Springfield, Ill., Charles C Thomas, 1973.
5. Galen: On Medical Experience, cited in Williams, L. P. and Steffens, H. J. The History of Science in Western Civilization. New York, University Press of America, 1978.
6. Beecher, H. K. Pain in men wounded in battle. Ann Surg 123:96–105, 1946.
7. Bernard, C. Cour de physiologie, cited in Williams, L. P. and Steffens, H. J. The History of Science in Western Civilization. New York, University Press of America, 1978.
8. Akil, H., Mayer, D. J., and Liebeskind, J. C. Antagonism as stimulation-produced analgesia by naloxone, a narcotic antagonist. Science 191:961–962, 1976.
9. Adams, R. D. and Victor, M.: Principles of Neurology, 3rd ed. New York, McGraw-Hill, 1985, p. 105.
10. Kelly, D. D. Pain inhibitory systems in the brain and the question of their behavioral purpose. In Levitan, S. J. and Berkowitz, H. L. (eds.). Pain Research and Treatment. Washington, D.C., American Psychiatric Press, 1985, pp. 18–34.
11. Foley, K. M. Pharmacological approaches to pain control. In Levitan, S. J. and Berkowitz, H. L. (eds.). Pain Research and Treatment. Washington, D.C., American Psychiatric Press, 1985, pp. 35–48.
12. Kantor, T. G. Control of pain by non-steroidal anti-inflammatory drugs. Med Clin North Am 66:1053–1059, 1982.
13. Bonica, J. J. Pain research and therapy: Past and current status and future needs. In Ng, L. K. Y., and Bonica, J. J. (eds.). Pain, Discomfort and Humanitarian Care. New York, Elsevier, 1980.
14. Ng, L. K. Y., and Bonica, J. J. (eds.). Pain, Discomfort and Humanitarian Care. New York, Elsevier, 1980.
15. Kornfeld, D. S.: Psychiatric factors in the management of pain. In Levitan, S.

J. and Berkowitz, H. L. (eds.). Pain Research and Treatment. Washington, D.C., American Psychiatric Press, 1985, pp. 50–77.
16. Hackett, T. P. The pain patient, the evaluation and treatment. In MGH Handbook of General Hospital Psychiatry. St. Louis, C. V. Mosby, 1978.

Suggestions for Further Reading

History of Medicine and Pain

Williams, L. P. and Steffens, H. J. The History of Science in Western Civilization. New York, University Press of America, 1978. Vol. 1–3. Includes original source material on Hippocrates, Epidemics, Case IV; Galen, On Medical Experience; Williams Harvey, Exercitatio Anatomica De Motu Cordis et Sanguinis Animalibus; Claude Bernard, Cours de physiologie, in Revue Scientifique.

Chambers, M., et al. The Western Experience, 3rd ed. Vol. 1–2. New York, Alfred A. Knopf, 1983.

Clinical Perspective

Diamond, S. and Dalessio, D. (eds.). The Practicing Physician's Approach to Headache, 4th ed. Baltimore, Williams & Wilkins: 1986.

Cailliet, R. Neck and Arm Pain, 2nd ed. Philadelphia, F. A. Davis, 1985.

Dalessio, D. (ed.). Wolff's Headache and Other Head Pain, 5th ed. New York, Oxford, 1985.

Neurology of Pain

Adams, R., and Victor, M. Principles of Neurology, 3rd ed. New York, McGraw-Hill, 1985.

Psychobiology of Pain

Adams, R., and Victor, M. Principles of Neurology, 3rd ed. New York, McGraw-Hill, 1985.

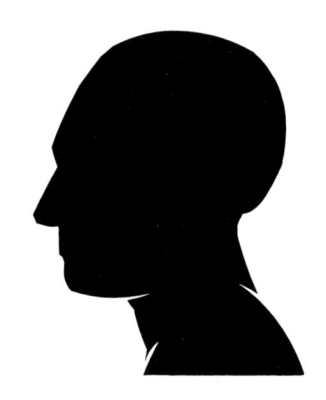

Chapter 2
Neurologic Causes of Head and Face Pain

Jeffrey T. Kessler

Pain in the head, neck, and face may be caused by a wide variety of disorders (Table 2–1).[1-4] Other sections of this book have dealt with a number of these disorders in considerable detail. It is the purpose of this chapter to discuss those entities that fall within the purview of the neurologist because the neurologist is usually not the first health professional contacted by the patient with complaints of this type of pain. Patients are often suspected of having and at times are treated for such conditions as sinusitis or dental disease, the symptoms of which may, at least in part, be mimicked by an underlying neurologic disorder.[5] We will discuss those disorders of primarily neurologic concern that can mimic oronasopharyngeal pathologic conditions. This differentiation is important for several reasons, including avoidance of destructive or other surgical procedures that may be done inadvertently on the basis of less than fully conclusive evidence for their performance. Another important reason is the avoidance of undue prescribing, in terms of extent and duration, of analgesics, in particular narcotic medications, for an undiagnosed condition. The third and obviously most important reason is proper identification and diagnosis so that definitive therapy can be given.

Many of the entities that cause head and neck pain most often present in a fashion that is sufficiently clear to allow them to be distinguished from the neurologic entities alluded to above, and the reverse is also true. For example, while sinusitis may be associated with headache in perhaps 10 percent of patients, it most often presents as facial pain and is associated with tenderness in the overlying tissues and straightforward radiographic findings. The symptom of headache is much more likely to prompt earlier

TABLE 2–1. Classification of Head and Face Pain

Vascular
    Migraine headache
    Cluster headache
    Carotidynia
    Temporal arteritis
    AV malformations
    Aneurysm
    Carotid cavernous fistula
Musculoskeletal
    Muscle contraction headache
    Cervical spondylosis
    TMJ (Costen's syndrome)
Infectious
    Sinusitis
    Osteomyelitis
    Dental disease
    Syphilis, leprosy, etc.
Neoplastic, inflammatory
    Tumors of extracranial tissues
    Intracranial tumors
    Sarcoidosis, orbital pseudotumor, histiocytosis, etc.
Trauma
Classic neuralgias
    Trigeminal
    Vagoglossopharyngeal neuralgia
Other neuralgias
    Postherpetic
    Sphenopalatine
    Geniculate
    Occipital
    Paratrigeminal syndrome of Raeder
Causalgia of the face
Atypical facial pain

referral in an unclear diagnostic situation than is facial pain for these reasons. It is, however, the circumstance in which there are no clearly evident symptoms and findings of sinus disease that the conditions to be discussed subsequently in this chapter should be considered.[1]

Headache arises from irritation of one of four general pain-sensitive structures in the head: (1) the scalp and its attached muscles, (2) the blood vessels, both intracranial and extracranial, (3) the skull and periosteum, and (4) the meninges. The parenchyma of the brain itself is not invested with pain-sensitive nerve endings. These facts and an understanding of the anatomy and physiology of head and face pain will aid in these distinctions.[6,7]

Headaches of a vascular nature are usually distinguishable by their clinical characteristics and unless associated with other symptoms, particularly in the face, are usually readily recognizable at least as vascular headaches. Vascular headaches are often pulsatile in quality, particularly when severe, and are usually increased by head movement, physical exertion, coughing or straining (Valsalva maneuver), or changes in position. The patient often complains of photophobia or sonophobia. The headaches generally increase in severity during a period of minutes to as long as an hour or two before reaching a peak. They may then last from hours to several days. Classic migraine can be distinguished from the foregoing, which is generally a description of common migraine, by the presence of preceding or accompanying focal neurologic symptoms and findings including visual loss, sensory loss, paralysis, or other symptoms and findings. Since 70 percent of patients with migraine have a family history and since such headaches often begin in adolescence and early adulthood and have a female preponderance, they are not usually confused with other causes of pain in the head and face.

Cluster headache, which at times may be confused with Raeder's paratrigeminal neuralgia, is a typical vascular throbbing, pounding headache located in the frontal and temporal regions and rarely lasts more than an hour. Although a Horner's syndrome can briefly appear during an attack, it is not present between attacks. The episodes may occur several times during the day and are associated with lacrimation and nasal stuffiness. They often occur at night and will awaken the patient from sleep, and are precipitated by the ingestion of vasodilating substances, particularly alcohol. The severity of the brief attacks lasting an hour or less without an intervening Horner's syndrome in a young adult male is usually sufficient to distinguish cluster headache from Raeder's syndrome.

Muscle contraction headache is often described as a "tight band around my head" or "a heavy hat." The pain is usually dull and aching, is located in the frontal and occipital as well as the nuchal and vertex regions, and generally develops in the morning and worsens as the day wears on. The pain tends to become maximal in the late afternoon or early evening and is generally relieved by recumbency and common analgesic medications. These headaches are not usually associated with focal neurologic complaints.

Headaches due to expanding intracranial lesions occur daily; they generally become worse with recumbency and will often awaken the patient at night. These headaches, like migraine, may be accompanied by nausea and vomiting, which does not usually characterize most other conditions causing head and face pain. The presence of specific or focal neurologic symptoms and findings usually prompts the institution of appropriate neurologic diagnostic testing.

The failure of apparent vascular or muscle contraction headache to respond to the usual remedies after one or two trials obviously raises the clinical index of suspicion, regardless of the absence of focal symptoms or findings, and requires the performance of CT or MRI scanning or other neurologic diagnostic testing. For further clinical description and evaluation the reader is referred to any of several simple standard neurologic texts on these headaches as well as headaches due to intracranial and extracranial disease states.[8-10] Similarly, the pain in the posterior neck and associated headache due to cervical spondylosis usually does not present with symptoms in the face or throat that would make this condition more difficult to distinguish from other entities. Temporomandibular joint disease is discussed elsewhere in this text. The main body of concern in this chapter, therefore, is with groups VI, VII, VIII, and IX in Table 2-1: the classic neuralgias, other neuralgias, facial causalgia, and atypical facial pain (Table 2-1).

Classic Neuralgias

This group encompasses chiefly trigeminal neuralgia and vagoglossopharyngeal neuralgia. The generally accepted criteria for a true or classic neuralgia are the following:

1. A paroxysmal, usually lancinating or searing pain that is markedly dysesthetic in quality in the known anatomic distribution of a cranial or peripheral nerve. This pain is usually measured in seconds, although an underlying persistent ache in the area is not uncommon.

2. The pain can be brought on by stimulation of trigger zones or areas within that anatomic distribution.

3. There is no objective sensory or motor loss in the distribution of that nerve.

Trigeminal Neuralgia

Possible clinical descriptions of trigeminal neuralgia have been ascribed to physicians such as Aretaeus and Caelius Aurelianus dating back as far as the first century A.D.,[11,12] but a number of authors[4,11-13] agree that the first accurate clinical description was made by the philosopher and physician John Locke in 1677 while attending the wife of the English ambassador during a visit to Paris. Since he did not think that bleeding the patient was likely to be of benefit, and other topical remedies had not succeeded, he consulted with colleagues in London for their further advice and sent them the following description:

> When the fit came, there was, to use my Lady's own expression of it, as it were a flash of fire all of a suddaine shot into all those parts and at everyone of those twitches, which made her shreeke out; her mouth was constantly drawn on the right side towards the right eare by repeated convulsive motions, which were constantly accompanied by her cries. . . . These violent fits terminated on a suddaine, and then my Lady seemed to be perfectly well, excepting only a dull pain which ordinarily remained in her teeth on that side, with an uneasinesse in that side of her tongue which she phansied to be swollen on that side, which yet, when I looked on it, as I often did, had not the least alteration in it in color, bignesse or any other way, though

it were one of her great complaints that there was a scalding liquor in her fits shot into all that half of her tongue.... With all this torment that she endured, when the fit was over there was not the least appearance of any alteration anywhere in her face, nor inflammation or swelling in her mouth, cheeke; very little deflection of rhewm more than what the contraction of those parts in those fits might cause. Speaking was apt to put her into these fits; sometimes opening her mouth to take anything, or touching her gums, especially on the places where she used to find throbbing; pressing that side of her face by lying on it were also apt to put her into fits. These fits lasted sometimes longer, sometimes shorter; were more or less violent, without any regularity, and the intervals between them at the longest not halfe an houer, commonly much shorter.[14]

Credit is usually given to the French physician Nicolaus André for first recognizing this condition as a clinical entity. He is also credited with coining the term *tic douloureux*. Although this term has come into common medical parlance, it literally means an unbearably painful twitch, which is much less specific than the preferred term *trigeminal neuralgia*. Thirteen years after the recognition of this entity by Nicolaus André, John Fothergill in England reported 14 patients who had it and recognized that this condition was chiefly present in the elderly.[13] Following the demonstration of localization of sensory function of the face to the trigeminal nerve by Bell in the first quarter of the nineteenth century, the localization of tic douloureux to the trigeminal nerve and the evolution of the term *trigeminal neuralgia* arose. From that time until the last 25 years many widely varied approaches to the problem were tried. Treatment with leeches, bleeding, various medicinal and surgical approaches, and psychic techniques were employed without reliable efficacy. Current effective medical and surgical approaches will be discussed later in this chapter.

Trigeminal neuralgia may be associated with various pathologies in various locations, beginning centrally and developing peripherally as well, as shown in Table 2–2.[4, 15, 16] Many of these conditions are often associated with signs of trigeminal neuropathy. In idiopathic trigeminal neuralgia various theories and accumulations of evidence supporting both central and peripheral causes have been advanced. The findings of arterial compression of the trigeminal nerve near its emergence from the pons, various pathologic changes in the trigeminal ganglion, stretching of the nerve root across the

TABLE 2–2. Pathology of Trigeminal Neuralgia

CONDITION	APPROXIMATE INCIDENCE (%)
Multiple sclerosis	2–6
Tumors	3–6
Aneurysm, arteriovenous malformation	1
Congenital anomaly	1
Arachnoiditis, adhesions	1
Vascular compression	Up to 90
No gross pathology (idiopathic)	Up to 40

petrous ridge, and central changes in the trigeminal tract in the pons have all been proposed.[17-20] Conclusive support for any of these positions is still lacking. Although it is clear that surgical intervention and manipulation of the nerve under direct visualization is a highly effective procedure, the exact mechanism of this benefit is unclear.

The recovery of herpes simplex virus from human trigeminal ganglia[21] and the association of herpes simplex virus with recurrent trigeminal neuralgia[22] have led to the speculation that herpetic infection of the ganglion may be a cause of idiopathic trigeminal neuralgia. Rothman and Monson[23] reviewed 526 patients admitted for neurosurgical relief of trigeminal neuralgia to Massachusetts General Hospital or the Lahey Clinic between 1955 and 1970 and compared them with a control group of 528 patients; they failed to find any significant correlation between cold sores or sore throats and trigeminal neuralgia. These data, although not excluding herpes simplex as a possible etiologic agent, do suggest that the presence of recurrent herpetic lesions in attacks of trigeminal neuralgia in a patient reported by Behrman and Knight is more likely to be coincidental than etiologic.[22,24]

In regard to etiology, a somewhat different approach has been recently advanced by Shaber and Krol,[25] who found localized areas of pathology in the jawbones of eight patients. In five patients they found bony "devoidation," described as a "non-epithelium-lined cavity containing either loosely adherent fatty-like tissue or no tissue whatsoever." In the other three patients there were areas of what they called "reactive bone," which appeared to have a consistency similar to that of normal bone but with a different color and character. After surgical treatment of these areas in these eight patients they reported total or near-total relief of pain in this somewhat limited series.

These findings and this theory, of course, do not account for the presence of trigeminal neuralgia that is clinically indistinguishable from idiopathic trigeminal neuralgia in patients with multiple sclerosis and other pathologic conditions as indicated above, which clearly involve the trigeminal nerve.

As suggested by Fothergill in the eighteenth century, trigeminal neuralgia is typically a disease of older people, with most series suggesting that symptoms begin after age 40 in 90 percent of patients. In a study done by Rothman and Monson,[23] of a variety of risk factors, the only ones that achieved clear statistical significance were a non-Jewish religion and birth in the United States. Other factors that did not reach statistical significance but were thought to be possibly associated included nonsmoking, nondrinking, and the presence of tonsils. Multiple sclerosis was, in addition, found to be a clear risk factor. The female-to-male sex ratio found by these authors was 1.7 to 1. Review of patient records at the Mayo Clinic[26] suggests an incidence of 4.3 cases per 100,000 people per year or approximately eight to nine thousand new cases per year in the United States. The rates, broken down by sex, were 5.0 for women and 2.7 for men, substantiating the increased incidence in women noted in other studies.[26] An increased incidence in patients with multiple sclerosis was also noticed in this series and appears to range generally from 2 to 5 percent in patients with multiple sclerosis. Conversely, approximately 2 or more percent of trigeminal neuralgia patients are suffering from multiple sclerosis.[27]

In 1974 Rothman and Wepsic presented a review of 508 patients with unilateral trigeminal neuralgia.[28] They found that the pain occurred on the left side in 38 percent of the patients and on the right side in 62 percent, confirming previous studies indicating a right-sided predominance. They were unable to find an association between the side of pain and handedness. In a smaller subgroup they were unable to find an association between an elevated ipsilateral petrous apex and the side of facial pain. Although there have been several reports of inherited or familial trigeminal neuralgia,[29] in these limited instances at least two different types of genetic transmission are described, and no such pattern has been noted in the many large series presented throughout the literature, which makes the presence of a specific inheritable factor for this condition unlikely.

As suggested in the above paragraphs the annual incidence of trigeminal neuralgia is 1 per 250,000 adults, according to Wepsic.[28] This means an estimated 10,000 people in the United States will develop trigeminal neuralgia every year. Thousands more will have facial pain of other types. It therefore becomes important to distinguish first whether the patient is suffering from trigeminal neuralgia and then whether this is idiopathic or symptomatic. The frequency with which symptomatic trigeminal neuralgia presents varies from author to author depending on one's theory of the origin of the pain. Jannetta has stated that tic douloureux is not an idiopathic disease but is always symptomatic. In 1976,[30] in a series of 100 consecutive surgical patients with trigeminal neuralgia, he found evidence of compression of the nerve in 94 percent of his patients. This compression was vascular in origin in 88 percent of patients and caused by tumors or vascular malformations in 6 percent of patients. He estimated that the other 6 percent of the patients in his series had multiple sclerosis, most probably with plaques at the root entry zone of the nerve in four patients and an atrophic nerve in two patients. The finding of an incidence of tumors in the posterior fossa in 5.6 percent of patients undergoing neurosurgical exploration for trigeminal neuralgia reported by Dandy[15] in 1934 agrees with Jannetta's data. In a more recent study[31] in which 2000 patients with facial pain were reviewed retrospectively during a 10-year period, the incidence of tumors was found to be 0.8 percent. This series included both patients with trigeminal neuralgia and "atypical facial pain," which was used to describe any other type of facial pain other than trigeminal neuralgia. It was suggested from this series that severe pain of an atypical nature associated with a progressive neurologic deficit was likely to be associated with a tumor of the middle cranial fossa, whereas tumors in the posterior fossa were more likely to cause trigeminal neuralgia and to be accompanied by more subtle neurologic deficits. The suggestion from the above studies is therefore that patients with facial pain that does not fit the clinical description of trigeminal neuralgia are not likely to have tumors unless there is an associated deficit on neurologic examination. On the other hand, patients with trigeminal neuralgia are less likely to have an associated neurologic deficit with an underlying tumor and are more likely to have an underlying cause of this nature, though these patients still constitute a small percentage of cases.

The distinction of trigeminal neuralgia can usually be made by a clear history and careful physical examination. The patient usually describes the pain as sharp, more like a "bolt of lightning." The patient often states that it feels as if "a red hot poker were placed against my face" or like a sharp current of electricity.[32] This lancinating pain is often described as "unbearable" and generally lasts no more than seconds to a minute or so. There may be an underlying dull, aching sensation between attacks, which may occur repeatedly with varying frequency throughout the day. The pain is limited to the trigeminal distribution, usually in a single division; the second and third divisions account for 95 percent of cases. As previously mentioned, trigeminal neuralgia occurs in women more often than in men (by a 3 to 2 ratio) and is more often on the right side than the left (by a 1.7 to 1 ratio).[26-28] In addition to paroxysmal lancinating pain limited to the known anatomic distribution of a peripheral or cranial nerve, the presence of trigger zones usually constitutes the definition of a true neuralgia. With trigeminal neuralgia these trigger zones are usually small, perhaps 2 to 4 mm in size, and are usually located at the bottom of the nose and the mouth and gums.[33] Pain may be brought on by washing the face, brushing the teeth, speaking, chewing, or other movements of the jaw and mouth. Dalessio[33] found in a study of ten patients that the application or release of pressure in a susceptible area frequently evoked attacks, as did vibratory but not thermal stimuli. In these patients, using a quantified light tapping stimulus of various frequencies and dimensions, Dalessio was able to show evidence of summation. Thus, the greater the frequency of stimuli, the more rapidly pain would be induced. In addition, a refractory period has been noted following the pain during which time a trigger zone can be touched without producing pain.[34] It has also been asserted that psychodynamic factors may play a role as trigger zones and can be altered by hypnosis. Finally, the finding that blocking the upper cranial nerve roots and the greater auricular nerves may prevent the pain of trigeminal neuralgia makes the genesis of trigger stimuli somewhat uncertain.[34]

It is generally accepted that medical therapy should be tried first in an effort to control trigeminal neuralgia and that surgery should be reserved for failure of medical therapies, which may take place with the passage of time because there is a tendency for the condition to have periods of pain come closer and sometimes last longer as the patient gets older (Table 2–3). Many such medical therapies have been proposed and tried. Stilbamidine, which appears to produce specific effects on the trigeminal structures, has been discarded because it produces hepatorenal toxicity and unwelcome facial tingling and numbness, and not infrequently has a protracted onset of action. Reported successes in small numbers of patients by Iannone et al.[35] led to initial enthusiasm for treatment with Dilantin. Other subsequent studies with this drug have shown efficacy in probably no more than 30 percent of patients, a rate that closely approximates the placebo effect. The

TABLE 2–3. Medical Treatment of Trigeminal Neuralgia

DRUG	EFFICACY (%)
Stilbamidine	50–60
Diphenylhydantoin	30
Mephenesin	60
Carbamazepine	80
Baclofen*	70–80
Sodium Valproate*	50
Clonazepam*	65
Tocainide	Not established
Tizanidine	Not established

*Should be considered in addition to or instead of carbamazepine when this drug fails prior to consideration of surgery.

role of Dilantin at this time is rather limited. It is used at times in association with other medications, although less frequently in recent years due to the appearance of more effective agents.

In 1966 King[36] reported on 52 patients who were treated with mephenesin carbamate during a 7-year period. He found a rather low incidence of side effects, and control of pain was sufficient in 60 percent of patients to make a surgical procedure unnecessary. He noted that patients with a more recent onset of pain tended to respond better. Patients who had relapses during oral therapy were often hospitalized for intravenous therapy. The need to administer the drug every 3 hours by mouth somewhat limits this treatment, which has not found great favor over the years.

In 1962 Blom[37] reported the trial of a new anticonvulsant drug (G-32883) and found that 6 of 11 patients became completely free of symptoms within 24 hours after the introduction of this agent, carbamazepine (Tegretol). Although initially there was concern about bone marrow and liver toxicity, careful monitoring of hepatic and hematologic function has significantly reduced the risk of the drug. It is currently considered the initial medical treatment of choice. Unfortunately, the incidence of these unwanted effects tends to be more common in the older group, the same group in whom there is the highest incidence of trigeminal neuralgia.[38] This drug is effective in 70 to 75 percent of patients,[39–41] although higher and lower rates of success have been reported. One of the chief difficulties in the use of carbamazepine, apart from its toxicity, is a tendency for the drug to induce its own metabolism, making achievement of steady blood levels somewhat more difficult.[38, 42] The correlation of serum levels with clinical efficacy has nevertheless been documented, levels in the generally accepted range for anticonvulsant activity being most suitable. The usual daily dosage reduced to achieve a therapeutic level ranges from 400 mg to as high as 1200 mg.

The most common side effects of nausea, drowsiness, and complaints of dizziness can often be avoided by gradually introducing the medication, beginning with 100 mg two or three times per day on the first day with increases of 100 mg per day every 12 to 24 hours until pain relief is obtained. Should side effects occur, the dose should be reduced to the previous highest tolerated level, and a serum drug level should be obtained before proceeding with higher doses at a slower rate. Liver function studies and complete blood counts should be obtained weekly in the first few weeks of therapy; the intervals of testing can be spread out as tolerance to the drug and lack of toxicity are demonstrated.

The report of Fromm et al.[43] in 1980 on the efficacy of baclofen in trigeminal neuralgia has added another drug to the armamentarium for medical management of trigeminal neuralgia. They found relief of pain in 10 of 14 patients receiving 60 to 80 mg of baclofen per day; they also found that a reduction of the dosage resulted in recurrence of pain in five of six patients. A number of patients were also receiving Dilantin or carbamazepine. Baclofen was effective in five patients who were taking no other medication. Side effects of mild sedation and mental dullness as well as mild incoordination were reported in this series. These side effects are not uncommon in the usual usage of this drug and can be avoided in a number of instances by beginning with low doses of 5 mg three times daily and increasing the dose by 5 to 15 mg every few days. The time required to build an effective dose of baclofen probably makes it second to carbamazepine for the treatment of trigeminal neuralgia, but it may be added to either carbamazepine or Dilantin for treatment of patients who previously responded to either of these agents and are losing that response.

In 1976 Court and Kase[44] reported on the efficacy of clonazepam, a new anticonvulsant drug, in 25 patients with trigeminal neuralgia. They reported complete control of neuralgia in 40 percent of patients and significant relief of pain in an additional 23 percent. Of some interest is the fact that 16 of these 25 patients had not responded to carbamazepine previously, and half of these patients were completely relieved by the clonazepam. There were significant side effects present in the great majority of patients, and these were severe in half of them. These included sedation and an unsteady gait. These undesirable effects were not noted in Smirne and Scarlato's[45] series of 14 patients, 64 percent of whom responded satisfactorily to clonazepam. They reported an effective dose range of between 6 and 9 mg per day.

A study by Peiris[46] and colleagues indicated a response to the use of sodium valproate in approximately 50 percent of patients in a series of 20. This drug may merit further study in larger groups of patients in whom serum levels are monitored. It, like baclofen and carbamazepine, requires monitoring for hepatic and hematologic toxicity.

New pharmacologic approaches are being pursued. A recent study of Tizanidine,[47] a new imidazole derivative with analgesic and myorelaxant properties, failed to demonstrate satisfactory efficacy in treatment of trigeminal neuralgia. Recently a trial of Tocainide, a lidocaine derivative that can be used orally, produced some potentially encouraging results in a small number of patients.[48] Recent reports of serious hematologic side effects with several deaths have limited further investigation.

The experiments of Bell and Magendie, in which the sensory function of the trigeminal nerve and motor function of the facial nerve were identified, allowed a rational approach to surgical management of trigeminal neuralgia.[11] A summary of these methods is presented in Table 2–4. Treatment throughout the nineteenth century, however, consisted chiefly of neurectomy of the peripheral branches of the trigeminal nerve, but because of frequent return of pain this gave way to direct alcohol injections by the first part of the twentieth century. In the last decade of the nineteenth century attempts were made by Hartley and Kraus to use an extradural approach, which was later improved by Spiller, Frazier, and Tiffany as well as Stookey. These technical developments formed the basis for modern intracranial technique, largely by means of a subtemporal approach. During this time Dandy pioneered a posterior fossa approach to the trigeminal root. His approach led to the development of a variety of procedures, the most popular of which is Jannetta's compression-decompression operation. Bulbar trigeminal tractotomy has the advantage of being able to selectively destroy pain-bearing fibers while preserving fibers responsible for light touch. Performance of this procedure in the lower medulla oblongata has been safely achieved. Unfortunately, when this selective destruction is not achieved with any of these procedures both anesthesia and analgesia may develop and may be accompanied by a severe constant facial pain known as anesthesia dolorosa in as many as 4 to 5 percent of patients.[49]

As stated by Sweet,[49] many of the tactile and kinesthetic fibers are well myelinated, whereas pain fibers tend to be relatively unmyelinated. The recognition of this anatomic fact led to the use of glycerol instillation or radiofrequency heating to produce selective damage to pain fibers. The development of the technique of radiofrequency thermocoagulation of the trigeminal ganglion and rootlets by Sweet and Wepsic[50] led to a procedure that preserved touch in some or all of a trigeminal division that had been rendered analgesic. Subsequently, a number of significant large series have been published by various other authors.[51-54] These data have been reviewed by Sweet.[49] The complication rate of this procedure has been low, sensory paresthesias being the most common side effect, occurring in 15 percent of patients; cranial nerve palsies, which are almost always transient, are

TABLE 2–4. Surgical Treatment of Trigeminal Neuralgia

Anterior fossa or peripheral
  Peripheral injection
  Neurectomy
Middle fossa
  Gasserman ganglion injections
  "Compression" and "decompression" procedures
  Thermocoagulation
  Trigeminal rhizotomy
Posterior fossa
  Trigeminal rhizotomy
  Bulbar trigeminal tractotomy

uncommon, occurring in 2 percent of patients.[55] An overall success rate of 90 to 95 percent can be anticipated in patients after the first procedure when it is performed by an experienced neurosurgeon. The recurrence rate varies from 10 to 30 percent. In addition to persistent paresthesias, anesthesia dolorosa may occur (it is rather uncommon) as may keratitis. Arrhythmias and hypertension may occur during the surgical procedure.[56] Other, less common complications are carotid-cavernous fistulas, which may require surgical repair, and meningitis. Cerebral hemorrhage and brain abscess have occurred rarely.

The use of retrogasserian injection of glycerol as reported by Nathanson[57] was initially embraced by Sweet and his colleagues[58] as possibly superior to radiofrequency thermocoagulation. The mechanism of action of this technique was thought to be due to disruption of abnormally myelinated nerve fibers because histopathologic evaluation revealed areas of focal demyelination, axonal swelling, and endoneural fibrosis with neuronal loss. In addition, abolition of evoked potentials was found.[59] None of the above anatomic or physiologic changes were noted in animals injected with saline. It has since been discontinued because of a higher initial failure rate, a higher frequency of later recurrences, and major sensory loss or dysesthesia (anesthesia dolorosa). In spite of recent efforts to treat anesthesia dolorosa,[60] this complication remains one of the most feared, unpleasant, and difficult to manage complications resulting from retrogasserian rhizotomy.

The finding of contact with an artery in only 14 of 40 nerves was noted by Jannetta and colleagues[61] when the trigeminal nerve root entry zones were examined bilaterally in 20 cadavers of people without a history of facial pain. Only four of these vessels actually produced compression or distortion of the nerve. This fact is in contrast with the vascular relationships of 40 nerves in individuals treated surgically for trigeminal neuralgia. In these 40 individuals, 31 nerves, or roughly 78 percent, showed evidence of compression by an adjacent blood vessel. In addition, another four cadaver nerves showed evidence of venous compression, whereas eight additional patients with trigeminal neuralgia showed evidence of venous compression. In microvascular decompression, if compression of the nerve by an artery is found following posterior fossa exploration by way of suboccipital craniectomy, a piece of material composed of polyvinyl alcohol is placed between the blood vessel and the nerve as a cushion or shock absorber. If venous compression is found, the vein is usually coagulated. If there is no evidence of neurovascular compression, that portion of the sensory nerve innervating the symptomatic trigeminal division is cut. This procedure, however, while relieving trigeminal neuralgia, does result in some degree of sensory loss similar to that occurring with percutaneous rhizotomy. The failure rate[62] for microvascular decompression ranges from 17 to 26 percent with generally a 1 percent morbidity and 1 percent mortality in experienced hands. There are almost no major dysesthesias. It has been suggested[63] that this procedure could be offered to younger patients who are able to undergo posterior fossa exploration and who wish to avoid possible anesthesia dolorosa and have failed to respond to medical therapy. Patients who have failed to respond both to medical therapy and to percutaneous rhizotomy may also be offered this procedure. However, except in the circumstances noted above, the consensus remains that percutaneous stereotaxic rhizotomy is the procedure of choice for most patients with trigeminal neuralgia,[64] many of whom are older and may have underlying cardiovascular or other conditions that would increase surgical risk.

Vagoglossopharyngeal Neuralgia

The recognition of vagoglossopharyngeal neuralgia is generally attributed to Weisenburg,[65-67] who in 1910 described it without attaching a specific label to it in a patient with a cerebellopontine angle tumor. It was not until 1921 that Harris first described the idiopathic type and not until 1926 that he first used the term *glossopharyngeal neuralgia*, which was later expanded to *vagoglossopharyngeal neuralgia* by White and Sweet in recognition of the role played by the vagus nerve in this condition. The pain follows the suggested definitions of a true neuralgia.[4, 7] It is sharp, lancinating or stabbing in quality, and can last from seconds to a few minutes. It may recur repeatedly throughout the day for hours or days on end. Occurring in the distribution of the somatosensory distribution of the vagus and glossopharyngeal nerves, the pain may involve one or a combination of the following regions: throat, ear, tonsillar region, posterior third of the tongue, larynx, external auditory canal, and eustachian regions (Table 2–5).

In the great majority of patients reported since Weisenburg's description the condition has been considered to be idiopathic. However, Laha and Jannetta[68] described six patients in 1977 and found that in five of them the ninth and tenth cranial nerves were compressed by a tortuous vertebral artery or posterior inferior cerebellar artery at the root entry zone. A cure resulted in these patients, who were treated with microvascular decompression without sectioning of the nerves, a procedure similar to those applied in patients with trigeminal neuralgia. Vagoglossopharyngeal neuralgia has also been described in association with metastatic laryngeal carcinoma and other head and neck tumors.[69-71] In 1958 Eagle[72] described his reported experience of the previous 20 years with elongated styloid processes, which can produce a clinical constellation very similar to that seen in vagoglossopharyngeal neuralgia. This condition often follows tonsillectomy. He estimated that 4 percent of the population have elongated styloid processes, and 4 percent of these become symptomatic. Treatment consists of surgical shortening of the offending process.

The pain can be precipitated by a variety of stimuli, the most common of which is swallowing, although chewing, coughing, touching the tragus of the ear, talking, or occasionally eating cold or highly spiced foods as well as turning the head and neck may be trigger factors. It has even been described in association with trigeminal neuralgia in a series of nine patients by Brzustowicz in 1955.[73]

Although most patients are older than age 50, the condition has been

TABLE 2–5. Vagoglossopharyngeal Neuralgia

Exceedingly uncommon (1% of the incidence of trigeminal neuralgia)
Equal sex incidence
90% of patients are over age 40
Left side is affected more than right side, with bilaterality in less than 2% of cases
Pain is sharp and burning, usually lasting seconds
Pain usually located in the throat or ear with radiation to:
   Posterior third of tongue
   Tonsillar pillars and fossae
   Nasopharynx, oropharynx, laryngopharynx
   Larynx
   Eustachian tube and middle ear
   External auditory canal
Trigger points or provocation
   Common—swallowing, talking, eating, and chewing
   Less common—nose blowing, sneezing, laughing, shouting, yawning, coughing, head turning
May occur at nght, which is very unusual in trigeminal neuralgia
May be accompanied by bradycardia with secondary syncope and convulsions
Treatment
   Medical—carbamazepine (Tegretol), baclofen, and clonazepam
   Surgical—Glossopharyngeal rhizotomy and upper vagal rootlet sectioning, compression, decompression, radiofrequency coagulation of the petrous ganglion

reported in young adults. Spontaneous remissions have been reported in the majority of patients, but as in trigeminal neuralgia these appear to become progressively shorter with increasing age. The relative incidence of vagoglossopharyngeal neuralgia is approximately 1 percent of that of trigeminal neuralgia. Bilateral involvement was reported in only 4 of 217 patients by Rushton et al.[65] in contrast to about 5 percent of their patients with trigeminal neuralgia who had bilateral involvement. They also reported a combined occurrence of vagoglossopharyngeal neuralgia and trigeminal neuralgia in 25 of their 217 patients, thereby extending the series of Brzustowicz.[65, 73] A left-sided preponderance has been suggested by Ross,[4] and, indeed, five of Laha and Jannetta's[68] six patients had left-sided involvement. Of some interest is the fact that in their 217 patients Rushton et al.[65] found no instances of multiple sclerosis, whereas this entity has a generally accepted incidence of 2 percent in patients with trigeminal neuralgia.

Although the pain of trigeminal neuralgia is thought to be more severe, a greater potential danger lies in the small percentage of patients with vagoglossopharyngeal neuralgia who may suffer syncope and possibly secondary convulsions. These episodes do not appear to occur as the result of hypersensitivity of the carotid sinus because massage and stimulation of this area does not usually result in syncope, convulsions, or asystole.

According to Rushton, "the usual mechanism proposed has been a spillover of impulses from the glossopharyngeal nerve via the tractus solitarius to the dorsal motor nucleus of the vagus nerve resulting in reflex bradycardia or asystole."[65] Reports of managing this condition with a pacemaker and medical treatment have been recorded.[74-76] Surgery has been reliably successful in preventing syncope and relieving pain.

The diagnosis of vagoglossopharyngeal neuralgia can be aided by performance of a cocaine test using a 10 percent solution applied to the regions of the tonsils and hypopharynx. The test is considered positive if stimuli that had formerly induced pain in these trigger areas are no longer successful. This test was performed by Rushton et al.[65] in a series of 125 patients and was found to be positive in 112. They found a good correlation between a positive test and the results of surgical treatment but also stated that a negative test does not preclude the diagnosis or successful surgical intervention.

Attempts at medical therapy prior to the advent of carbamazepine were uncommon, and medical therapy in general is less successful for this condition than it is for trigeminal neuralgia. Some early success was reported by Ekbom and Westerberg,[77] who tried carbamazepine in four patients. In the large series from the Mayo Clinic reviewed by Rushton and colleagues,[65] partial or complete benefit with the use of Dilantin was noted in nine patients, four of whom eventually had return of pain that could not be managed. Nine patients failed to benefit from the use of Dilantin. Similarly, whereas ten patients initially benefited in part or wholly with carbamazepine, six eventually experienced return of pain. An additional three patients had sufficient relief to avoid surgery, and seven patients were not benefited. There was no greater success when the two drugs were used together. The results of medical treatment for this condition are, as suggested above, less encouraging than they are for trigeminal neuralgia, and carbamazepine is probably the drug of choice. More recently, Ringel and Roy[78] have reported successful treatment of vagoglossopharyngeal neuralgia with baclofen. Clonazepam has been used in a single patient.[45]

In the large series of Rushton et al.,[65] 129 patients were eventually treated surgically; of these, 110 patients obtained good relief of pain, 13 patients experienced no relief, and 6 patients required reoperation. A 5 percent mortality in the immediate postoperative period was reported in this series. These patients had undergone sectioning of the upper rootlets of the vagus nerve and the pharyngeal nerve. Approximately 20 percent had difficulty swallowing or an unpleasant sensation in the throat as a postoperative complication. These authors recommend surgical sectioning of the glossopharyngeal nerve and the upper two or three rootlets of the vagus nerve. When pain involves the inner portions of the ear and the cocaine test is negative, sectioning of the nervus intermedius should be considered. Possible hypotension due to manipulation of the ninth and tenth cranial nerves during surgery has been noted. Further experience with microvascular decompression needs to be obtained to determine whether this will prove superior to a destructive procedure.[68, 79] In addition, the use of radiofrequency coagulation of the petrous ganglion has been proposed as a treatment for this condition, but it requires further experience and exploration.[80]

Other Neuralgias

Neuralgia of the Nervus Intermedius (Geniculate Neuralgia)

This condition, originally described by J. Ramsay Hunt, has been called the intermedius neuralgia of Hunt, tic douloureux of the nervus intermedius, and geniculate neuralgia. In its classic form the pain is sharp, lancinating, and severe and involves the distribution of the nervus intermedius in the internal and middle ears as well as the upper eustachian and mastoid areas.[81, 82] A careful history and a negative cocaine test of the hypopharynx will help distinguish this condition from vagoglossopharyngeal neuralgia. Geniculate neuralgia, however, may take the form of a dull aching pain of gradual onset punctuated by paroxysms of sharp shooting, lancinating, or burning pain superimposed on the background of a dull ache. There does not appear to be a sex or side preference, and thus far most reported patients have been young to middle-aged adults. A careful history and physical examination will help distinguish this condition from carcinoma of the nasopharynx or external auditory canal region, and simple radiographs will identify an elongated styloid process.[83] The presence of identifiable trigger phenomena has not been reported. A careful search for herpetic vesicles should be made.

There are no reports of successful medical therapy. A trial of carbamazepine with or without baclofen is warranted before considering a surgical approach. The largest recent series was reported by Pulec,[84] who reported excision of the nervus intermedius and geniculate ganglion through a middle cranial fossa approach. No instances of facial paralysis were noted. All patients experienced loss of tearing on the involved side after surgery, which produced no problem. At times, selective section of portions of the trigeminal nerve were included to produce a successful result in these 15 cases. Intracranial sectioning of the nerve of Wrisberg has also been reported to be successful.[85, 86]

Postherpetic Neuralgia

Postherpetic neuralgia is a condition of the elderly, with over 90 percent of cases occurring after age 60; it is common after age 70.[87] When the cranial nerves are affected, producing head or face pain, the trigeminal nerve is involved in the overwhelming majority of instances. Involvement of the geniculate ganglion is associated with a rash in the external auditory canal and weakness of the face ipsilaterally. Although it may be difficult to find the herpetic vesicles unless one looks carefully in the external ear canal, the association between this pain, the vesicles, and facial weakness usually identifies the rather rare Ramsay Hunt syndrome. The ophthalmic division of the trigeminal nerve is affected in 80 percent of instances, and the ganglion is affected in approximately 20 percent.[88] The pain may precede the development of the rash by as much as 2 weeks, although a typical eruption does occur eventually in almost all instances. Subsequent scarring and sensory loss in the distribution of the affected part of the ophthalmic division of the trigeminal nerve is typically seen. The pain, which has been likened to causalgia,[87] may be a continuation of the initial pain. The condition appears to develop somewhat more frequently in women than in men (by a 3 to 2 ratio). It has even developed in the trigeminal ganglion 10 years after retrogasserian rhizotomy for trigeminal neuralgia.[89]

The incidence of postherpetic neuralgia following herpes zoster infection of the trigeminal ganglion or its first division varies from 2 to 10 percent but clearly increases with increasing age. It has been suggested[90,91] that early treatment with steroids during the infective stage will significantly reduce the incidence of postherpetic neuralgia, particularly in elderly patients with no increased incidence of disseminated herpes.

Russell et al.[87] initially suggested treatment consisting of procaine block of the nerve supplying the affected area combined with massage of the area for 10 to 15 minutes several times per day. Topical spray with ethyl chloride (which may be hazardous in the region near the eye) may allow this massage, which should take place with a cloth having the texture of a Turkish towel. Application of a mechanical vibrator has also been advocated by Russell but is probably of limited benefit, as are local saline injections.

In keeping with Russell's assertion that "postherpetic neuralgia resembles causalgia,"[87] Milligan and Nash[92] found that stellate ganglion block produced benefit in three-quarters of patients who had had pain for less than 1 year, and nearly half became pain-free. This benefit was observed in a series of 77 patients, a number of whom had failed to respond to pharmacotherapy with fluphenazine, amitriptyline, or carbamazepine. Ekblom and Hansson[93] produced relief in 10 of 30 patients with orofacial pain through the use of transcutaneous electrical nerve stimulation (TENS), whereas only 4 of 20 patients taking placebos responded. They concluded that TENS is of minor value in this unselected group. Its value in treating postherpetic neuralgia is therefore uncertain.

The use of psychotropic drugs for the treatment of postherpetic neuralgia is well established.[88,94] Treatment should be started initially with amitriptyline, beginning with 25 mg per day and gradually increasing the dose to a range of 100 to 150 mg per day. Woodforde et al.[95] produced good or complete relief of pain in 11 of 14 patients treated with amitriptyline. In the elderly or those with significant medical disease a beginning dose of 10 mg should be considered. Addition of a phenothiazine may also be tried. Other medical treatments such as vitamin B_{12} injections, carbamazepine, and Dilantin have been of questionable value.

Hitchcock and Schvarcz,[96] citing their own experience that "peripheral neurectomy or posterior rhizotomy has been helpful in relieving the hyperpathia of post-herpetic neuralgia without affecting the deep background pain, which may actually get worse," have advocated stereotaxic trigeminal tractotomy for postherpetic facial pain. They advocate destruction of the spinal trigeminal nucleus and descending tract and have reported relief of both the hyperpathia and deep pain in three patients. Sensory loss in the ipsilateral entire face, neck, and arm in one patient and contralateral body below D10 in another patient accompanied this procedure. Siegfried reported significant benefit in a series of 10 patients, noting complete relief in five patients and significant relief in three other patients treated with chronic stimulation of the ventral posterior medial thalamic nucleus.[97] This technique involved continual stimulation using a monopolar electrode. It should be remembered, however, that surgical procedures should generally be considered last in patients with this condition, given the limited experience and potential risks involved.

Sphenopalatine Neuralgia

Sphenopalatine neuralgia or Sluder's neuralgia was named for the sphenopalatine ganglion, which lies in the sphenopalatine fossa adjacent to the sphenoid and posterior ethmoidal sinuses. Because of its location Sluder believed that it could be affected by inflammatory processes in the nasal passages. He found evidence of congestion of the turbinates and other nasal mucosal surfaces. Eagle[98] found an intranasal deformity in 80 percent of his patients, which was relieved by submucous resection of the nasal septum. The pain described by both authors is not typically neuralgic in nature but rather constant, and, although at times burning, it is usually a persistent aching sensation, generally behind the eyes or in the region of the upper jaw or hard or soft palate. This pain is often associated with a variable headache. The painful episodes, which may be bilateral, may follow a dental or sinus infection and may last from an hour to several days. During the acute phases, injection of the conjunctivae, lacrimation, and facial erythema can be noted on the affected side. Ryan and Facer[99] found a greater frequency in women (2 to 1 ratio) compared with men and a preponderance of cases in the age range from 30 to 50. Attacks could be brought on by exposure to drafts, changes in climate, and use of alcohol or tobacco. They confirmed the effectiveness of the use of topical cocaine in this region, which had originally been suggested by Eagle and which is also helpful in confirming the diagnosis. This condition has been lumped with "atypical trigeminal neuralgia," and the possibility that it may be part of a vascular compression syndrome has been raised.[100]

The importance of distinguishing sphenopalatine ganglion neuralgia from cluster headache was addressed by Ryan and Facer.[99] A careful history alone should suffice because cluster headache occurs predominantly in men (80 to 90 percent of cases). The attacks, which are usually frontal and temporal in location, generally are throbbing and pounding in character and may be associated with nausea and vomiting.[101] The pain is generally severe but usually does not last more than 30 to 60 minutes, although it may recur a number of times during the day and may even awaken the patient from sleep at night. It is frequently precipitated by alcohol ingestion and may recur on a daily basis for a number of weeks and then remit for periods of several months to a year or longer. The various medical and surgical treatments offered for cluster headache are outside the scope of this chapter. Ross et al.[4] consider the entities petrosal neuralgia and erythroprosopalgia to be synonymous with cluster headache, also referred to as migrainous neuralgia.

Occipital Neuralgia

Occipital neuralgia has been thought to arise from varied causes.[4, 102, 103] It has been divided into primary and secondary types.[4] The primary type is regarded as more of a true neuralgia and consists of severe unilateral, lancinating pain in the distribution of the greater occipital or lesser occipital nerves. The neurologic examination is generally normal in these areas with no sensory loss or other findings, and definite trigger phenomena are present such as combing the hair or direct stimulation of the hair and scalp. An underlying ache may persist during the periods that are punctuated by more acute pain. The secondary type of occipital neuralgia is a more persistent dull, aching discomfort that is more chronic and may be bilateral. It is associated with underlying conditions such as Arnold-Chiari malformations, cervical spondylosis, primary and metastatic tumors, and mastoid infection as well as trauma to the subgaleal space in that region. The role of psychogenic muscle contraction has been debated. The role of C1–C2 arthrosis has been recently discussed by Ehni and Benner.[102, 103]

Treatment of the primary type of occipital neuralgia may be attempted first with the use of amitriptyline and is often successful (unpublished personal data). Should that fail, local blockade of the occipital nerve may result in a cessation of attacks. Persistent symptoms may need to be dealt with by surgical intervention. A trial of Dilantin prior to such surgery has been recommended.[4] Treatment of the secondary type is, of course, based on treatment of the underlying condition. The recent surgical results in the management of seven patients with C1–C2 arthrosis syndrome[102] suggests that an aggressive surgical approach in patients who fail to respond to medical treatment or local steroids and anesthetic injections may be warranted (Table 2–6).

Raeder's Paratrigeminal Syndrome

In 1962 Boniuk and Schlezinger[104] collected, in addition to Raeder's original five cases, 12 additional cases from the English language literature and added nine patients of their own. They proposed that patients with Raeder's syndrome be divided into two groups (Table 2–7). Group I would include patients with neuralgia in whom pain occurred in the ophthalmic and to some extent maxillary divisions of the trigeminal nerve. Pain in such

TABLE 2–6. Occipital Neuralgia

Primary type
    Severe unilateral electric shocklike pain
    Definite trigger zones activated by wearing a hat, use of a comb, or direct touching
    Treatment
        Amitriptyline
        Local steroid and anesthetic injections
        C2 dorsal rhizotomy
Secondary type
    Pain in same distribution (suboccipital, occipital and posterior parietal areas) but usually present for hours, days, or longer
    Usually associated with nuchal muscle spasm
    Associated with cervical spondylosis, craniocervical malformations, syringomyelia, and Arnold-Chiari malformations

patients is associated with Horner's syndrome without facial anhidrosis but with involvement of one or more other cranial nerves, chiefly parasellar. Group II would include patients with Raeder's syndrome as described but without parasellar cranial nerve involvement. All of Boniuk and Schlezinger's nine cases as well as the other 12 cases that they found belonged in group II, whereas neoplasm and trauma accounted for three of Raeder's original five cases. Two years later Minton and Bounds[105] added five more cases. Of the 27 patients considered to belong in group II, 26 were male and the left side was involved twice as often as the right side. Nonspecific associated inflammatory conditions, pneumonia, chronic sinusitis, dental abscesses, otitis media, and upper respiratory infections were found in eight of Minton and Bound's group II cases. There was a history of hypertension in nine patients, and six patients had migraine headaches. Head trauma was also thought to be a possible etiologic factor in Minton and Bound's series. The subsequent demonstration in 1968 of an internal carotid aneurysm in a patient with group II Raeder's paratrigeminal syndrome without evidence of other cranial nerve or parasellar involvement was reported by Law and Nelson,[106] who recommended that carotid arteriography be considered in all cases, group I or group II. A group I presentation of intracranial internal carotid artery aneurysm has also been described.[107] Inflammation of the adjacent wall of the carotid artery due to inflammation of the sphenoid sinus[108] has led to the suggestion that "the underlying pathology of group II cases may be compression of the internal carotid sympathetic fibers caused by swelling of the internal carotid arterial wall."[4]

Confirmation of a Horner's syndrome should be carried out by means of

TABLE 2–7. Paratrigeminal Syndrome of Raeder

> Throbbing headache in the distribution of the ophthalmic
> and upper maxillary divisions of the trigeminal nerve
> Ipsilateral Horner's syndrome with preserved sweating
> Two groups
>   Group I "symptomatic" with parasellar cranial nerve
>   involvement
>   Group II without parasellar cranial nerve involvement
> Etiologies or associated conditions
>   Group I
>   Metastases to middle cranial fossa
>   Calcification of internal carotid artery
>   Infections or trauma to petrous apex
>   Meningioma of gasserian ganglion
>   Group II
>   Upper respiratory infection
>   Chronic sinusitis and otitis media
>   Dental abscesses
>   Hypertension
>   Migraine headache
>   Aneurysm of the supracavernous portion of the internal
>   carotid artery
> Sex and side ratios
>   Over 90% of cases occur in males
>   Occurs on left side rather than right by a 2 to 1 ratio

an appropriate cocaine test with instillation of a 4 percent solution, which will produce no response in a second- or third-order neuron Horner's syndrome. Prompt dilatation will occur in a normal eye or a first-order Horner's syndrome. The use of Paredrine can help to carry the distinction further and identify a third-order Horner's syndrome.

Some disagreement about the criteria of Raeder's paratrigeminal syndrome has been recently raised by Mokri,[109] who considers the syndrome to be defined by evidence of trigeminal nerve involvement in addition to the complete Horner's syndrome. In addition, his definition requires the presence of true neuralgic pain in the distribution of the trigeminal nerve. It is our experience that the pain in Raeder's paratrigeminal syndrome is often a persistent severe ache, and a careful history will often distinguish it from cluster or other vascular headache.

The treatment of group I patients in Boniuk and Schlezinger's classification depends on identification of the underlying pathologic process, which may include primary and metastatic tumors of the middle cranial fossa, calcification of the internal carotid artery, infection or trauma of the petrous apex, and other conditions. Although group II cases often have a self-limited course, amitriptyline may be of benefit in relieving pain in these patients.

Reflex Sympathetic Dystrophy (Causalgia) of the Face

Reflex sympathetic dystrophy of the face has been reported following penetrating trauma, head injury, difficult dental procedures, maxillofacial surgery for cancer, and other facial trauma. It is characterized by a constant burning, at times searing, pain that is similar to reflex sympathetic dystrophy elsewhere in the body and is increased by local tactile or thermal stimuli and emotional stress. The usual trophic vascular and osseous changes noted with reflex sympathetic dystrophy of the extremities have not been seen in the facial region, although some localized rubor, calor, and turgor have been noted. Other stimuli of the face such as smiling, chewing, and other movements may increase or exacerbate the pain. The diagnosis is suggested by the presence of a constant burning pain. Successful treatment in recent cases with sympathetic blockage of the stellate ganglion has been reported.[110-112] Sympathectomy has been performed in patients in whom blockade of the stellate ganglion has provided only temporary relief.[113]

Atypical Facial Pain

Atypical facial pain appears to include those patients in whom structural pathology and other specific causes of facial pain have been investigated and ruled out. In addition, patients whose symptoms do not fit any of the classically accepted clinical entities are usually grouped in this category (Table 2–8). The syndrome was initially named *atypical facial neuralgia* by Fraser and Russell in 1924 and later modified to *primary atypical facial neuralgia* by Glazer[114] in his description of 245 patients in 1940. He noted at least 70 descriptive terms used by his patients to describe the sensations they experienced and added that they usually had difficulty describing it accurately. Engel in 1951[115] described a series of 20 such patients, 19 of whom were women. He noted there seemed to be a female preponderance in the literature at that time. He also found that patients were generally unable to describe their pain clearly and that they used a variety of descriptive terms. He noted pain on the right in eight patients and pain on the left in five; seven had bilateral pain, although not always simultaneously. Three-quarters of the patients had had pain for at least 1 year, and five had had pain for more than 15 years. Two of the twenty patients reported vasomotor changes including edema and vasodilatation in the skin during the attacks, but these changes disappeared when the pain abated. He remarked on the striking incidence of other somatic symptoms in addition

TABLE 2–8. Atypical Facial Pain

Pain is usually aching, poorly localized, and diffuse without neuritic character or correspondence to known neuroanatomy
Pain lasts for hours, days, or months and is variable in intensity and duration
No trigger zones or provocative factors
Depression and neurotic (obsessive-compulsive) traits are important factors in causation. Hysterical features common
Insomnia, fatigue, mood changes, and weeping spells also common
Frequent association with gastrointestinal complaints, dizziness, fainting and obviously hysterical sensory and motor deficits
Relief obtained with antidepressants in a large percentage in controlled studies

to the face pain in all but 1 of the 20 patients. He noted that "no patient could be described as having enjoyed good health until the face pain developed or as being well except for the face pain." Seventeen of the twenty patients had experienced pain at other times and in other parts of the body, at times similar to the facial pain. Many patients had had dental procedures. Two-thirds of the patients had had one form of surgery or another, and 52 surgical procedures had been performed on those 14 patients. Evidence of psychological difficulty was present in all of Engel's patients, who had poor marital, work, and social relationships. He termed them generally a "uniformly unhappy and unsatisfied group of people." He noted a long history of suffering and misfortune involving illness, injury, and life situation failures as a frequent concomitant. It was his opinion that primary atypical facial neuralgia was a hysterical conversion symptom, although that did not necessarily indicate that the correct psychiatric diagnosis was conversion hysteria. He found a consistent character structure of persistent masochism. Smith et al.[116] subsequently found deviant MMPI profiles, especially involving the hysterical scale, in 32 such patients.

Engel's opinion, drawn from his and later[117] studies, was later shared by Miller,[118] who stated that "the typical patient is female, middle-aged, edentulous, haggard, and importunate." He and others[119] have noted that these patients had often had a variety of dental or otolaryngologic procedures, often without a firm basis for their performance. He noted a lack of response to analgesic drugs and failure to respond to anything except antidepressant agents, although there was a tendency in some instances toward spontaneous remission.

The role of depression in patients with head and face pain that defies etiologic classification was emphasized by Dalessio.[120] Lascelles[121] had shortly before recommended a regimen of Nardil and Librium after finding frequent depressive symptoms in 93 such patients. However, Dalessio suggested the use of Elavil, feeling that monoamine oxidase inhibitors were too dangerous for use in these circumstances. The addition of Librium, especially at bedtime, was also recommended. The role of depression in head and face pain and the use of tricyclic antidepressant medications have also been addressed by others.[122, 123]

As summarized by Friedman,[124] the typical patient with atypical facial pain describes a discomfort that may vary in severity and character and does not follow any known anatomic distribution. The pain often is present for hours or days and lacks clear trigger zones or other precipitating factors. The patients are generally middle-aged women, and there are no specific findings on neurologic evaluation or subsequent neurologic, dental, or ear, nose and throat (ENT) evaluation. It is our experience that these patients respond to a confident approach by the physician coupled with an understandable explanation of the role of endorphin depletion in the genesis of chronic pain and the expected role of tricyclic antidepressants, particularly Elavil, in the restoration of this biochemical lack.

References

1. English, G. M. Pain of the head and neck. In English, G. M. (ed.). Otolaryngology. Philadelphia, Harper & Row, 1979, pp. 1–19.
2. Donlon, W. C. and Jacobson, A. L. Maxillofacial pain. Am Fam Pract 30:151–163, 1984.
3. Chasin, W. D. Facial pain, neck pain and headache. In Katz, A. E. (ed.). Manual of Otolaryngology—Head and Neck Therapeutics. Philadelphia, Lea & Febiger, 1986, pp. 313–333.
4. Ross, G. S., Wolf, J. K. and Chipman, M. The Neuralgias. In Baker, A. B. and Joynt, R. J. (eds.). Clinical Neurology. Philadelphia, Harper & Row, 1985, pp. 1–33.
5. Lazar, M. L., Greenlee, R. G. and Naarden, A. L. Facial pain of neurologic origin mimicking oral pathologic conditions: Some current concepts and treatment. JADA 100:884–888, 1980.
6. Smith, B. H. Anatomy of facial pain. Headache 9:7–13, 1969.
7. Arieff, A. J. Neurologic substance of pain (neuralgia). Headache 9:14–19, 1969.
8. Raskin, N. H., and Appenzeller, O. Headache. Philadelphia, W. B. Saunders Co., 1980.
9. Diamond, S. and Friedman, A. P. Headache. New Hyde Park, Medical Examination Publishing Co., 1980.
10. Diamond, S. and Dalessio, D. J. The Practicing Physician's Approach to Headache, 4th ed. Baltimore, Williams & Wilkins, 1986.
11. McMurtry, J. G. The history of medical and surgical interests in facial pain. Headache 9:1–6, 1969.
12. Stookey, B. and Ransohoff J. Trigeminal Neuralgia: Its History and Treatment. Springfield, Ill., Charles C Thomas, 1959.
13. Fields, W. S. and Lemak, N. A. Trigeminal neuralgia: Historical background, etiology, and treatment. BNI Quart 3:47–56, 1987.
14. Locke, J. Letter to Dr. Maplelott, as quoted in Stookey, B. and Ransohoff, J. Trigeminal Neuralgia: Its History and Treatment. Springfield, Ill., Charles C Thomas, 1959, pp 8–10.

15. Dandy, W. E. Concerning the causes of trigeminal neuralgia. Am J Surg 24:447–455, 1934.
16. Jannetta, P. J. Neurovascular compression in cranial nerve and systemic disease. Ann Surg 192:518–525, 1980.
17. Jannetta, P. J. Arterial compression of the trigeminal nerve at the pons in patients with trigeminal neuralgia. J Neurosurg 26:159–162, 1967.
18. Kerr, F. W. L. Evidence for a peripheral etiology of trigeminal neuralgia. J Neurosurg 26:168–174, 1967.
19. Malis, L. I. Petrous ridge compression and its surgical correction. J Neurosurg 26:163–167, 1967.
20. King, R. B. Evidence for a central etiology of tic douloureux. J Neurosurg 26:175–182, 1967.
21. Baringer, J. R. and Swoveland, P. Recovery of herpes simplex virus from human trigeminal ganglions. New Engl J Med 288:648–650, 1973.
22. Behrman, S. and Knight, G. Herpes simplex associated with trigeminal neuralgia. Neurology 4:525–530, 1954.
23. Rothman, K. J. and Monson, R. R. Epidemiology of trigeminal neuralgia. J Chron Dis 26:3–12, 1973.
24. Wepsic, J. G. Tic douloureux: Etiology, refined treatment. New Engl J Med 288:680–681, 1973.
25. Shaber, E. P. and Krol, A. J. Trigeminal neuralgia—a new treatment concept. Oral Surg 49:286–293, 1980.
26. Yoshimasu, F., Kurland, L. T. and Elveback, L. R. Tic douloureux in Rochester, Minnesota, 1945–1969. Neurology 22:952–956, 1972.
27. Rovit, R. L. Trigeminal neuralgia: Observations on etiology and treatment strategies. Neuroview 3:13–16, 1987.
28. Rothman, J. J. and Wepsic, J. G. Side of facial pain in trigeminal neuralgia. J Neurosurg 40:514–516, 1974.
29. Daly, R. F. and Sajor, E. E. Inherited tic douloureux. Neurology 23:937–939, 1973.
30. Jannetta, P. J. Microsurgical approach to the trigeminal nerve for tic douloureux. Prog Neurol Surg 7:180–200, 1976.
31. Bullitt, E., Teu, J. M. and Boyd, J. Intracranial tumors in patients with facial pain. J Neurosurg 64:865–871, 1986.
32. Amols, W. Differential diagnosis of trigeminal neuralgia and treatment. Headache 9:50–53, 1969.
33. Dalessio, D. J. A re-appraisal of the trigger zones of tic douloureux. Headache 9:73–76, 1969.
34. Cave, B. L., Shelden, C. H., Pudenz, R. H. and Freshwater, D. B. Observations on the pain and trigger mechanism in trigeminal neuralgia. Neurology 6:196–207, 1956.
35. Iannone, A., Baker, A. B. and Morrell, F. Dilantin in the treatment of trigeminal neuralgia. Neurology 8:126–128, 1958.
36. King, R. B. The value of mephenesin carbamate in the control of pain in patients with tic douloureux. J Neurosurg 25:153–158, 1966.
37. Blom, S. Trigeminal neuralgia: Its treatment with a new anticonvulsant drug (G-32883). Lancet I:839–840, 1962.
38. Green, M. W. Medical treatment of trigeminal neuralgia and cluster headache. Psychosomatics 26 Suppl.: 19–23, 1985.
39. Nicol, C. F. A four year double-blind study of tegretol in facial pain. Headache 9:54–57, 1969.

40. Davis, E. H. Clinical trials of tegretol in trigeminal neuralgia. Headache 9:77–82, 1969.
41. Marotta, J. T. A long term study in trigeminal neuralgia. Headache 9:83–87, 1969.
42. Tomson, T., Tybring, G., Bertilsson, L., Ekbom, K. and Rane, A. Carbamazepine therapy in trigeminal neuralgia: Clinical effects in relation to plasma concentration. Arch Neurol 37:699–703, 1980.
43. Fromm, G. H., Terrence, C. F., Chattha, A. S. and Glass, J. D. Baclofen in trigeminal neuralgia: Its effect on the spinal trigeminal nucleus: A pilot study. Arch Neurol 37:768–771, 1980.
44. Court, J. E., Kase, C. S. Treatment of tic douloureux with a new anticonvulsant (Clonazepam). J Neurol Neurosurg Psychiatr 39:297–299, 1976.
45. Smirne, S. and Scarlato, G. Clonazepam in cranial neuralgias. Med J Aust I:93–94, 1977.
46. Peiris, J. B., Perera, G. L. S., Devendra, S. V. and Lionel, N. D. W. Sodium valproate in trigeminal neuralgia. Med J Aust II:278, 1980.
47. Vilming, S. T., Lyberg, T. and Lataste, X. Tizanidine in the management of trigeminal neuralgia. Cephalgia 6:181–182, 1986.
48. Lindstrom, P. and Lindblom, U. The analgesic effect of tocainide in trigeminal neuralgia. Pain 28:45–50, 1987.
49. Sweet, W. H. The treatment of trigeminal neuralgia (tic douloureux). New Engl J Med 315:174–177, 1986.
50. Sweet, W. H. and Wepsic, J. G. Controlled thermocoagulation of trigeminal ganglion and rootlets for differential destruction of pain fibers. Part I: Trigeminal neuralgia. J Neurosurg 39:143–156, 1974.
51. Nugent, C. R. and Berry, B. Trigeminal neuralgia treated by different percutaneous radiofrequency coagulation of the Gasserian ganglion. J Neurosurg 40:517–523, 1974.
52. Onofrio, B. Radiofrequency percutaneous Gasserian ganglion lesions. J Neurosurg 42:132–139, 1975.
53. Siegfried, J. 500 percutaneous thermocoagulations of the Gasserian ganglion for trigeminal pain. Surg Neurol 8:126–131, 1977.
54. Tew, J. M., Lockwood, P. and Mayfield, F. H. Treatment of trigeminal neuralgia in the aged by a simplified surgical approach (percutaneous electrocoagulation). J Am Geriatric Soc 23:426–430, 1975.
55. Mittal, B. and Thomas, D. G. T. Controlled thermocoagulation in trigeminal neuralgia. J Neurol Neurosurg Psychiatr 49:932–936, 1986.
56. Samuels, S. I., Brodsky, J. B., Kehler, C. H. and Britt, R. H. Trigeminal neuralgia: Treat but do not prolong. Br Med J 283:987–988, 1981.
57. Nathanson S. Trigeminal neuralgia treated by injection of glycerol into the trigeminal cistern. Neurosurgery 9:638–646, 1981.
58. Sweet, W. H., Poletti, C. E. and Macon, J. B. Treatment of trigeminal neuralgia and other facial pains by retrogasserian injection of glycerol. Neurosurgery 9:647–653, 1981.
59. Lunsford, L. D., Bennett, M. H. and Martinez, A. J. Experimental trigeminal glycerol injection, electrophysiologic and morphologic effects. Arch Neurol 42:146–149, 1985.
60. Hasobuchi, Y., Adams, J. E. and Rutkin, B. Chronic thalamic stimulation for the control of facial anesthesia dolorosa. Arch Neurol 29:158 161, 1973.
61. Haines, S. J., Jannetta, P. J. and Zorub, D. S. Microvascular relations of the trigeminal nerve: An anatomical study with clinical correlation. J Neurosurg 52:381–386, 1980.

62. Piatt, J. H. and Wilkins, R. H. Treatment of tic douloureux and hemifacial spasm by posterior fossa exploration: Therapeutic implications of various neurovascular relationships. Neurosurg 14:462–471, 1984.
63. Tew, J. M. and Van Lovern, H. Surgical treatment of trigeminal neuralgia. Am Fam Pract 31:143–150, 1985.
64. Menzel, J., Piotrowski, W. and Penzholz, H. Long-term results of Gasserian ganglion electrocoagulation. Neurosurg 42:140–143, 1975.
65. Rushton, J. G., Stevens, J. C. and Miller, R. H. Glossopharyngeal (vagoglossopharyngeal) neuralgia: A study of 217 cases. Arch Neurol 38:201–205, 1981.
66. Chawla, J. C. and Falconer, M. A. Glossopharyngeal and vagal neuralgia. Br Med J 3:529–531, 1967.
67. Bohm, E. and Strang, R. R. Glossopharyngeal neuralgia. Brain 85:371–388, 1962.
68. Laha, R. K. and Jannetta, P. J. Glossopharyngeal neuralgia. J Neurosurg 47:316–320, 1977.
69. Giorgi, C. and Broggi, G. Surgical treatment of glossopharyngeal neuralgia and pain from cancer of the nasopharynx. J Neurosurg 61:952–955, 1984.
70. Dykman, T. R., Montgomery, E. B. Jr., Gersttenberger, R. D., et al. Glossopharyngeal neuralgia with syncope secondary to tumor: Treatment and pathophysiology. Am J Med 71:165–168, 1981.
71. MacDonald, D. R., Strong, E., Nielsen, S., et al. Syncope from head and neck cancer. J Neuro-Oncology 1:257–267, 1983.
72. Eagle, W. E. Elongated styloid process. Arch Otolaryngol 67:172–176, 1958.
73. Brzustowicz, R. J. Combined trigeminal and glossopharyngeal neuralgia. Neurology 5:1–10, 1955.
74. Jamshidi, A. and Masroor, M. Glossopharyngeal neuralgia with cardiac syncope: Treatment with a permanent cardiac pacemaker and carbamazepine. Arch Intern Med 136:843–845, 1976.
75. Jackson, R. R. and Russell, R. W. R. Glossopharyngeal neuralgia with cardiac arrhythmia: A rare but treatable cause of syncope. Br Med J I:379–380, 1979.
76. Alpert, J. N., Armbrust, A., Akhair, M., et al: Glossopharyngeal neuralgia, asystole and seizures. Arch Neurol 34:233–235, 1977.
77. Ekbom, K. A. and Westerberg, C. E. Carbamazepine in glossopharyngeal neuralgia. Arch Neurol 14:595–596, 1966.
78. Ringel, R. A. and Roy, E. P. Glossopharyngeal neuralgia: Successful treatment with baclofen. Ann Neurol 21:514–515, 1987.
79. Wilkins, R. H. Neurovascular compression syndromes. Neurol Clin North Am 3:359–372, 1985.
80. Lazorthes, Y. and Verdie, J. C. Radiofrequency coagulation of the petrous ganglion in glossopharyngeal neuralgia. Neurosurgery 4:512–516, 1979.
81. Furlow, L. T. Tic douloureux of the nervus intermedius (so-called idiopathic geniculate neuralgia). JAMA 119:255–259, 1942.
82. Sachs, E., Jr. The role of the nervus intermedius in facial neuralgia. J Neurosurg 28:54–60, 1968.
83. Hora, J. F. and Brown, A. K. Obscure otalgia. Laryngoscope 74:122–133, 1964.
84. Pulec, J. Geniculate neuralgia: Diagnosis and surgical management. Laryngoscope 86:955–964, 1976.
85. Wilson, A. A. Geniculate neuralgia. J Neurosurg 7:473–481 1950.
86. Sachs, E., Jr. Further observations on surgery of the nervus intermedius. Headache 9:159–161, 1969.

87. Russell, W. R., Espir, M. L. E. and Morgansern, F. S. Treatment of post-herpetic neuralgia. Lancet I:242–245, 1957.
88. Diamond, S. Post-herpetic neuralgia prevention and treatment. Postgrad Med 81:321–322, 1987.
89. Teng, P. and Papatheodorou, C. Post-herpetic trigeminal neuralgia: Ten years after retro-Gasserian rhizotomy. J Neurosurg 28:61–62, 1968.
90. Elliott, F. A. Treatment of herpes zoster with high doses of prednisone. Lancet II:610–611, 1964.
91. Eaglstein, W. H., Katz, R. and Brown, J. A. The effects of early corticosteroid therapy on the skin eruption and pain of herpes zoster. JAMA 211:1681–1683, 1970.
92. Milligan, N. S. and Nash, T. P. Treatment of post-herpetic neuralgia: A review of 77 consecutive cases. Pain 23:381–386, 1985.
93. Ekblom, A. and Hansson, P. Extrasegmental transcutaneous electrical nerve stimulation and mechanical vibratory stimulation as compared to placebo for the relief of acute oro-facial pain. Pain 23:223–229, 1985.
94. Taub, A. Relief of post-herpetic neuralgia with psychotropic drugs. J Neurosurg 39:235–239, 1973.
95. Woodforde, J. M., Dwyer, B., McEwen, B. W., et al: Treatment of post-herpetic neuralgia. Med J Aust II:869–872, 1965.
96. Hitchcock, E. R. and Schvarcz, J. R. Stereotaxic trigeminal tractotomy for post-herpetic facial pain. J Neurosurg 37:412–417, 1972.
97. Siegfried, J. Monopolar electrical stimulation of nucleus ventroposteromedialis thalami for post-herpetic facial pain. Appl Neurophysiol 45:179–184, 1982.
98. Eagle, W. W. Sphenopalatine ganglion neuralgia. Arch Otolaryngol 35:66–84, 1942.
99. Ryan, R. E. and Facer, G. W. Sphenopalatine ganglion neuralgia and cluster headache: Comparisons, contrasts and treatment. Headache 17:7–8, 1977.
100. Jannetta, P. J. Cranial nerve vascular compression syndromes (other than tic douloureux and hemifacial spasm). Clin Neurosurg 28:445–456, 1981.
101. Duvoisin, R. C. The cluster headache. JAMA 222:1403–1404, 1972.
102. Ehni, G. and Benner, B. Occipital neuralgia and the C1/2 arthrosis syndrome. J Neurosurg 61:961–965, 1984.
103. Ehni, G. and Benner, B. Occipital neuralgia and C1/3 arthrosis. New Engl J Med 310:127, 1987.
104. Boniuk, M. and Schlezinger, N. S. Raeder's paratrigeminal syndrome. Am J Ophthalmol 54:1074–1084, 1962.
105. Minton, L. R. and Bounds, G. W. "Raeder's Paratrigeminal Syndrome." Am J Ophthalmol 58:271–275, 1964.
106. Law, W. R. and Nelson, E. R. Internal carotid aneurysm as a cause of Raeder's paratrigeminal syndrome. Neurology 18:43–46, 1968.
107. Jain, D. C., Ahoja, G. K. and Goulaim, R. K. Intracranial internal carotid artery aneurysm as a cause of Raeder's paratrigeminal syndrome. Surg Neurol 16:357–359, 1981.
108. Nolph, M. B. and Dion, M. W. Raeder's syndrome associated with internal carotid artery dilation and sinusitis. Laryngoscope 92:1144–1148, 1982.
109. Mokri, B. Raeder's paratrigeminal syndrome: original concept and subsequent deviations. Arch Neurol 39:395–399, 1982.
110. Jaeger, B., Singer, E. and Kroening, R. Reflex sympathetic dystrophy of the face: Report of two cases and a review of the literature. Arch Neurol 43:693–695, 1986.

111. Khoory, R., Kennedy, S. F. and MacNamara, T. E. Facial causalgia: Report of a case. J Oral Surg 38:782–783, 1980.
112. Hanowell, S. T. and Kennedy, S. F. Phantom tongue pain and causalgia: Case presentation and treatment. Anesthesiol Analg 58:436–438, 1979.
113. Bingham, J. A. W. Causalgia of the face. Br Med J I:804–805, 1947.
114. Glazer, M. A. Atypical facial pain diagnosis, cause and treatment. Arch Intern Med 65:340–367, 1940.
115. Engel, G. L. Primary atypical facial neuralgia: an hysterical conversion symptom. Psychosom Med 13:375–396, 1951.
116. Smith, D. P., Pilling, L. F., Pearson, J. S. et al. A psychiatric study of atypical facial pain. Can Med Assoc J 100:286–291, 1969.
117. Engel, G. L. Psychogenic pain and the pain-prone patient. Am J Med 26:899–918, 1959.
118. Miller, H. Pain in the face. Br Med J 2:577–580, 1968.
119. Patten, J. P. Typical-atypical facial pain. Anesthesiol Prog 18:32–35, 1970.
120. Dalessio, D. J. Some reflections on the etiologic role of depression in head pains. Headache 8:28–31, 1968.
121. Lascelles, R. G. Atypical facial pain and depression. Br J Psychiat 112:651–659, 1966.
122. Kienast, H. W. Psychological aspects of facial pain. Headache 9:31–35, 1969.
123. Gayford, J. J. The aetiology of atypical facial pain and its relation to prognosis and treatment. Br J Oral Surg 7:202–207, 1970.
124. Friedman, A. P. Atypical facial pain. Headache 9:27–30, 1969.

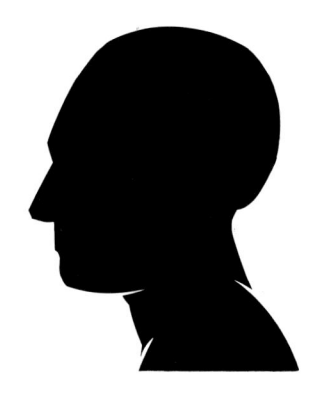

Chapter 3
Otalgia

Kenneth F. Mattucci and Young B. Choo

Ear pain (otalgia) is a very common symptom and is one of the most frequently encountered facial, head, and neck pains. It is often associated with hearing loss, tinnitus, fullness in the ears, and disorders of balance, and it is the presence or absence of these associated symptoms that frequently allows the physician to arrive at a possible diagnosis. However, a significant number of these complaints, or "ear pain" itself, may be nonotogenic in origin.

The clinician must first determine if the otalgia is actually caused by an ear disorder, and if so, must correctly locate the anatomical site of pathology.

Sensory innervation of the ear is derived from branches of the fifth, seventh, ninth, and tenth cranial nerves. The mandibular division (V3) of the fifth cranial nerve, by way of the auriculotemporal nerve, supplies sensation to the tragal skin and superior-anterior wall of the external auditory canal and contiguous portion of the tympanic membrane. The auricular branch (nerve of Arnold), a division of the vagus nerve, communicates with branches of the glossopharyngeal nerve and branches of the facial nerve to supply the inferior posterior portion of the external auditory canal and the contiguous portion of the tympanic membrane.

Innervation of the middle ear occurs through the tympanic plexus (Jacobson's nerve), which is composed of branches of the glossopharyngeal nerve and branches of the sympathetic plexus of the internal carotid artery. The tympanic branch of the glossopharyngeal nerve also supplies the inner surface of the tympanic membrane.

As a guide to organizing the clinician's approach to *otalgia*, we have found it helpful to think in terms of traumatic, inflammatory, and neoplastic causes of pain in each of the well-defined anatomic regions of the ear—namely, the pinna (external ear), external auditory canal, tympanic mem-

TABLE 3–1. Causes of Ear Pain

I. Otogenic causes
   A. External ear (pinna, external auditory canal, periauricular area)
      1. Trauma
         a. Pinna—hematoma, seroma, laceration, abrasion, burn, frostbite
         b. External auditory canal—abrasion, foreign body, cerumen, fracture of temporal bone
      2. Inflammation
         a. Pinna—cellulitis, dermatitis (psoriasis, seborrhea, neurodermatitis, contact dermatitis), abscess, perichondritis
         b. External auditory canal—furuncle, external otitis, osteoma, exostoses, malignant external otitis (necrotizing otitis externa)
      3. Neoplasm
         a. All regions—both benign and malignant tumors, often with associated inflammation
   B. Tympanic membrane
      1. Trauma—barotrauma, perforation, foreign body
      2. Inflammation—bullous myringitis, myringitis
      3. Neoplasm—usually part of an extension from another region
   C. Middle ear
      1. Trauma—temporal bone fracture, barotrauma, foreign body
      2. Inflammation—otitis media, serous otitis media, cholesteatoma
      3. Neoplasm—primary carcinoma of temporal bone, metastatic carcinoma, glomus jugulare and glomus tympanicum. Extension of nasopharyngeal carcinoma to middle ear
   D. Temporal bone (mastoid and inner ear)
      1. Trauma—temporal bone fracture, barotrauma
      2. Inflammation—mastoiditis (acute and chronic), mastoid abscess, cholesteatoma, lateral sinus thrombosis and thrombophlebitis, complications of ear disease with central nervous system extension
      3. Neoplasm—glomus jugulare, carcinoma, sarcoma, histiocytosis, metastatic disease, acoustic neuroma[7]

II. Nonotogenic causes
   A. Neurologic and referred pain
      1. Tonsillitis and post-tonsillectomy pain
      2. Oral and dental disease (dental caries, abscess, periodontal disease, ulcerations)
      3. Teeth eruption
      4. Lesions of hypopharynx, laryngopharynx (foreign body, carcinoma, ulcers), cricoarytenoid joint arthritis
      5. Nasosinus complex
      6. Nasopharyngeal disease—carcinoma, Tornwaldt's disease
      7. Eagle's syndrome (elongated styloid process)
      8. Neuralgias—glossopharyngeal neuralgia, sphenopalatine neuralgia, trigeminal neuralgia, and vidian neuralgia
      9. Cervical arthritis
     10. Cardiac (ischemic cardiac episodes)

TABLE 3–1. Causes of Ear Pain *Continued*

  B. Parotid gland disorders—inflammation with or without stones, benign and malignant neoplasms
  C. Miscellaneous—vascular abnormalities (temporal arteritis, carotidynia, aneurysms, collagen disorders)
  D. Psychogenic
  E. Myofacial pain dysfunction syndrome (MPD), temporomandibular joint syndrome, rheumatoid arthritis, osteoarthritis, primary muscle spasm

brane, middle ear space, intratemporal bone region (mastoid and inner ear), and the middle and posterior cranial fossae (see Table 3–1).

The history must be thorough and accurate. The characteristics of the pain should be reviewed as well as its intensity, frequency, duration, and area of radiation. Is the pain throbbing or steady? What brings it on—chewing? Swallowing? Yawning? Pressure? Traction on the ear? What were the circumstances immediately preceding the onset of pain? Was the patient flying, diving, swimming, using Q-tips, undergoing dental procedures? Did the patient have a preceding upper respiratory infection? Were there prior attempts to remove wax or a foreign body?

One must also question the patient about the presence of known, prior, or pre-existing otologic disease such as prior episodes of external otitis, cerumen accumulations, perforation of the tympanic membrane, intermittent discharge (watery, mucinous, or foul-smelling), previous operations on the ear, and the presence of associated symptoms such as pressure, fullness, tinnitus, vertigo, and hearing loss.

The presence of an underlying systemic disorder may be related directly or indirectly to otalgia. Does the patient have diabetes, arteriosclerotic cardiovascular disease, hypertension, allergy, collagen disorders, a previous diagnosis of malignant disease, or arthritis? The physician must be aware of the medications, both topical and systemic, that have been administered to the patient both prior to the onset of symptoms and currently.

As the patient relates the history, the physician should listen attentively and let that information guide the selection of further questions. During the examination the findings or lack of findings will also act as a guide to selection of appropriate questions. Talking to and questioning the patient or the parent during the examination relaxes the patient, is time efficient, and provides ongoing feedback. The patient's general hearing abilities can be appraised in this way, and the degree of relative discomfort can be assessed.

The examination of the ear should be approached anatomically. Visual inspection of the pinna, anteriorly and posteriorly, as well as palpation of the ear and periauricular region should be done. Skin should be assessed in regard to warmth, texture, and color. Inspect the opening of the external auditory canal. Using light traction on the pinna posteriorly, the clinician can evaluate the degree of discomfort elicited, if any. The ear canal is inspected next, using the appropriate size of speculum. By visually spiraling down the ear canal, one should attempt to inspect 360 degrees of the canal, especially near the tympanic membrane and annulus. Very often this is not possible owing to angulation of the external canal or exostoses. The canal and tympanic membrane region should be debrided. The presence of significant disease may be obscured by an insignificant appearing piece of cerumen, crust, or accumulation of epithelial debris. One should be conscious of any foul or unusual odor from the ear canal.

The tympanic membrane should be studied and its anatomic characteristics noted. Attention should be directed toward its integrity, clarity, color, presence of scars, and presence or absence of a light reflex. Special attention should be paid to the region of the "pars flaccida" and the attic and the presence of debris, retraction, or perforation noted. Pneumatic otoscopy (Fig. 3-1) is very useful in assessing the relative mobility of the tympanic membrane and the relative middle ear and eustachian tube function. Is there a middle ear effusion present with bubbles, retraction, or perforation? Does the Valsalva maneuver cause tympanic membrane motion?

The presence of a tympanic membrane perforation is occasionally difficult to recognize. A very thin, healed perforation may appear to be open. A small and light insufflation of powder (boric acid powder) and a second look may show that the perforation is indeed closed if powder granules are present on the healed membrane. Lack of powder granules in the region of the suspected perforation contrasted with the presence of granules on the tympanic membrane surface confirms the suspicion of perforation.

In studying the middle ear mucosa, which may be visible through the perforation, the presence and characteristics of exudate should be noted. Does the mucosa appear edematous, moist, dry, or erythematous? Do the findings represent the possibility of underlying chronic disease? If so, the patient may be questioned as the examination proceeds about prior ear or mastoid infection or prior operations. Reinspection of the postauricular region for the confirmatory scar of prior mastoidectomy may be desirable. The patient's memory may be refreshed by such questions.

Although one must and should always perform a complete head and neck examination as part of the assessment for otalgia, the history and physical findings will direct the selection of the *extent* of head and neck

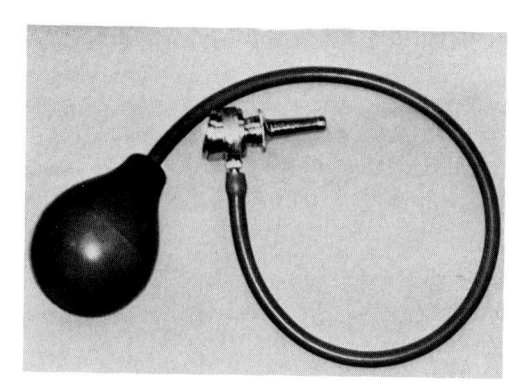

FIGURE 3-1. Pneumatic otoscope.

assessment. The presence of a suspected neoplasm of the ear or periauricular area may suggest that more time be spent in careful palpation of the neck to rule out gross cervical adenopathy, whereas the presence of middle ear disease may direct attention primarily to the nose and nasopharynx and may require nasoendoscopy or perhaps biopsy of the nasopharynx.

The examination should continue until the diagnosis is complete and assured. If the degree of discomfort is great, this initial evaluation may be stopped when the presenting cause of pain is discovered and therapy instituted. Since the patient will most likely return for re-examination and evaluation of the therapeutic response, a *complete* head and neck evaluation may be deferred until the patient is more comfortable and cooperative. It must be stressed, however, that it is the clinician's responsibility to perform a complete examination of the head and neck before the patient is discharged from his care for the presenting complaint of otalgia.

At times it will be necessary to perform further diagnostic tests to confirm or document one's diagnostic suspicion and to assess the patient's course and response to instituted therapy. Disease processes may progress despite the improvement of symptomatology. Unsuspected and significant hearing loss may be detected. In today's litigious society it is imperative to identify and document *objectively* existing problems prior to the institution of therapy, especially if one must use potentially ototoxic systemic or topical therapy. Underlying nonrelated sensorineural hearing losses are often discovered in patients who are being treated for disease that causes overwhelmingly conductive hearing loss. Impedence audiometry and tympanometry are not only extremely useful in documenting middle ear pathology but are also useful in monitoring the continued patency of tympanostomy tubes or in raising the index of suspicion of retrocochlear pathology. Is there significant reflex decay? By studying and comparing the volume recordings during impedence audiometry, one can determine if the ventilation tube is patent or blocked and can assess the integrity of the tympanic membrane. If the volume recorded is the volume of the external auditory canal only, one can be fairly certain that the tympanic membrane is intact or that a tube, if present, is blocked. If the tympanostomy tube is patent or if a tympanic membrane perforation exists, the volume of air recorded will be a measure of the volume of the external auditory canal, middle ear, and mastoid. Occasionally, a seal will be impossible to maintain because of a functioning eustachian tube. Therefore, documentation of the patency and function of a tube may help the clinician to consider or rule out the possibility of a whole spectrum of causes of otalgia.

The history, findings on physical examination, and results of audiometric and tympanometric tests may in some instances require the performance of radiographic imaging studies. The classic and routine radiographic studies, depending on the disorder being considered, the examining physician, the radiologist, and the patient, may be the most cost-effective means of securing a diagnosis. The suspected disease process itself, the results of the basic radiographic studies, or the progression of disease may suggest the need for computed tomography (CT) with or without enhancement, magnetic resonance imaging (MRI), or more invasive dye studies, including angiography.

In most instances, following a thorough history, a careful and complete physical examination, and selected appropriate audiometric, tympanometric, and radiographic studies, the complaint of otalgia will be found to be caused by primary otogenic disease. Occasionally, one must be prepared to requestion, re-examine, or retest the patient and to "rethink" the problem to achieve a proper diagnosis. If all the preceding measures have been accomplished to the best of one's abilities and no primary otologic cause is discovered, the physician must then proceed to consider the nonotogenic causes of ear pain. At this point the clinician must be prepared to explain to the patient that although the complaint is ear pain, the pain may originate from some other region. The patient must understand *why* the physician is examining the nose or the larynx or *why* he or she is ordering radiographic studies of the airway or scheduling a biopsy of the nasopharynx or tonsil.

A close working relationship and coordination of effort must exist between the primary care physician, the dentist, the neurologist, and the otologist. It is extremely important that examination, testing, and consultations be closely related temporally because the timing and pattern of otalgia and ear disease, and for that matter, nonotogenic pathology, can change quickly and dramatically.

The otogenic and nonotogenic causes of ear pain (Table 3-1) will be reviewed, and some of the associated signs and symptoms and the diagnostic and therapeutic approaches to each will be briefly described.

Otogenic Causes of Ear Pain

External Ear and Ear Canal

Pain arising from the external ear structures is usually not difficult to recognize. Frequently the history is sufficient to raise the index of suspicion. Often, there is a history of trauma or manipulation of the ear (use of Q-tips, blunt trauma) or water exposure. Inspection alone may make a diagnosis obvious, as in cases of auricular hematoma, seroma, laceration, perichondritis, or frostbite.

An auricular *hematoma* resulting from trauma is caused by an accumulation of blood and serum between the perichondrium and the cartilage of the external ear; these in turn lead to localized swelling with fluctuation and discoloration. Because cartilage receives its blood supply from the perichondrium, a separation of the perichondrium from cartilage may lead to aseptic necrosis and contraction and deformity. Aspiration of the hematoma using careful aseptic techniques followed by a pressure dressing is most often sufficient to prevent complications. Recurrent aspirations and occasionally incision and drainage may be necessary. Prophylactic antibiotics should be administered to prevent secondary infection, perichondritis, and auricular deformity (cauliflower ear).

Burns of the external ear are common when patients have received generalized head burns. These burns may be caused by fire, sun exposure, or electrical current and frequently progress to suppurative perichondritis. First-degree burns may be treated conservatively and supportively with analgesics only. Second-degree burns are treated by lavage and irrigation with saline or liquids to neutralize the offending agent. Reconstructive surgery and grafting may be necessary with severe burns.[1]

The anatomic location of the auricle, its extension from the head, and its exposure circumferentially to the environment make it very susceptible to temperature fluctuation. The initial phase of *frostbite* produces vasoconstriction and pallor; ice crystals then form in the extracellular fluid, resulting in a hypertonic state in the remaining fluid and intracellular dehydration. As the affected area thaws, edema develops, occasionally accompanied by bulla formation followed by erythema. Treatment should be directed at rewarming the area with moist cotton or gauze at a temperature of 38° to 42° C. The application of ice or snow or exposure to radiant heat is contraindicated.[2,3]

Perichondritis may be the result of either blunt trauma or infected hematoma, as noted, or of laceration or surgical procedures on the auricle or mastoid. There may be localized or generalized erythema, swelling, tenderness, and pain. Cultures of the area of infection should be made, and specific chemotherapy should be instituted promptly. Cephalosporins or aminoglycosides are the most effective agents.

The external ear may be involved by localized circumscribed neurodermatitis or contact dermatitis or by a systemic dermatologic disorder such as psoriasis or seborrhea with infection, or it may manifest local changes secondary to diffuse viral or bacterial illness such as herpes simplex or herpes zoster. The presence of discharge from the ear canal and its characteristics (purulent, hemorrhagic, serumucinous) and/or the presence of edematous skin may suggest acute infection. The infectious process may progress to include the entire external ear and face, scalp, occiput, and neck, and it may produce cellulitis in varying degrees of severity. Hearing may be affected if the disorder causes occlusion of the external auditory canal with obstruction of sound transmission down the canal to the tympanic membrane surface, as may occur with a foreign body, cerumen, secretions, edematous canal skin, or a tumor mass.

A variety of *foreign bodies* may be found in the external auditory canal including metallic and glass items, animal and insect material, and plant protein. Very often by the time the patient is seen by the ear specialist several attempts to remove the object have been made by the patient, the patient's family, or other physicians. The ear canal may be traumatized, swollen, or bleeding, making removal much more difficult. As with cerumen, removal with a pick, cerumen curette, alligator forceps, or suction tip is most often successful. Microscopic guidance can be invaluable. Rarely, irrigation will be necessary.

Insects can be removed piecemeal or whole with forceps. Live insects may be killed first by applying mineral oil and then removing them with a suction tip or alligator forceps. Vegetable matter (bean, peas, and seeds) may swell if saturated with water or blood, producing much tissue reaction and making removal very difficult. Occasionally, treatment with topical steroids or antibiotic drops or systemic antibiotics will be necessary to control the skin reaction and infection in the ear canal, after which the foreign body is removed.

Inflammation within the external auditory canal with or without impaired hearing may be suspected when pain is increased by traction of the pinna. Palpation of the auricle and preauricular region may also produce or increase pain and will help to localize the site, for instance, with a furuncle of the tragus or canal, inflammation of the concha, or inflamed preauricular or postauricular adenopathy.

Circumscribed external otitis (*furunculosis*) is an infection of the skin of the hair-bearing area of the cartilaginous portion of the external ear and ear canal. It is an infection of hair follicles caused by *Staphylococcus aureus*. Localized swelling and erythema, exquisite tenderness and pain, and occasional narrowing of the external auditory canal with hearing loss may exist. There may be periauricular tenderness and swelling due to lymphadenopathy. Warm soaks and antibiotics (penicillin, Staphcillin) are very beneficial.

External otitis is treated effectively by frequent and careful débridement of the external auditory canal and maintenance of an acid pH by the introduction of a topical agent such as Burow's solution or acetic acid drops. If there is significant edema or swelling of the skin of the ear canal, introduction of a gauze wick will be necessary to allow the medication to penetrate deep into the ear canal. A one-eighth or one-quarter inch piece of gauze or length of umbilical tape is inserted gently and atraumatically, and the patient is instructed to keep the gauze saturated with the prescribed drops. As the swelling and edema subside, the wick either will spontaneously fall from the ear canal or can be removed by the patient or physician and the drops continued. Occasionally one must elect to treat the infected ear canal in a "dry" fashion by instilling powder (boric acid) into the ear canal. This treatment can be very useful in patients with a large tympanic membrane perforation and intermittent drainage. A technique used decades ago and still quite effective is direct topical application of an antibiotic powder such as Chloromycetin or sulfa into the ear canal or open mastoid cavity. The patient should not allow water to get in the ears and should avoid self-cleaning the ears. Refractory cases of otitis externa often are caused by less common bacterial or fungal pathogens and may necessitate culture and sensitivity testing to determine a specific therapeutic approach. Specific systemic or topical antibiotics may be necessary at times, as may dermatologic and allergy consultations. In addition, one may need to resort to surgical drainage, aspiration, or biopsy to accomplish a specific diagnosis.

External otitis occurring in a diabetic patient should be a cause of major concern, like all infections occurring in the diabetic. The presence of a *Pseudomonas* external otitis associated with granulation tissue on the floor of the external auditory canal, most often at the junction of the bony and

Otalgia

cartilaginous portions of the canal, and very often accompanied by a significant degree of pain, may indicate *malignant external otitis (necrotizing otitis externa)*, which is a disorder associated with a high degree of morbidity and significant mortality.

It is believed that the *Pseudomonas* organism produces an endotoxin, including a neurotoxin, which is capable of producing peripheral polycranial neuropathy[1] and enzymes that cause a necrotizing vasculitis. The problem is compounded by the peripheral vasculitis that is secondary to diabetes mellitus. The disease may spread from the external auditory canal through the fissures of Santorini to the periauricular tissue, neck, parotid gland, temporomandibular joint, and soft tissues at the base of the skull. The most common cranial nerves involved are the facial, glossopharyngeal, hypoglossal, and vagus nerves.[4, 5]

Aggressive medical management consisting of control of diabetes, frequent débridement, curettage of granulation tissue with microscopic and histologic evaluation,[6] cultures and sensitivities, and institution of high-dose intravenous chemotherapy (cephalosporin, aminoglycosides) is mandatory. Surgical intervention may occasionally be necessary. Therapy should be continued until there is clinical, radiographic, and bone scan (Fig. 3–2) evidence of control and resolution of infection.

Open mastoid cavity infections in patients who have had the classic "canal down" modified radical mastoidectomy or radical mastoidectomy are similar to external otitis in symptomatology and treatment. In these circumstances one must always be suspicious of underlying recurrent

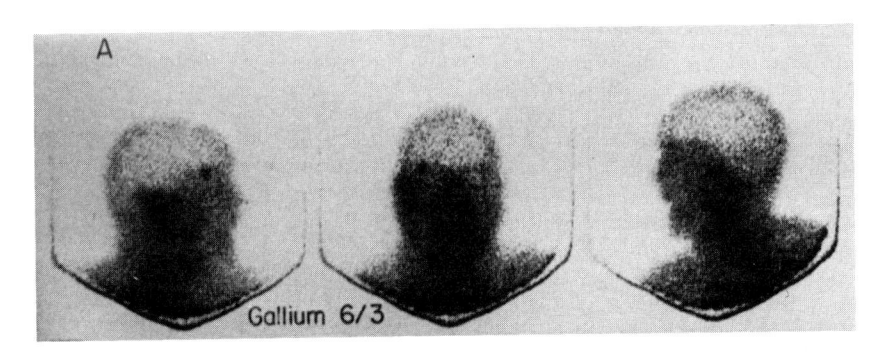

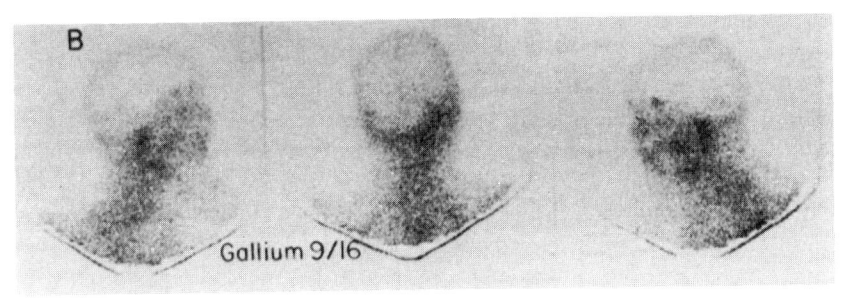

FIGURE 3–2. Gallium scan demonstrating bone infection (*A*) and resolution of infection following 3 months of therapy (*B*).

mastoiditis or recurrent disease. The most important aspect of diagnosis is adequate débridement and inspection. These procedures occasionally must be performed under general anesthesia, especially in children, and revision mastoid surgery may be indicated. All aspects of the mastoid cavity must be well aerated and exteriorized. An intermittently discharging and recurrently moist or infected open mastoid cavity may result from areas of "mucosalization" of the skin-lined cavity or from an open eustachian tube. Patches of mucosa within a skin-lined mastoid cavity may need to be cauterized or curetted to allow adequate epithelialization. Regularly scheduled periodic and routine cavity inspections and cleansing are mandatory, and occasional treatment with topical medication, as in patients with external otitis, is very effective.

Tympanic Membrane

Otoscopy is necessary to evaluate the tympanic membrane and the middle ear space. It is surprising how often tympanic membrane and middle ear disease is diagnosed *without* visualization of the tympanic membrane because a foreign body, cerumen, or infection of the canal makes inspection of the tympanic membrane impossible.

Perforations themselves are painless. The problem that caused the perforation is frequently also the cause of the pain, as in cases of blunt trauma to the ear, barotrauma, otitis media, and mastoiditis. Acute perforations frequently heal spontaneously. If the perforation occurred in a dry or clean environment, antibiotics are usually not necessary. Perforations are much more likely to heal spontaneously, in relatively short periods of time, when there is no infection. It is often necessary to initiate antibiotic therapy if the perforation occurred in an unsterile or nonclean environment, as, for instance, during swimming or diving accidents, in blunt water skiing injuries, or in circumstances that demonstrate or are suspicious for contamination, as with a traumatic perforation of the eardrum occurring during an episode of external otitis. Antibiotics chosen in these circumstances should either cover a broad spectrum of potential pathogens or be organism specific if the pathogen is known. Careful avoidance of water entering the ear and the "tincture of time" may be all that are necessary to promote healing. Cauterization of the perforation margin with trichloroacetic acid may help to stimulate spontaneous closure. Larger perforations may require patching or surgical grafting. Following freshening of the edges of the perforation by surgical débridement or cauterization, or after unfolding the tympanic membrane remnants, a patch (made of cigarette paper) may be applied to serve as a template to allow either epithelialization or reapproximation of the torn tympanic membrane edges and subsequent healing. Very large perforations or chronic thick perforations of the tympanic membrane may require tissue grafting (tympanoplasty, myringoplasty). The most common tissue presently used for this purpose is temporalis muscle fascia. Homograft tympanic membranes are also available but are infrequently necessary.

Severe pain may be caused by a blister or bleb on the tympanic membrane (bullous myringitis). Bullous myringitis is usually associated with a viral upper respiratory infection and otitis. The patient often is afebrile and the hearing may be normal, or testing may demonstrate a conductive or mixed hearing loss. Single or multiple vesicles or bullae are usually found and are usually hemorrhagic or hemorrhagic–clear fluid-filled. Often no specific therapy is necessary for the bullae, and the problem resolves in several days. Therapy directed toward the upper respiratory infection at times may include antibiotics. If the pain is severe, the bleb may be aspirated or excised, care being taken not to perforate the tympanic membrane. Erythromycin has been recommended by some clinicians.

Middle Ear

All ear pain associated with an upper respiratory infection is an acute otitis media until proved otherwise. On the other hand, one must not assume that otalgia in patients with nasal congestion or upper respiratory infection is due to otitis media. Examination of the patient is critical, and otoscopy is most often diagnostic, provided the tympanic membrane can be visualized.

One must take the time to débride the canal of cerumen and secretions to accomplish inspection of the tympanic membrane. Débridement should proceed carefully and atraumatically by using cotton wire applicators (not Q-tips), ring curette, or suction. I prefer to use a flexible wire loop ring curette when the cerumen or epithelial–cerumen debris is hard and dry, and various "middle ear" suction tips, usually a No. 5 or No. 7 aspirator, to aspirate the loose or liquid–oily type of cerumen. Unless we are familiar with the patient and know that the tympanic membrane is intact, we rarely use irrigation. Lavaging an ear canal occluded with wax in a new patient or a patient in whom the integrity of the tympanic membrane is not known can lead to serious complications. Significant morbidity and extension of disease into the middle ear or mastoid may result from irrigation in the presence of perforation.

If the history is compatible with a middle ear infection and it is impossible to examine the tympanic membrane and assess the middle ear because of total occlusion of the canal with edema, swelling, or cerumen that cannot be removed, then therapy must be directed at both (1) the external canal infection and (2) the *potential* middle ear or mastoid infection. Once the canal obstruction and inflammation subside and the tympanic membrane can be inspected, treatment of the middle ear space infection can be continued or terminated depending on the clinical circumstances.

Tympanometry may be complementary to otoscopy in documenting a middle ear effusion, but this does not necessarily confirm infection. When a middle ear effusion, purulent or not, is present, a type B tympanogram is often obtained; there is usually an associated conductive hearing loss. Hearing loss may be documented by routine clinical tests of awareness of loudness, tuning forks, or conventional audiometry, but audiometry is usually not necessary in the presence of acute infection.

When tuning forks are used it is preferable to use forks of three different frequencies (250, 500, and 1000 cycles per second). Tuning fork testing is easy to perform and plays a very important role in the assessment of hearing. Although conventional audiometry may be performed, the *Weber* and *Rinne* tests are complementary to electrical testing and can be clinically useful.

Broad-spectrum antibiotics sufficient to cover the usual causative gram-positive organisms and *Haemophilus influenzae* in the very young patient along with decongestants and antihistamines are very effective in controlling the infection and allowing proper ventilation of the middle ear space through a functioning eustachian tube. Occasionally, myringotomy is necessary to alleviate pain or, in difficult cases or immunocompromised patients, to obtain a specimen of the middle ear effusion for appropriate culture and sensitivity testing for specific chemotherapy. Sudden relief from ear pain in patients with acute purulent otitis media is usually caused by spontaneous rupture of the tympanic membrane with evacuation of the purulent middle ear contents from the middle ear space into the external auditory canal. Spontaneous healing most often occurs.

Nonpurulent middle ear effusion is rarely the cause of ear pain. Although children and adults may complain of hearing loss, fullness, or pressure, young children and infants most often are asymptomatic. A slowly progressive effusion may occur without any realization of hearing loss and is frequently first detected by screening audiometric and tympanometric tests or screening otoscopic examination. Once detected, treatment is very effective. The proper management of nasosinus and nasopharyngeal disease and the maintenance of normal and adequate eustachian tube function will clear most cases of middle ear effusion. Decongestants, antihistaminics, humidification, and occasional steroids and topical vasoconstrictor agents will, in most instances, restore adequate middle ear ventilation. Treatment is continued for a period of 8 to 12 weeks, and the patient is monitored during this period of time for objective signs of improvement. If there is no improvement of hearing function or if the tympanic membrane architecture is not restored, the patient is considered for myringotomy with or without tube insertion. If there is evidence of adenoid obstruction of the fossa of Rosenmueller, either by direct inspection with a mirror or endoscope, by palpation, or radiographically, adenoidectomy may be necessary in addition to myringotomy. If adenoidectomy has previously been performed, reinspection of the nasopharynx is necessary to rule out adenoid regrowth or scarring in the fossa that is restricting mobility of the cartilaginous eustachian tube or causing obstruction of the lumen of the tube. Digital inspection of this area with finger lysis of adhesions at the time of myringotomy may provide much useful information and may be therapeutic. Tonsillectomy is rarely indicated in patients with middle ear disease and eustachian tube dysfunction. The indications for tonsillectomy and for adenoidectomy are independent of one another but may coexist.

Rapid changes in pressure, negative or positive (barotrauma), such as may occur during flying or diving, may also produce acute and sudden ear pain, as may acute eustachian tube dysfunction (tubotympanitis, eustachian tube salpingitis).

Air travel should be discouraged in patients with acute respiratory infection or acute nasal congestion. In patients who are frequently bothered by ear pains when they fly, an oral decongestant may be administered one-half to 1 hour before takeoff; this is combined with use of a topical nasal decongestant when seatbelts are fastened prior to takeoff and again just prior to descent. Because alcoholic beverages may produce nasal congestion, their use is discouraged prior to and during flight.

Primary eustachian tube dysfunction, whether chronic or longstanding, usually does not produce pain. Patients usually complain of fullness or pressure in the ear or have some unusual "awareness" of the ear. The clinical history of surrounding events and confirmatory pneumatic otoscopy or tympanometry helps in the diagnosis. When the usual techniques of yawning, swallowing, and chewing do not relieve the pressure or pain, decongestants, steroids, nosedrops, anti-inflammatory agents, or the Valsalva maneuver may relieve the symptoms. Rarely must one resort to myringotomy or myringotomy with tube insertion for relief.

Cholesteatomas, whether they are (1) large congenital growths, (2) primary acquired or attic retraction cholesteatomas, or (3) secondary acquired cholesteatomas of the pars flaccida or pars tensa, may produce pain but usually only in the presence of infection. Chronic otitis media and chronic mastoiditis usually do not produce ear pain.

In chronic otitis media with or without cholesteatoma the presence of pain or a change in the character of the symptoms may indicate an impending or evolving complication or progression of the disease process, and may indicate a need for immediate intervention. Although the presence of pain may indicate that there may be a serious complication of *chronic* ear disease, the *absence* of pain should not denote a "safe lesion."

Erosion of the bony plate covering the middle fossa dura, sigmoid sinus, or posterior fossa is frequently noted during mastoidectomy for cholesteatoma. Slowly progressing bony erosion may not produce noticeable symptoms.

There may be discharge from the ear, hearing loss, or pressure, or, more ominously, vertigo, facial weakness, or evidence of intracranial extension causing meningitis, temporal lobe or cerebellar abscess, or increased intracranial pressure.

In the presence of cholesteatoma, hearing loss may not be noticed by the patient unless the ossicles are involved in the disease process and there is loss of continuity of a sound-conducting mechanism. Sound may be transmitted directly across the mass of the cholesteatoma, and even when the ossicles are absent or eroded, audiometric testing may reveal no detectable or measurable hearing loss (Fig. 3–3).

Erosion of the horizontal semicircular canals by cholesteatoma may produce vertigo and this erosion is not infrequently encountered during mastoid surgery for cholesteatoma disease. When a semicircular canal fistula is suspected, pressure against the tragus toward the tympanic membrane

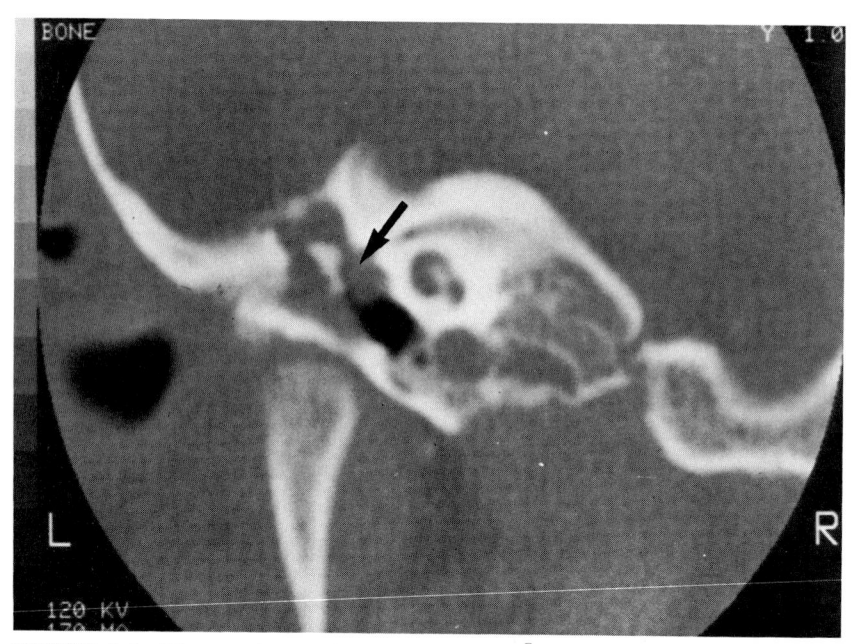

FIGURE 3–3. CT scan of mastoid. Dense mass filling attic and middle ear (see arrow) surrounding an ossicle and possible eroding of horizontal semicircular canal suggest cholesteatoma.

may induce sudden, violent vertigo and nystagmus. Pneumatic otoscopy may produce the same findings, which can be documented by electronystagmography. The cochlea may be eroded, and a profound sensorineural hearing loss may occur.

Diagnosis in chronic ear disease is achieved by otoscopy with supportive and confirmatory audiometric, tympanometric, and radiographic studies. Cholesteatoma (Fig. 3–4) most often must be controlled by surgical excision, but occasionally only exteriorization, debridément, and debulking are necessary. Careful follow-up is required to be sure of its ultimate control.

Neoplasms of the middle ear (Fig. 3–5) are rare and may produce pain. Pain in these instances is usually due to secondary inflammation and infection or erosion into contiguous structures with neural irritation. Diagnosis is achieved by otoscopy, radiographic studies, or biopsy.

Caution is needed when selecting biopsy because one must be sure that a careful clinical and laboratory evaluation is done prior to surgical exploration to avoid performing a biopsy of extensive vascular lesions such as glomus jugulare tumors, aneurysms of the carotid artery, abnormally positioned carotid artery or sigmoid sinus, or a high arched jugular bulb. Herniated brain tissue from the middle cranial fossa or middle ear extension of a brain tumor may also exist with or without signs of meningitis or meningismus.

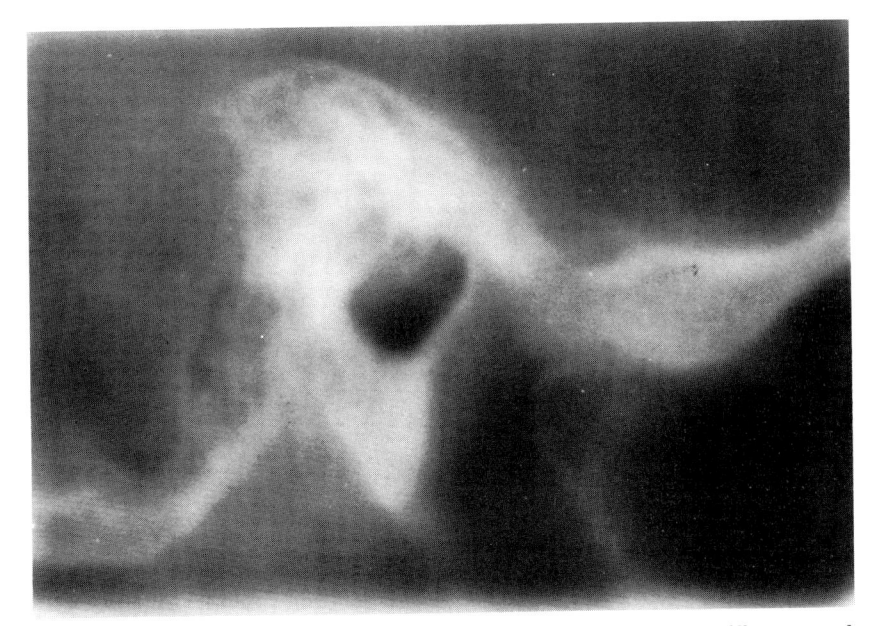

Otalgia

FIGURE 3–4. Mastoid tomogram of cholesteatoma showing sclerotic mass filling mastoid antrum and attic.

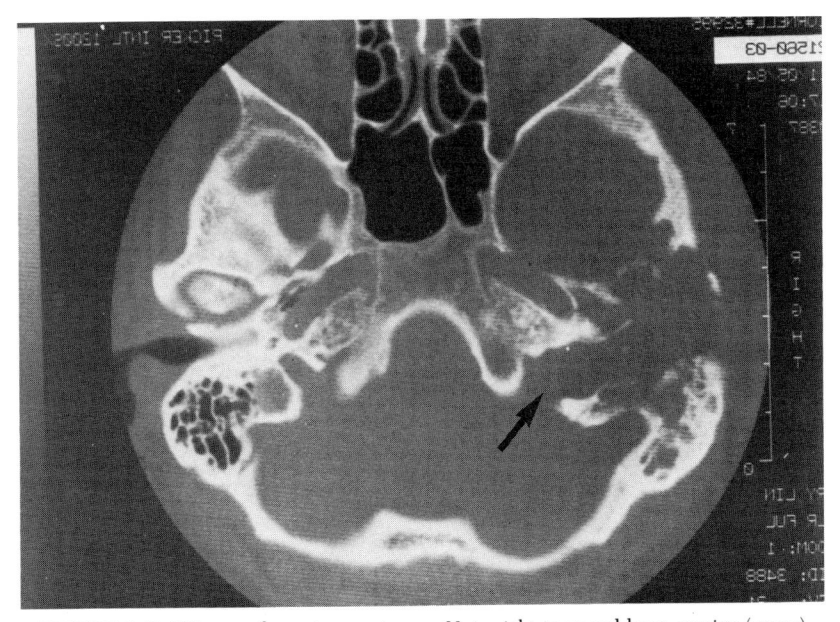

FIGURE 3–5. CT scan of massive carcinoma. Note right temporal bone erosion (arrow).

Temporal Bone (Mastoid and Inner Ear)

The history and physical findings may indicate that an intratemporal bone lesion may be the site of ear pain. Radiographic studies may delineate a *temporal bone fracture*. A *longitudinal fracture* may involve the squamous portion of the temporal bone (Fig. 3–6), ear canal, and middle ear and may demonstrate a ruptured tympanic membrane or hemotympanum and a conductive hearing loss. It frequently responds to conservative treatment and follow-up. A *transverse fracture* of the temporal bone usually courses through the petrous portion of the temporal bone and therefore may produce a total sensorineural hearing loss, acute vertigo, and nystagmus, and even facial paralysis secondary to laceration of the nerve in its bony canal. Conservative treatment again is most often all that can be offered for this type of fracture. Surgical decompression of the facial nerve, suturing, or grafting of the damaged seventh nerve may be necessary. Significant temporal bone trauma frequently produces a *mixed type* of fracture, with elements of both the longitudinal type and the transverse type of fracture of the temporal bone.

Herpes zoster oticus (Ramsay Hunt syndrome) is caused by herpetic inflammation of the geniculate ganglion and is characterized by facial paralysis, vesicular eruption (herpetic) of the external auditory canal, concha, and tympanic membrane, severe otalgia, sensorineural hearing loss, and vertigo. There may be oral manifestations of this disease, including vesicles in the oropharynx and hypopharynx. Ear pain may precede the skin eruption and may persist after the skin lesions abate. Pain is usually intense and focuses on the external auditory canal, concha, tragus, antitra-

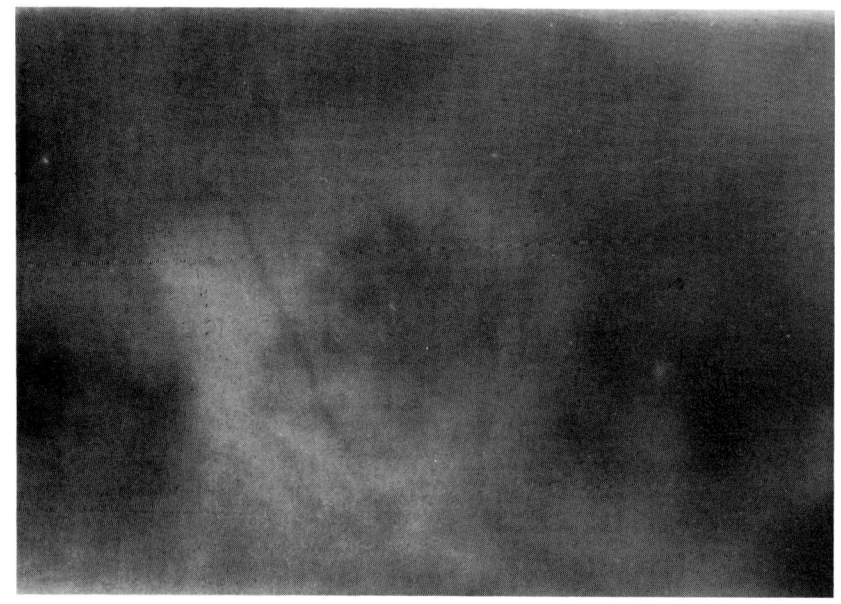

FIGURE 3–6. Temporal bone fracture, longitudinal type.

Otalgia

gus, antihelix, and lobule. It is the presence of pain and multiple cranial nerve involvement (cranial nerves V, VII, and VIII) that differentiates this disease from idiopathic Bell's palsy.

Although the predominant effects of Bell's palsy are *motor*, there may be a neuritic type of burning pain in the ear region as well. The presence of severe pain is considered by many to be a poor prognostic sign for spontaneous recovery. No definite medical or surgical treatment is universally agreed upon. The role of steroids or conventional surgical decompression of the facial nerve continues to be debated. Many clinicians believe that decompression of the seventh cranial nerve from the stylomastoid foramen to the level of the geniculate ganglion may be necessary if nerve excitability tests demonstrate significant or progressive impairment of facial nerve function.[7]

Acute mastoiditis (Fig. 3–7) usually follows acute otitis media and often is accompanied by otitis media. However, the possibility of mastoid disease in the presence of a normal tympanic membrane and middle ear cannot be ignored. The middle ear space communicates with the mastoid by way of the aditus and aditus-ad-antrum. If the aditus region is obstructed by edematous tissue, scar tissue, polyps, or secretions, mastoid disease may progress in spite of an improving middle ear space or a normal middle ear space. The middle ear may heal because a myringotomy or spontaneous perforation occurred or because eustachian tube function is improved. Pain and tenderness, swelling, erythema, and displacement of the auricle down-

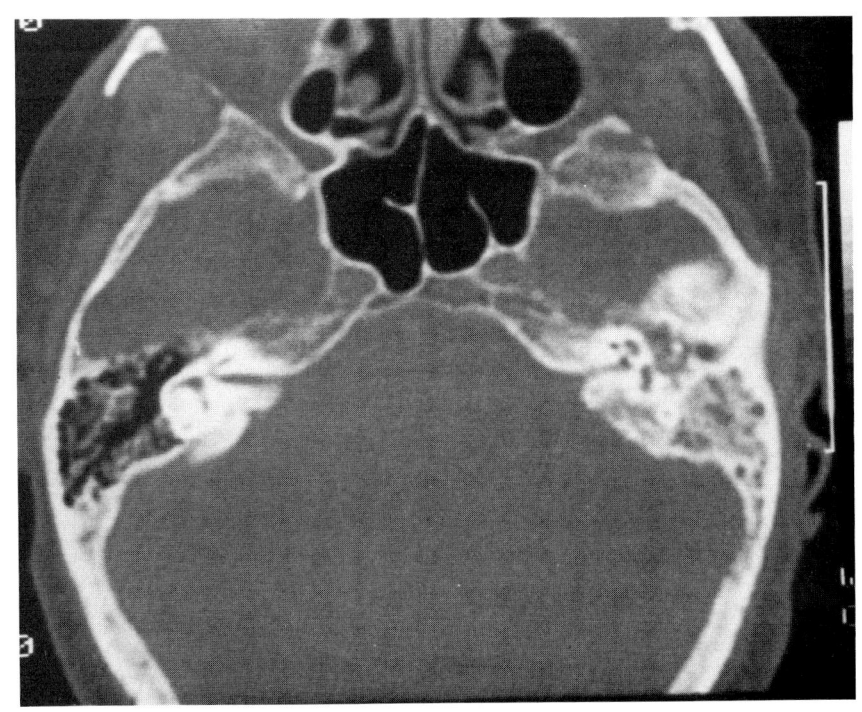

FIGURE 3–7. CT scan showing clouding of mastoid cells indicative of mastoiditis.

ward and outward may be the first sign of acute mastoiditis. It is not uncommon early in its development for pain to be present in the mastoid region (Macewen's triangle). The pain is usually throbbing or progressive in character with radiation to the mandible or neck. Increasing or persistent pain or the recurrence of pain in the presence of appropriate antibiotic therapy may indicate progression of disease. Sudden relief from pain during documented acute mastoiditis is most often due to decompression of the subperiosteal space into the mastoid air cells, subcutaneous region, or by tympanic membrane perforation by way of the middle ear and does not necessarily indicate a cessation of the pathologic process.

With temporal bone neoplasms, benign and malignant, and mastoiditis, pain arises from periostitis secondary to underlying bone disease, inflammation of the dura due to intracranial extension, or extension into the region of the lateral sinus. The mastoid bone itself is insensitive to pain. All too often, intracranial signs and symptoms may be the first indication that mastoid disease exists (Fig. 3–8). Meningitis, increased intracranial pressure, severe and diffuse headaches, seizure, coma, or death may occur. Often the presence of severe progressive or recurrent headache is the first symptom of an otogenic brain abscess, venous sinus thrombophlebitis, otitic hydrocephalus, or meningitis, and headaches developing in a patient with previous otitis media or mastoiditis, whether acute or chronic, can be very significant. Unilateral deep-seated pain in the face and ear in the presence of diplopia may indicate an extension of infection from the more lateral mastoid air cells to the petrous apex cells with involvement of the ipsilateral sixth cranial nerve (Gradenigo's syndrome). Immediate surgical intervention is necessary. Radiographic studies may show opacification of the mastoid

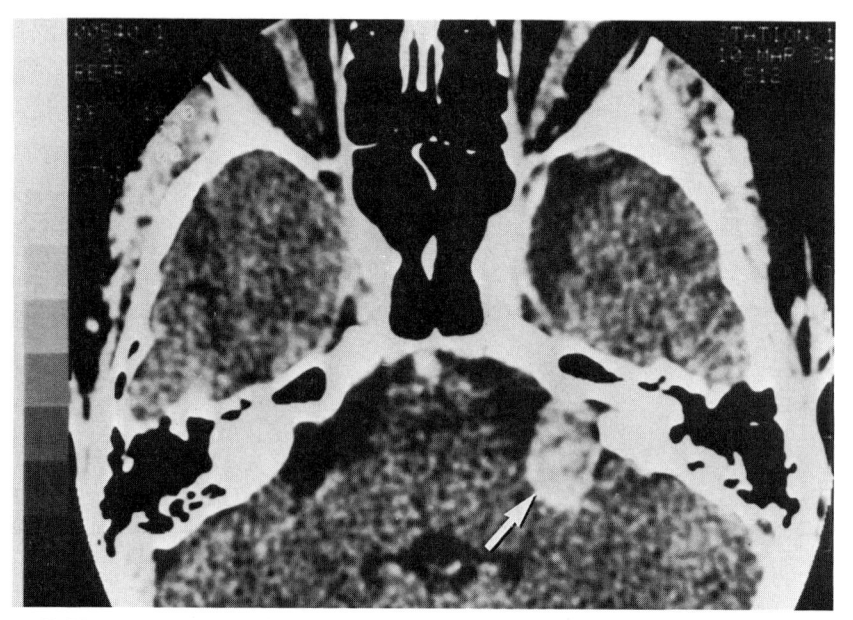

FIGURE 3–8. CT scan of acoustic neuroma in the right cerebellopontine angle (see arrow).

air cells, loss of intercellular septa, or erosion through the bony confines of the mastoid. Antibiotic treatment, occasionally in combination with myringotomy, usually controls early mastoiditis, but more extensive mastoid surgery may be needed if the disease progresses in spite of adequate antibiotic and chemotherapeutic agent administration.

When the history, physical examination including otoscopy and pneumatic-otoscopy, impedance audiometry, audiometry, and, when indicated, radiographic studies demonstrate that the ear is *not* the cause of pain, one must consider the nonotogenic factors.

Nonotogenic Causes of Ear Pain

Pain, as defined in Dorland's Illustrated Medical Dictionary,[8] is a localized sensation of discomfort, distress, or agony resulting from the stimulation of specialized nerve endings. Referred pain is pain experienced at sites other than the one of primary stimulation and is neurologically related, occurring at sites supplied by the same or adjacent neural segments. Referred pain may or may not be accompanied by primary site pain. Primary pain may be modified or inhibited or suppressed unconsciously until it is not felt by the patient.

Referred pain to the ear is a common cause of otalgia. Tonsillitis, the post-tonsillectomy fossa, carcinoma of the tonsil and oropharynx, sharp foreign bodies in the pharynx and palate such as bones or wood splinters, chancres, and burns in the pharynx, hypopharynx, and laryngopharynx may cause ear pain by way of the glossopharyngeal nerve and nerve of Arnold.

Glossopharyngeal neuralgia is characterized by intermittent, unilateral stabbing pains lasting several seconds, followed by a burning sensation lasting several minutes located in the region of the posterior aspect of the tongue, lateral wall of the pharynx and hypopharynx, and soft palate, with radiation to the ear. Frequently there is a trigger zone located at the base of the tongue and tonsil region or lateral pharyngeal wall. A prominent elongated styloid process may be one cause of glossopharyngeal neuralgia (Eagle's syndrome) (Figs. 3–9 and 3–10). Styloid process pain may be identified by palpation of the styloid process through the tonsillar fossa and can be confirmed radiographically. Treatment consists of transoral surgical resection of the styloid process. The pain of glossopharyngeal neuralgia may be associated with tearing and increased salivation. Cocainization of the lateral pharyngeal wall may stop the attack of pain and is a good diagnostic tool. Longer lasting relief may be obtained by blocking the trigger zone (tonsil region) or the glossopharyngeal nerve with a local anesthetic, or by avulsion of the glossopharyngeal nerve at the jugular foramen. Intracranial section of the glossopharyngeal nerve has also been performed.

Sphenopalatine neuralgia (lower-half headache, Sluder's syndrome) is characterized by intermittent deep pain similar to that of tic douloureux, noted in the region of the ethmoid, orbit, nose, cheek, or ear. The pain is

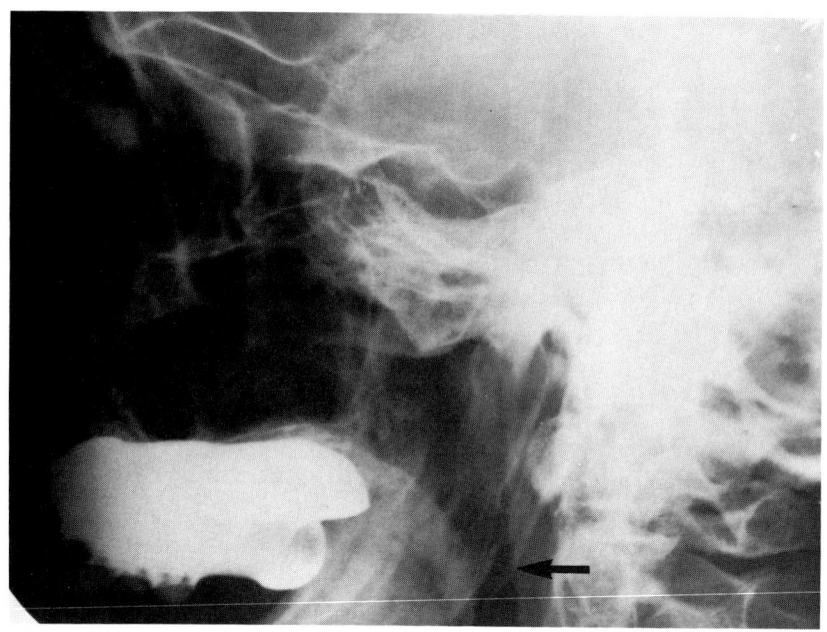

FIGURE 3–9. Eagle's syndrome. Lateral view showing elongated styloid process (arrow).

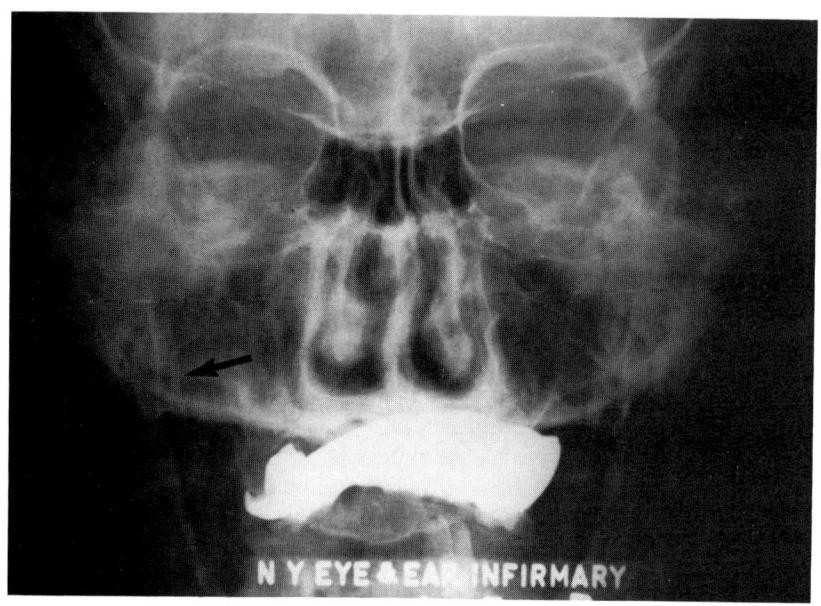

FIGURE 3–10. Eagle's syndrome. Anteroposterior view showing elongated styloid process (arrow).

sudden in onset, unilateral, intermittent, and lasts several minutes to a few hours. This disorder is very often secondary to intranasal pathology, such as a septal spur, nasal or sinus infection, or tumor, and may serve as a trigger zone. Cocainization of this trigger zone, or nerve block by way of the greater palatine foramen, is a good diagnostic tool; occasionally resection of the sphenopalatine ganglion is necessary. If otalgia is present at the time of the examination and a central spur is impinging on the turbinate and is the cause of this pain, a 5 to 10% cocaine solution applied to the discrete septal spur and turbinate area will alleviate the pain. Submucosal reconstruction of the nasal septum may be curative. If the patient has no pain at the time of the examination, he or she should be told to return for the diagnostic cocainization procedure when the same type of pain and headache recur. This can be most effective in establishing a good rapport and in effectively managing this difficult and complex problem.

Vidian neuralgia most often occurs following infection in the sphenoid sinus and is caused by inflammation of the vidian nerve in the vidian canal. Typically, severe attacks of unilateral pain in the nose, face, ear, head, and neck are found. Some believe that this disorder actually is a vascular syndrome produced by a dilated, tortuous, pulsating, or inflamed third portion of the internal maxillary artery adjacent to and lying against the vidian nerve and sphenopalatine region. This neuralgia may be successfully treated by addressing the primary sphenoid sinus disorder, by treating with antibiotics or performing a sphenoid sinus wash or sphenoid sinusotomy, or by exploration of the region of the vidian canal in the pterygopalatine fossa. The artery may be clipped and transected or merely cushioned from the underlying neural tissue. The long-term beneficial response from the last procedure has not met expectations.

Neoplastic, inflammatory, and traumatic lesions of the larynx (Fig. 3–11), similarly, by way of the vagus nerve and nerve of Arnold, may refer pain to the ear. Foreign bodies in the hypopharynx and laryngopharynx such as fish bones and chicken bones may, on swallowing, cause otalgia with or without associated throat pain. Carcinoma of the larynx occurring in the supraglottic, epiglottic, or postcricoid region may produce pain in the ear or neck without other laryngeal symptoms. The usual complaint of hoarseness may not be present if vocal cord mobility and free margin are normal. Time must be taken with the patient to explain why indirect or direct laryngoscopy is being performed and why attention is being directed to the larynx and throat when the patient is complaining of ear pain.

The chief mediator of somatic pain to the head and neck is the fifth cranial nerve. *Trigeminal neuralgia* (tic douloureux) is not often a cause of otalgia. There is usually recurrent severe, unilateral, often radiating pain, distributed over one or more branches of the trigeminal nerve. These pain episodes may occur spontaneously or after stimulation of a trigger zone located along one of the branches of the trigeminal nerve. *Trotter's syndrome* (sinus of Morgagni syndrome) is caused by invasion of the trigeminal nerve in the lateral wall of the nasopharynx (sinus of Morgagni) by a nasopharyngeal carcinoma. This syndrome consists of unilateral con-

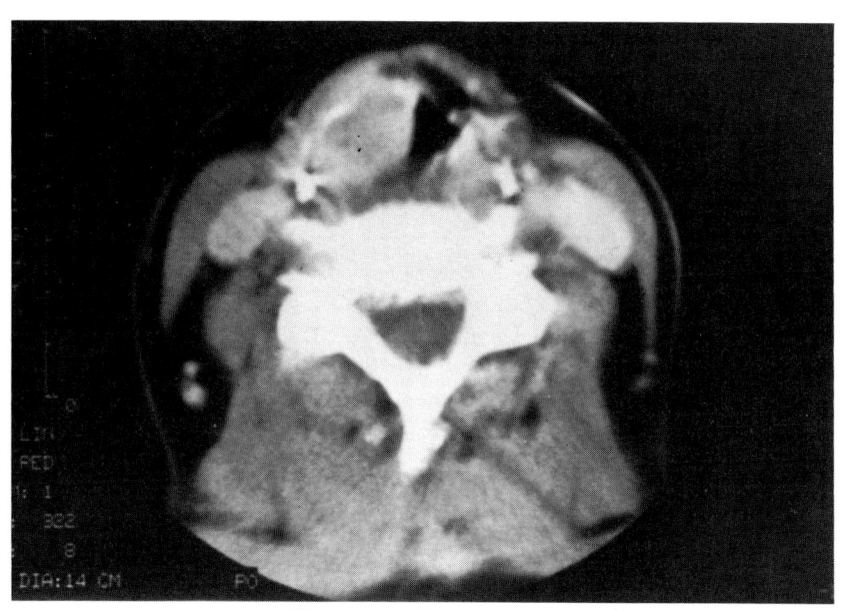

FIGURE 3–11. CT scan of large laryngeal carcinoma filling entire right hemilarynx.

ductive deafness caused by eustachian tube obstruction, trismus, and altered palate mobility due to muscle invasion by tumor, and pain is distributed to the ear, tongue, mandible, and teeth.

Many of us have experienced ear pain as a result of dental problems (abscess, eruption of teeth, dental extractions). Pain of dental origin frequently is unilateral. The pain may extend to the molar region or radiate to the occipital or parietal region. It may be constant or intermittent and may or may not change with mastication. Nasopharyngeal carcinoma, Tornwaldt's bursa and abscess, acute nasopharyngitis, and adenoiditis may also refer pain to the ear.

A complete examination of the ear, nose, throat, and head and neck is therefore necessary to evaluate patients with ear pain. Inspection and palpation of the periauricular region (parotid gland, mastoid area, temporomandibular joint, and cervical region) are critical to rule out disorders of the major salivary glands and vascular causes such as carotodynia and temporal arteritis. Temporal arteritis is an inflammatory disorder of the superficial temporal artery possibly due to an autoimmune or collagen disease. The pain is thought to be due to distention of the artery. There is marked tenderness on palpation. The headache is of a deep throbbing character with a burning component, and there is frequently hyperalgesia of the scalp. It is a self-limited condition with a tendency to recur. Biopsy of the superficial temporal artery is frequently necessary to establish a diagnosis. Ocular symptoms often accompany this disorder and may be described as diplopia and photophobia. Approximately one-third of patients with temporal arteritis may suffer from partial or complete loss of vision believed to be due to occlusion of the central retinal artery. Treatment consists of very careful follow-up and occasionally introduction of steroids.

Carotodynia is characterized by tenderness and a pulsatile pain in the region of the common carotid artery and external carotid artery that may be referred to the ipsilateral eye, ear, and neck; deep-seated intracranial pain may also be present, perhaps by way of the vagus nerve. The pain is intermittent and self-limiting and usually lasts 10 days to 2 weeks. The cause is unknown but is believed to be a result of inflammation. Treatment is generally supportive. Salicylates are helpful, but corticosteroids have not been found very useful.

Intraoral palpation of the muscles of mastication, temporomandibular joint, and floor of the mouth and tongue and the study of occlusion are necessary to rule out the possibility of myofacial pain dysfunction or temporomandibular joint syndrome. The temporomandibular joint receives sensory fibers from the fifth and seventh cranial nerves. The posterior part of the temporomandibular joint capsule is innervated by the auriculotemporal nerve. A "ligamentlike" structure extends from the temporomandibular joint capsule to the neck of the malleus that is contiguous with the fibrous layer of the tympanic membrane, and it is therefore theorized that spasm in the temporomandibular joint region may "pull" the anterior malleolar ligament. Because of these neuroanatomic relationships, it is fairly well established that myofacial pain dysfunction can cause otalgia.

There is no objective evidence that hearing loss is related to disorders of the temporomandibular joint, nor is there any objective evidence that hearing is improved following therapy for temporomandibular joint dysfunction. Very often subjective improvement is noted and may be secondary to general well-being and emotional improvement provided by emotional support and relief of pain by muscle relaxation.

Also, no pathophysiologic correlations have been proved between the symptoms of tinnitus or vertigo and disorders of the temporomandibular joint or myofacial pain dysfunction. Symptoms have been ascribed, primarily by dentists, to the "mandibular-malleolar ligament," as described above. It is felt by most investigators that these complaints are psychogenic in origin or are due to a concomitant nonrelated disorder.

Ear pain due to psychogenic causes is a diagnosis of exclusion and must be considered in patients with the appropriate personality and in those for whom there are possible social and/or monetary gains. Psychiatric referral for evaluation and therapy is indicated. There may be concomitant emotional and physical dysfunction, and to succeed in therapy both must be treated. In the complete assessment of the patient with otalgia, one must be prepared to consult with and consider other specialists. Many difficulties coexist, and it may not be clear which disorder is the primary cause of the problem. For example, otitis media or stress may "trigger" a temporomandibular joint syndrome, or acute otitis media with perforation may cause a secondary external otitis, dermatitis, and cellulitis of the face, all of which may cause ear pain. A close cooperative effort between the various disciplines must exist and must be temporally related. It is for this reason that a multidisciplinary team approach to the diagnosis and treatment of facial, head, and neck pain has proved to be the most cost-effective manner of dealing with this symptom.

Clinicians must always keep in mind that most ear pain has a pathologic cause but that the disorder may not arise from the ear. All *otalgia* is not *otitis*, nor is it *otogenic*!

Ear pain (otalgia) with or without tinnitus, hearing complaints, fullness in the ear, and disorders of balance are symptoms most commonly due to primary disorders of the ear. However, a significant percentage of these subjective complaints may be nonotogenic in origin.

It is important for the clinician to characterize these symptoms as to their site of origin and distinguish between otogenic and nonotogenic otalgia. Such a distinction is usually possible after performing a careful physical examination of the head and neck and related areas, taking a careful history, and selecting a battery of objective tests to determine whether or not the presenting complaints are due to primary ear pathology. The physician must be aware of the anatomic, muscular, and neuroanatomic relationships of the ear, head, and neck.

A clinical approach to the patient with otalgia is presented in this chapter. There must be a close working relationship and coordination of effort between the primary treating physician, otolaryngologist, neurologist, dentist, ophthalmologist, and psychiatrist. The etiology of ear pain may be so multifactoral that virtually all disciplines of medicine and dentistry may be needed to obtain the proper diagnosis and treatment.

References

1. Grant, D. A., et al. Early management of the burned ear. Plast Reconstr Surg 44:161, 1969.
2. Sessions, B. G., et al. Frostbite of ear. Laryngoscope 81:12–23, 1971.
3. Holms, P. C. and Vangaard, L. Frostbite. Plast Reconstr Surg 54:544–551, 1974.
4. Chandler, J. R. Malignant external otitis. Laryngoscope 78:1257–1294, 1968.
5. Parisier, S. Malignant external otitis. Ann Otolarngol 86:417–428, 1977.
6. Mattucci, K. F., Setzen, M. and Galantich, P. Necrotizing otitis externa occurring concurrently with epidermoid carcinoma. Laryngoscope 96:264–266, 1986.
7. Giancarlo, H. R. and Mattucci, K. F. Facial palsy (facial nerve decompression). Arch Otolaryngol 91:30–36, 1970.
8. Dorland's Illustrated Medical Dictionary, 27th ed. Philadelphia, W. B. Saunders Co., 1988.
9. Mattucci, K. F., et al. Childhood acoustic neuroma. NY State J Med 87:665–666, 1987.

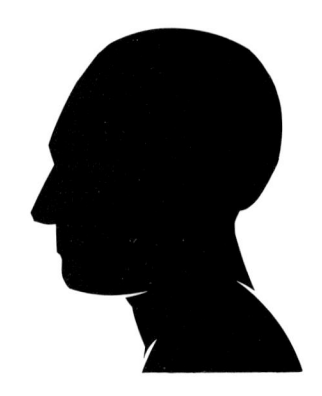

Chapter 4
Head Pain Associated With the Eye

Kevin C. Greenidge and Monica Dweck

Head pain can be the presenting symptom of many disorders, of which only a few should be the cause of alarm. From an ophthalmologic point of view, head pain can be divided into three categories: (1) pain arising from the eye without obvious signs of ocular involvement; (2) pain arising from the eye with signs of ocular involvement; and (3) pain associated with nonocular etiologies that may involve the eye. Often the most difficult diagnoses for the nonophthalmologist to make are those arising from the eye without signs of inflammation. Therefore, this chapter will discuss these entities in the greatest detail.

The Eye Examination

In order to diagnose ocular problems, the examiner must be able to perform an adequate eye examination. A routine ophthalmologic examination must include a careful elicitation of the patient's history, a physical examination of the eyes, and an assessment of visual function. The history should reveal general information about the patient, including age, occupation, visual requirements, allergies, and previous personal as well as family history. Additional information should include whether or not the patient works with small objects, works with objects at unusual distances, or uses the eyes for long periods of time. The family history can be useful, especially if it includes a history of glaucoma, cataracts, retinal detachments, or poor vision of undetermined cause. Specific questions related to the patient's present ocular history include onset of symptoms, duration, intensity, location, aggravating factors, methods of alleviating symptoms, and a prior history of similar complaints.

Visual acuity testing should be a part of the routine examination for every patient, especially those with head pain. If the patient normally wears glasses, visual acuity testing should be done both with and without corrective lenses. Preschool children or illiterate patients can be tested with special charts. To determine the distance visual acuity, the patient should read a chart that has been adjusted to be the equivalent of reading a chart at 20 feet. Near vision is ascertained by reading a near chart at 12 to 14 inches. Under normal circumstances, distance and near vision should be similar.

The pupils should be inspected for size, shape, reaction to light, effect of accommodation, and the presence or absence of an afferent pupillary defect. Pupils are usually 3 mm bilaterally. Unequal pupil size (anisocoria) may be suggestive of neurologic disease. The pupils may be constricted (miotic) from bright illumination, narcotics, central nervous system syphilis, or parasympathomimetic drugs. They may be dilated as a result of myopia, systemic poisoning, dim illumination, sympathomimetic drugs, ocular contusion, or neurologic disease of the midbrain. The shape of the pupil or its ability to move at all may be affected by congenital abnormality or scarring from iritis, trauma, or intraocular surgery. Absence of an equal response in both eyes to light stimuli is indicative of a prechiasmal lesion, most often involving the optic nerve or the retina. On fixating an object 12 inches from the eye (accommodation), both eyes should look inward (converge), and both pupils should constrict. Syphilis should be suspected if the pupils do not react to light stimulation but do constrict on accommodation. A swinging light test is performed to determine if there is symmetrical optic nerve function. When the patient is fixated on a distant object, a light that is rapidly moved from eye to eye should cause immediate pupillary constriction. Immediate dilatation is indicative of optic nerve or extensive retinal disease (Marcus-Gunn pheonomenon).

The movement of the eyes in all fields of gaze should be examined. Gross disorders of eye movements can be observed by having a patient follow a moving object while holding the head in a fixed position. A penlight can be used to determine asymmetrical positioning of the light reflex, which indicates a deviation.

Confrontation fields examination provides an estimate of the patient's visual field by comparing it with the examiner's visual field. The patient is asked to fixate on the examiner's one open eye while the examiner slowly brings an object from the periphery toward his open eye, in a plane midway between the patient and himself. The patient should note the object at the same time as the examiner. If this test is repeated in all quadrants, gross alterations of the visual field can be detected. Disorders to be suspected if a defect is identified include retinitis, advanced glaucoma, optic nerve disease, or intracranial disease.

Inspection of the external ocular structures, lids, conjunctivae, corneas, sclerae, and lacrimal apparatus should be next. With good lighting, the lashes and eyebrows should be inspected for signs of inflammation and scaling. Missing lashes, the presence of more than one row of lashes, and the turning in or out of the lashes are very important signs. The lid margins should be examined for changes in color, texture, swelling, position, motility, inflammation, and the ability to close completely. The lid margins should meet the cornea in the same place bilaterally. Less coverage in one eye may indicate exophthalmos (a protruding eye forcing the lids apart) or lid laxity (a drooping lower lid resulting from decreased muscle tone). More coverage of the cornea may be due to ptosis. Since it is difficult to determine if one lid is down or the contralateral lid is up, a comparison with a normal subject may prove helpful. All acute changes in lid position require evaluation. The main lacrimal gland is located anteriorly in the superotemporal quadrant of the orbit, beneath the upper lid; it is lobulated, pink in color, and should not be confused with an abnormal growth. It is most easily seen when the patient looks inferonasally and traction is placed on the upper-outer eyelid. Both glands are equal in size, and any change in color, size, or tenderness should be a cause of concern.

The conjunctivae should be examined for hyperemia, foreign bodies, pterygium, scarring, and inflammation. The presence of conjunctival hyperemia may indicate conjunctivitis, or it may be a clue to other ocular disorders. If there are atypical findings, additional investigation is warranted. Cavernous sinus thrombosis may initially present as unilateral engorged conjunctival blood vessels.

The cornea, which is a smooth transparent structure, can be examined adequately with the aid of only a penlight. A well-defined light reflex should be seen when a penlight is directed at its surface. Absence of this crisp reflex may indicate a corneal surface abnormality. This abnormality may be due to primary corneal disease, acute glaucoma, or inflammation within the eye. Most acute eye diseases are associated with conjunctival hyperemia, the absence of which indicates chronicity. Corneal sensitivity should be determined prior to instillation of topical anesthetics, especially if the examiner suspects herpetic disease. Corneal sensitivity is determined by lightly touching the cornea with a piece of cotton as the lids are held apart. This contact should elicity symmetrical responses from each eye.

Finally, direct ophthalmoscopy should be performed. Ideally, this is done through a dilated pupil and in a darkened room. However, with practice this can be accomplished without dilatation; also, dilation should be avoided in eyes that have a shallow anterior chamber. An estimation of the depth of the anterior chamber can be made by illuminating it from the side with a penlight. If a shadow is cast on the opposite side of the pupil, the eyes should not be dilated; a horizontal corneal diameter of less than 11 mm is also a risk factor for angle closure. The examiner should determine whether the media (aqueous, lens, vitreous) are clear. A clear ophthalmoscopic view of the posterior aspect of the eye indicates the absence of any significant media opacity, and a reasonable assumption can be made that the patient should have good visual acuity. If this is not the case, the patient should be referred to an ophthalmologist for further evaluation. The optic disc should be examined to ensure that the disc margins are sharp and that the cup within the disc (central pale area) comprises less than 50 percent of the disc tissue. A larger pale area may indicate neurologic or glaucomatous disease.

Ocular Conditions That Cause Head Pain Without Ocular Findings

Optics

A majority of headaches that occur without visual evidence of active eye disease are related to optical errors of the eye. It is the patient's frustrated attempt to correct these refractive errors internally and the resultant muscular fatigue that cause pain. A basic knowledge of the optical system of the eye is helpful in understanding these disorders.[1]

Light enters the eye through the cornea, traverses the anterior chamber, enters the pupil, penetrates the crystalline lens, and is focused through the vitreous cavity onto the retina in the area of the fovea (Fig. 4–1). The light is altered at each tissue or fluid interface, both on entering and leaving. In an optically corrected eye, each tissue or fluid interface plays a role in focusing (refracting) the light on the retina.

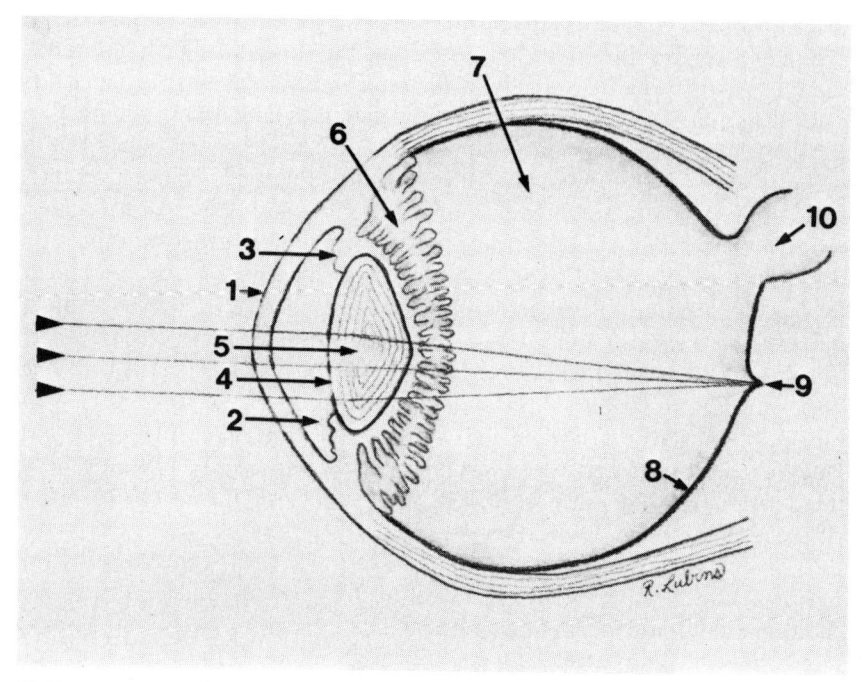

FIGURE 4–1. Optical system of the eye. (1) Cornea, (2) anterior chamber, (3) iris, (4) pupillary aperture, (5) crystalline lens, (6) ciliary body, (7) vitreous cavity, (8) retina, and (9) fovea.

If the eye is too long or too short (axial myopia or hyperopia), if the crystalline lens is too large or too small (lenticular myopia or hyperopia), or if the corneal surface is not regular (astigmatism), a refractive error results. Internal adjustments in the power of the crystalline lens or external additions to the natural refracting system can compensate for these errors.

Even if the optical system was functional during childhood and early adulthood, aging may have an adverse effect on the refracting system. As one approaches 40 years of age, the refractive power of the crystalline lens becomes limited (presbyopia), and reading glasses are needed; as one approaches the mid-fifties, the lens continues to change, and increased myopia, dazzling from lights, or blurred vision may result from cataracts.[1]

Visualization of objects requires that each eye be oriented in the same direction. As in refractive errors, problems in malalignment (phorias, tropias) may be compensated for by ocular regulatory systems or corrective lenses or may require surgical intervention.

Asthenopia

When the eye can fully compensate for a refractive error or malalignment, the system works well, and there are no symptoms of pain. When the eye cannot compensate at all, the system does not function optimally but is symptom-free. When the eye can partially correct for refractive and alignment errors and this compensation is at the expense of increased ocular muscle tone, the system becomes fatigued, and symptoms arise. Asthenopia is a specific group of disorders of the eye that result from strain and subsequent fatigue of the muscles associated with vision.[2] Asthenopic symptoms occur when the optical system of the eye attempts to increase the power of the crystalline lens by contraction of the ciliary muscle (accommodation) or to align the eyes by contraction of the medial rectus muscles (convergence). Unfortunately, the convergence center, which has yet to be anatomically located, simultaneously controls accommodation. The most severe asthenopic symptoms occur when there is a desire to increase accommodation greatly and simultaneously limit convergence. Since these two functions occur simultaneously, multiple conflicting demands are made on a small group of muscles, leading to fatigue and muscle spasm. In some individuals, spasms of the pupillary aperture may be noted. The specific complaint relates to the muscle group involved and its function. Symptoms are usually absent on awakening and increase during the day; they are aggravated by close work and relieved by rest. These symptoms include pain within the eye, pain surrounding the eye globe, episodic blurring of vision, lack of stamina for near work, pulling, pressure behind the eyes, deep pain within the skull, vertigo, and even vomiting.

ACCOMMODATIVE ASTHENOPIA
Hyperopia
Hyperopia, or farsightedness, occurs when the eye is too short for the refractive system (Fig. 4–2). This refractive error can be offset by accom-

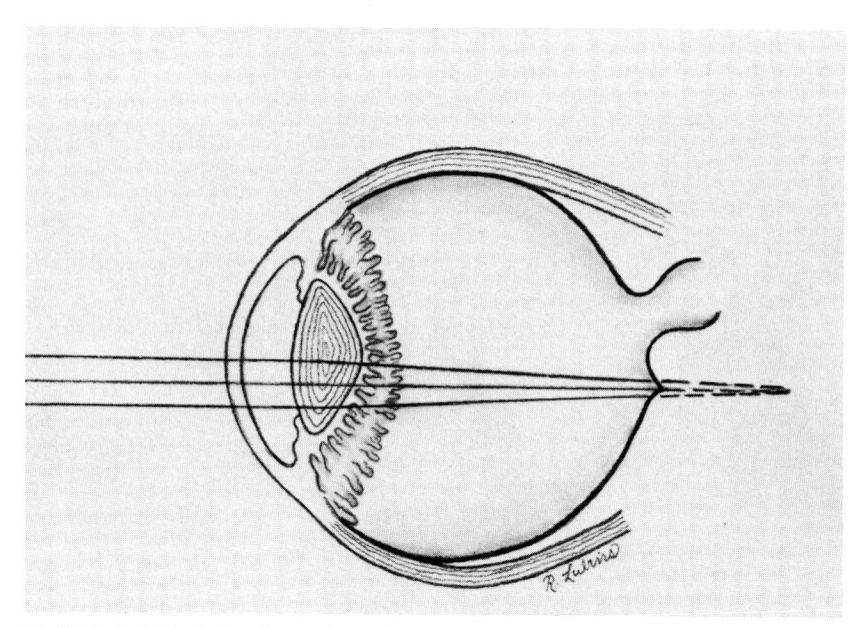

FIGURE 4–2. The light is focused at a theoretical point behind the eye, and a blurred image reaches the fovea (hyperopia).

modation. However, if one must accommodate to see at a distance, the eyes will converge, and diplopia or blurring of distant objects will occur. The negative feedback from the secondary blur will eventually cause fatigue, and symptoms will result. These symptoms will increase during the day, and the greater power required for near vision will make these symptoms worse following concentrated near work. As the patient adjusts for the amount of accommodation required to see, he may experience blurring of the objects of regard as well as their surroundings. As the system fatigues, these blurring episodes may be uncontrollable and may be associated with severe head pain or pulling behind the eyes. Paradoxically, some patients will hold items excessively close in order to obtain larger, albeit blurred, images. Some individuals find viewing a larger image with greater blur more comfortable than viewing a smaller image with less blur. These compensatory methods often lead to severe symptoms and cannot be maintained except for short periods of time (1).

Presbyopia

In young children the accommodative amplitude of the eye may be as great as 40 diopters, which decreases gradually throughout life, approximating 10 diopters at age 40. In a stable, mildly hyeropic individual, symptoms occur only when one's accommodative needs exceed reserves. Over the age of 40, there is a significant reduction in the amplitude of accommodation due to a decrease in the flexibility of the lens. Since the shape of the lens must change to increase its refractive power, a stiffer lens will not focus well at near, requiring the individual to wear additional corrective lenses. Most individuals hold reading material approximately 14 inches from their eyes. As the accommodative reserve decreases, objects are held further away from the eye. If one continues to hold items at 14 inches, asthenopic symptoms may occur owing to the increased accommodative effort required to read at this distance.

Astigmatic Asthenopia

Normally the corneal surface is not round but has greater dimensions in its vertical meridian than in its horizontal meridian. Light entering the eye on the vertical meridian is focused at a different point than that entering on the horizontal meridian. If this distance is greater than 0.5 diopters, the patient is said to have a clinically significant astigmatism.[2] When an astigmatism exists, the eye may make attempts at adaptation. With a mild astigmatism, the eye will adapt in such a way that part of the object appears in focus with other parts of the object out of focus. If the astigmatism is large and a great amount of blur is present in one meridian, the eye may select a midpoint so that the entire object is slightly blurred (point of least confusion) rather than one part being very blurred and the other part being in focus. In severe astigmatism, the eye may focus alternately on different parts of the object, and the whole object comes in and out of focus. This resultant confusion may eventually cause symptoms. These symptoms usually respond well to corrective lenses that can focus light waves differently in separate meridians. If the patient does not have an astigmatism and is given a pair of glasses with an astigmatic correction (induced astigmatism), symptoms may ensue. Sunglasses that are purchased without meeting optical standards may be etiologic in this process. Symptoms include a dull headache, dizziness, and even vomiting.

Anisometropic Asthenopia

If there is a difference of more than 2 diopters in the refractive errors of each eye, anisometropia exists. Sustained efforts to reduce the resultant monocular blur may give rise to symptoms. These complaints consist of a dull ache about the eye and in the eyebrow; pupillary spasm may also be seen.

Myopia

Since there is no attempt by the ocular system to correct for a required decrease in refractive power, myopia (nearsightedness) does not cause the classic asthenopic symptoms (Fig. 4–3). Nearsighted individuals bring items of regard close to their eyes to obtain a clear image. If the object has to be held extremely close, the myopic individual may be required to maintain an uncomfortable position, which may lead to neck, back, or shoulder pain that may radiate to the head. If a myopic individual is given an overcorrection, the eye can compensate by increasing its refractive power, and asthenopic symptoms may then occur. The symptoms are worse at near distances because the accommodative effort is greater than the requirement for convergence, leading to possible dizziness, vomiting, and deep head pain.

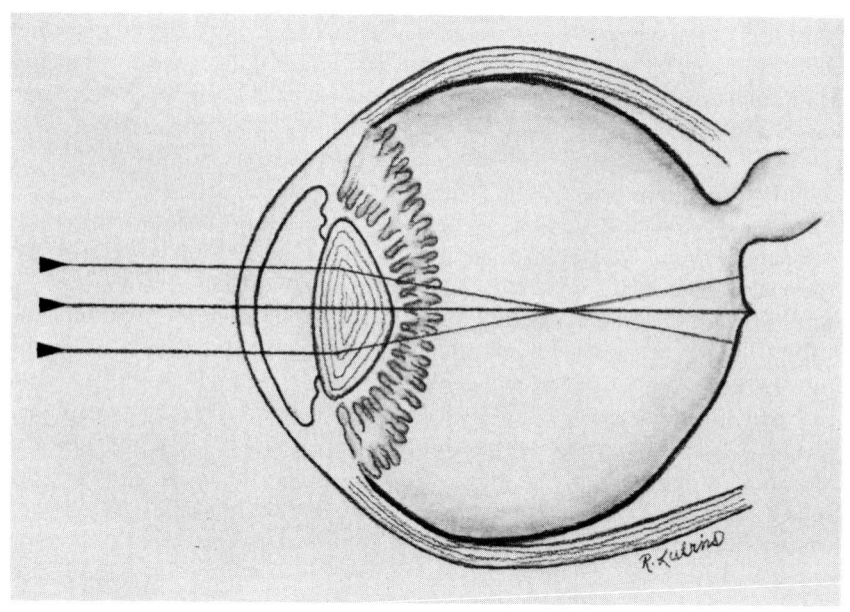

FIGURE 4-3. The light is focused within the eye, and a blurred image reaches the fovea (myopia).

Paresis of Accommodation
Paresis of accommodation can occur in pharmacologic mydriasis or in internal ophthalmoplegia. Attempts to accommodate despite the paralysis of the accommodative muscles lead to increased convergence. The continued effort fatigues the muscles of convergence and causes symptoms such as dull brow pain, increased light sensitivity, and rapid tiring.

PSYCHOLOGICAL FACTORS
Approximately 20 per cent of the population suffers from disorders that can produce asthenopic symptoms; however, only a small percentage of these affected individuals actually have symptoms. It has been shown in one study of 2316 such patients that only 5.7 per cent had complaints.[4] Patients with anemia and physical fatigue and those who are under unusally high stress have a higher level of asthenopic symptoms. In the majority of patients with asthenopic symptoms, either the underlying disorder is most significant or emotional factors are present. Most patients with asthenopia should be able to relate their symptoms to increased eye work at near distances; however, patients under stress may not be able to determine the cause of discomfort, thereby making the diagnosis more difficult. The patient in this category may deny stress, despite its obvious presence, confusing the symptoms in the denial process. In these individuals the treatment as well as the diagnosis may be quite complex.

TREATMENT
Accommodative asthenopia is treated by eliminating the need for sustained accommodative effort that is greater than the accommodative reserve.

Corrective lenses should be prescribed that allow the muscles of accommodation to relax and work within the limits of their reserve. Since the accommodative reserve is so great in young individuals, it is difficult to get their muscles to relax completely. A cycloplegic agent that causes a pharmacologic relaxation of the ciliary muscle as well as dilatation of the pupil is administered prior to refraction in these individuals. Once the proper prescription is given, reversal of symptoms may be gradual. Some patients must learn to relax while they concentrate on near activity. Even though symptoms are not completely eliminated as soon as the glasses are worn, some immediate improvement should be noted.

Muscular Asthenopia

As in accommodative asthenopia, increased muscle tone can also be utilized to offset minor deviations in ocular alignment. However, this can be accomplished only as long as the requirement to maintain proper fusion is not greater than the fusional reserve.[3] If a deviation can be corrected by utilizing the fusional reserve, a latent strabismus (heterophoria) exists. Depending on the degree of concentration and fatigue, a heterophoria may become overt (heterotropia). Symptoms vary depending on the type of heterophoria–heterotropia that is present (Fig. 4–4 and 4–5). Esotropia is the manifest inward turning of the eyes; exotropia exists when the eyes manifest an outward turn. As the fusional reserve limit is approached, symptoms of brow ache and a pulling sensation behind the eye may evolve. Once the fusional limit is exceeded, the patient's pain symptoms may resolve.

The patient with a heterotropia may or may not experience diplopia. If

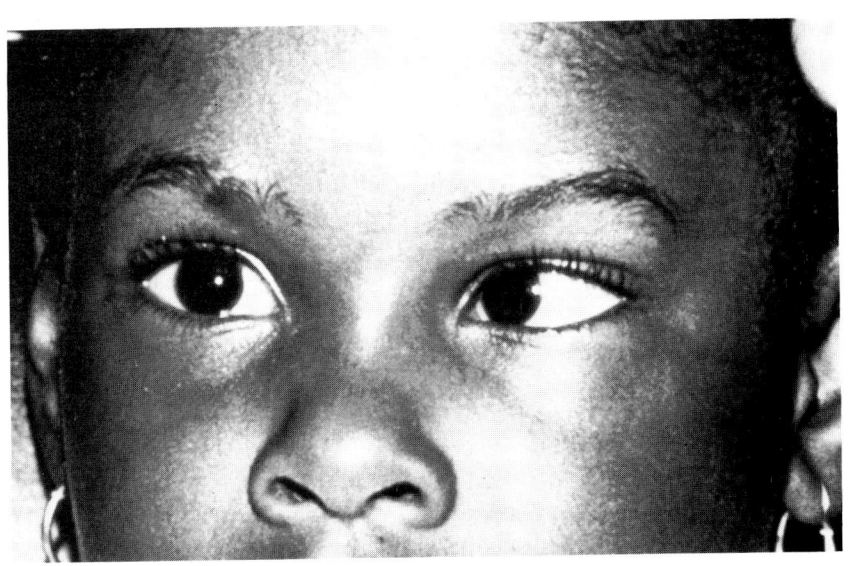

FIGURE 4–4. A child with an esotropia due to an uncorrected hyperopia. Note that the light reflex is central in the fixating right eye and is off center in the inwardly deviated left eye.

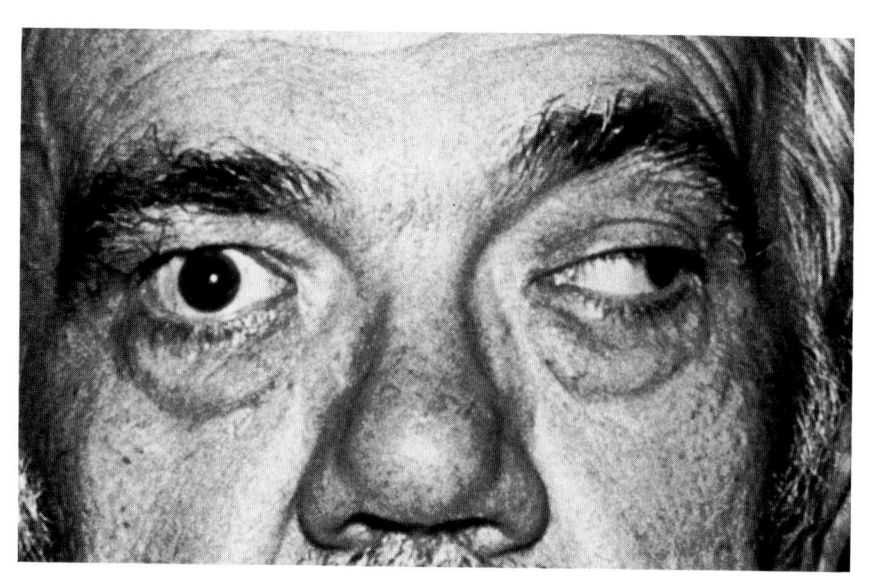

FIGURE 4–5. An adult with an acquired exotropia, the etiology of which requires neurologic investigation.

the deviation has been present since birth, diplopia does not exist. In congenital heterotropias, the image from the deviating eye is suppressed, the eye does not develop central vision (amblyopia), and double vision is avoided. If there is an acquired deviation, as in a muscle paresis, the patient does experience diplopia. Asthenopic symptoms may occur as the patient tries to eliminate the diplopia by forced convergence. Another compensatory mechanism is to tilt the head to avoid double vision; even though this mechanism may be cosmetically unpleasing, it rarely leads to asthenopic symptoms.

DIAGNOSIS

Heterophorias and heterotropias can be diagnosed by the nonophthalmologist. The patient is asked to look at an object across the room; while he is looking at the object, the examiner notes whether a light reflex strikes both eyes at the same point. If the light does not strike both eyes at the same point, a tropia exists. If no tropia is found, an occluder is placed over one eye, and the other eye is observed for motion; when the occluder is removed, the covered eye is again observed to see if it moves (the examiner may note a return to its original position). The same procedure is then performed on the other eye. If the eye wanders while occluded and then returns to its normal position when the occlusion is eliminated, a heterophoria is present. These deviations may change if the patient is asked to observe near objects at 14 inches; the cover-uncover test (Fig. 4–6) should be repeated at this distance.

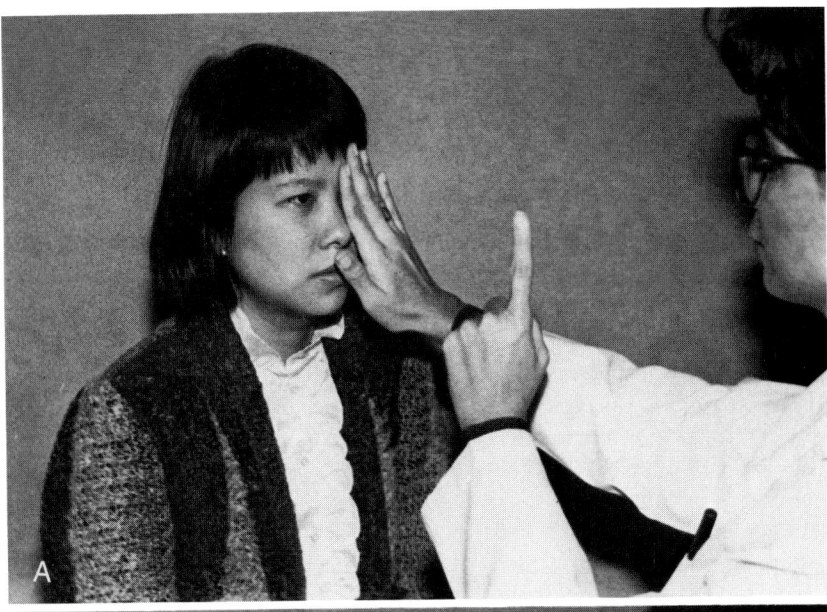

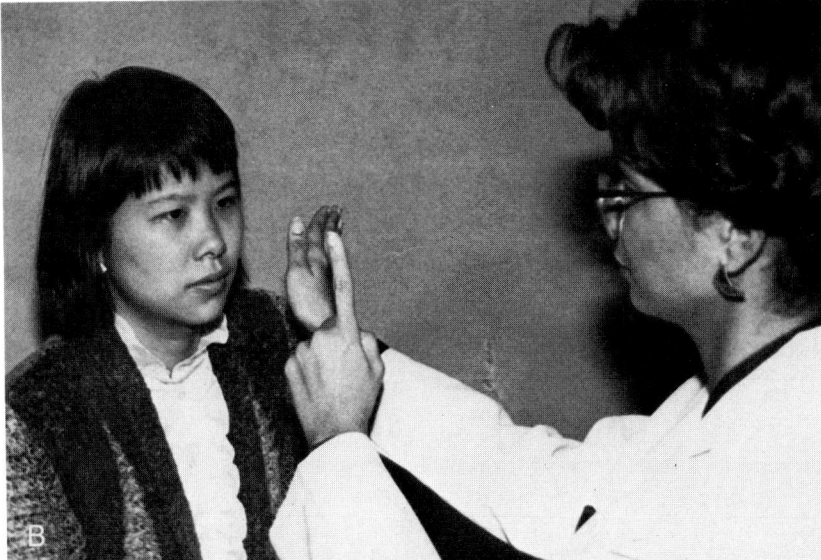

FIGURE 4–6. For assessing alignment of the eye, the cover-uncover test can be used to determine heterophoria and heterotropia. *A*, One eye is covered while the patient fixates on an accommodative target. The examiner observes for movement in the uncovered eye. *B*, The examiner then uncovers the occluded eye, observing for movement in the same eye.

Convergence Insufficiency

A common problem that can be most symptomatic in all age groups is the inability to maintain fusion on an object at 14 inches.[5] This abnormality can be due to an exophoria (eyes deviated outward), an abnormal accommodation–convergence ratio (which does not allow for the appropriate convergence), a basic weakness of the convergence amplitudes, or an uncorrected high hyperopia. Complaints are related to the fatigue experienced while reading and include a burning sensation in the eyes, brow ache, pulling on the eye, and occasionally neck pain.

Convergence amplitude can also be checked by the nonophthalmologist. The patient is asked to stare at a pen top at 20 inches from the nose. The top is slowly moved toward the nose, and the patient is asked to watch it carefully. The observer notes whether the patient can maintain fixation with both eyes on the pen top as it approaches the tip of the nose. The patient should be able to perform this procedure without difficulty or strain. If a convergence insufficiency is noted, one eye will break fusion and deviate outward; the patient usually experiences diplopia as the eye breaks convergence.

TREATMENT

When there is no underlying disease causing a muscular asthenopia, the most important treatment for this problem is proper refraction and the subsequent prescribing of corrective lenses. An artificial hyperopia can be produced by improperly fitting spectacles that cause a prismatic effect. When the muscular problem is overt, surgery may sometimes be necessary to obtain the correct alignment of the eyes. Symptoms related to convergence insufficiency can most often be alleviated by a short course of ocular exercises. It should be determined whether a muscle imbalance is congenital or acquired. The cause of an acquired deviation may include stroke or tumor.

Ocular Conditions That Cause Head Pain With Ocular Findings

In this section, diseases of the various parts of the eye that cause pain will be discussed in anatomic sequence.

Skin Surrounding The Ocular Region

Herpes Zoster. The red, weeping pustules that outline the distribution of the trigeminal nerve are quite characteristic and make this diagnosis less difficult (Fig. 4–7). However, the prodrome to herpes zoster can be quite painful, and in the absence of skin lesions the diagnosis may not be readily apparent. The limitation of the pain to one side of the face and the trigeminal distribution of the pain serve as clues. The classic pustules present within 7 days of the onset of pain, clarifying the diagnosis. Internal ocular involvement must be suspected if the skin lesions are present on the tip of the nose, indicating involvement of the nasociliary ganglion

Head Pain Associated With the Eye

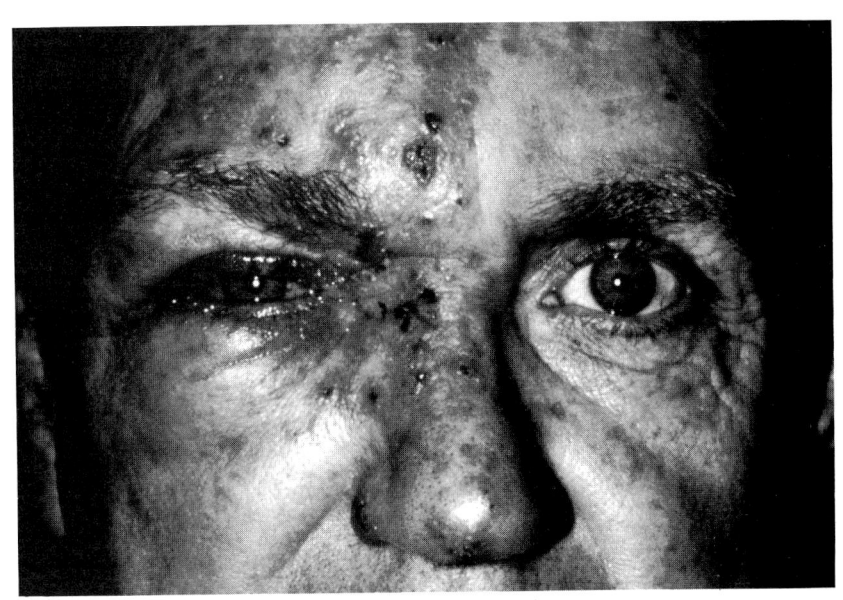

FIGURE 4–7. Herpes zoster involving the right trigeminal nerve. The lesion at the tip of the nose indicates ipsilateral intraocular involvement (Hutchinson's sign).

(Hutchinson's sign). Systemic steroids have been recommended as part of the treatment regimen to prevent postzoster neuralgias, which can be quite painful.[6–9]

Eyelids

Blepharitis. Each individual has a specific threshold for light, and when this threshold is exceeded, the patient may have symptoms of pain. Irregularities of the refractive media may generate symptoms even in the presence of normal light levels. Blepharitis, an infection of the lid margins, can cause such abnormalities.[7, 10] Staphylococci, the major cause of blepharitis, produce toxins that disrupt the tear film, leading to drying of the cornea. Once dry spots are present, the corneal epithelium becomes irregular, causing the defraction of light. This sparkling of light, alone or with the associated squinting, may cause muscle fatigue and create symptoms. In addition to asthenopic symptoms, the patient may also complain of lid discomfort, puffiness, and redness. On evaluation, the eyelid margins are usually inflamed, and crusting may be seen at the base of the cilia (Fig. 4–8). Cleansing of the eyelids with warm water and a cotton-tip applicator, followed by administration of a broad-speculum ophthalmic ointment, may prove beneficial. Unfortunately, in the elderly this condition may become chronic, and the antibiotic regimen may only control rather than eradicate the symptoms.

Entropion–Ectropion. Abnormal lid position also leads to tear film abnormalities, since proper lid movement is involved in tear secretion, tear movement, and tear removal.[11, 12] If this function is not carried out in an

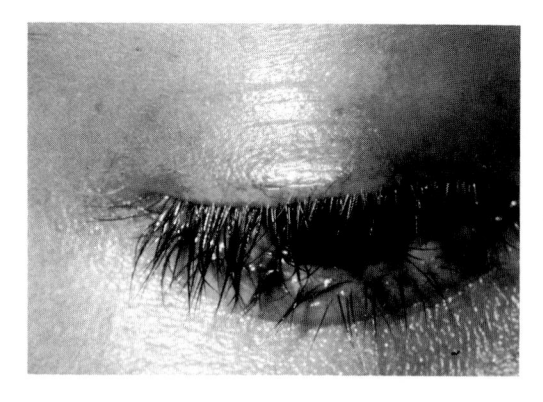

FIGURE 4–8. Blepharitis. The lid margins are inflamed and the cilia are misdirected.

efficient manner, corneal epithelial disruption may ensue. If the eyelids are turned toward the eye (entropion), the eyelashes may rub the cornea directly, causing surface abnormalities. If the eyelids are turned out (ectropion), the tears will not be kept against the cornea, allowing it to dry. Artificial teardrops can be helpful if the eyes become dry as a result of lid abnormalities. Surgical correction may be indicated in some cases (Fig. 4–9).

Conjunctiva

The goblet cells of the conjunctiva are mainly involved in the production of mucin, which serves to maintain corneal wetness between blinking. Chronic inflammation due to bacterial or viral infection, or to autoimmune

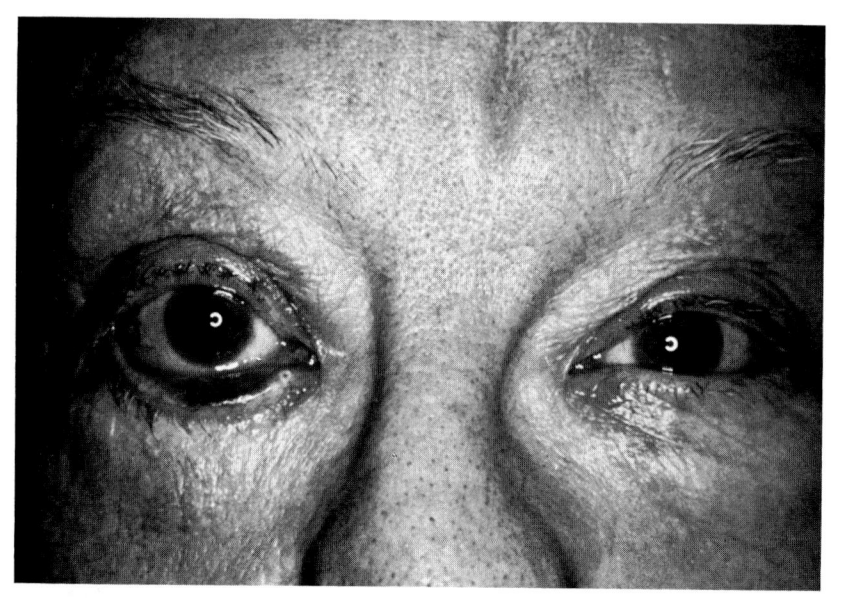

FIGURE 4–9. Ectropion. The lower right lid is turned outward, preventing proper lubrication of the cornea.

diseases (pemphigoid, Stevens-Johnson syndrome) may compromise the conjunctiva's ability to produce mucin.[7] The degree of severity of symptoms is usually related to the pathogenesis of the lid abnormality. Palpebral conjunctival abnormalities may not be readily apparent, and it may be necessary to pull down the inferior lid to examine its inner surface. Generalized erythema will be present if there is significant conjunctival involvement. Loss of the inferior fornix and scarring may be seen in conditions that adversely affect the basement membrane. If onset is acute and is associated with a watery discharge, a viral etiology should be suspected (Fig. 4–10), although *Chlamydia* infections in adults may present as a chronic follicular conjunctivitis. Ocular decongestants should be prescribed in acute viral conjunctivitis. A mucopurulent discharge usually suggests bacterial conjunctivitis, and a broad-spectrum antibiotic such as sulfacetamide 10 percent every 6 hours should be administered. If the complaints are severe and there is scarring of the conjunctiva, an autoimmune disease should be considered, and consultation with an ophthalmologist should be sought. Unfortunately, these disease processes can lead to severe visual impairment, and the recommended treatment may be quite complex.

Cornea

The cornea is the most powerful refracting surface of the eye. As such, disorders of the cornea have the greatest impact on vision. Irregularities caused by drying and secondary conditions give rise to symptoms as outlined previously. Primary diseases of the cornea include corneal ulcers, which

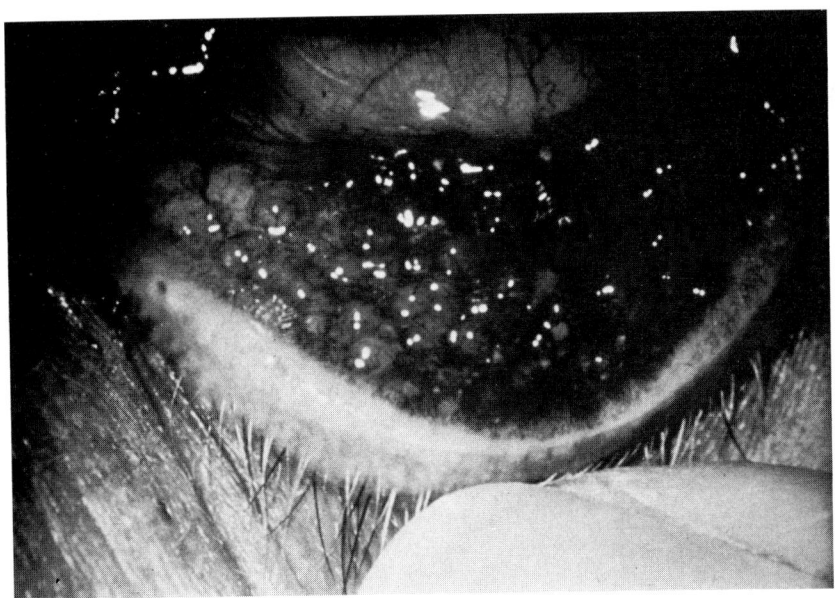

FIGURE 4–10. Viral conjunctivitis. Retraction of the lower lid reveals multiple follicles and a watery discharge.

represent invasion of the cornea by infectious agents.[13] These infiltrates are usually associated with marked pain and conjunctival hyperemia. Bacterial (*Pseudomonas, Staphylococcus*) and viral (herpetic) infections are more common than fungal infections, which create a less severe inflammatory response and are indolent in nature. Most corneal infections occur in individuals who have lost the normal protective mechanism of the cornea, such as tear secretion and lid movement, or have had longstanding periocular infections. It should be recognized that corneal infections can lead to total loss of vision and must be treated as ophthalmic emergencies (Fig. 4–11).

Sudden ocular pain may be the result of a corneal foreign body. The history and symptoms are usually suggestive, and copious irrigation with normal saline may be curative. If the foreign body has become embedded, removal may require biomicroscopic techniques. Staining of the cornea with fluorescein dye and subsequent examination with a blue light may reveal the secondary epithelial defect. Occasionally, the corneal epithelium may cover the foreign body, and the patient will complain of less severe ocular discomfort that lasts for a longer period of time (Fig. 4–12).

Primary degeneration of the cornea may also occur, causing symptoms of asthenopia. These symptoms are secondary to corneal opacities that can defract light and cause dazzling. These eyes are usually not inflamed, and examination of the cornea with a penlight may illustrate the corneal opacities associated with these diseases. These degenerations may require corneal transplantation, depending on the degree of visual compromise.

Glaucoma

Primary open-angle glaucoma, the most common form of glaucoma, does not present with pain. These patients are usually asymptomatic until there is significant loss of the peripheral visual field and early loss of the central field. If risk factors such as family history of glaucoma or diabetes are present, the patient should receive annual eye examinations.

Acute angle closure glaucoma is a disease of the elderly and rarely presents prior to age 55.[14,15] These patients complain of a sudden onset of eye pain associated with an acute diminution of vision. There is usually a

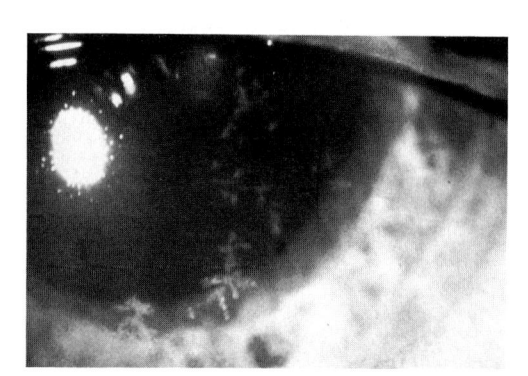

FIGURE 4–11. Herpes simplex. Multiple dendritic lesions involving the corneal epithelium. A mild foreign body sensation may be associated with conjunctival hyperemia.

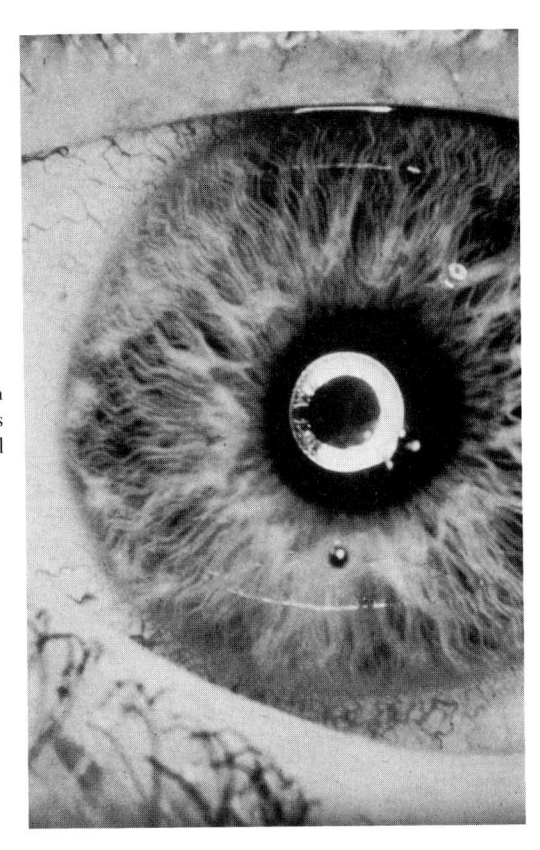

FIGURE 4–12. Corneal foreign body. A metallic foreign body is seen within the superficial corneal stroma.

history of farsightedness (hyperopia), which predisposes these individuals to an attack. Signs include conjunctival hyperemia, a dull corneal reflex, and a mid-dilated pupil (4 to 5 mm), which does not constrict with light stimulation. The cornea usually measures 11 mm or less in the horizontal meridian.

Treatment of these patients should include a drop of timolol (a beta blocker) if there are no contraindications. In addition, 500 mg of acetazolamide is given orally. These medications are utilized to decrease the intraocular pressure. These patients should then be referred to an ophthalmologist for continued care. They usually require laser surgical intervention in the acute stage of the disease process.

Uveitis

Uveitis is a general term used to indicate inflammation of the uvea within the eye.[16] Inflammation within the eye may be limited to the iris (iritis) or the retina (retinitis) (Fig. 4–13) with secondary involvement of other parts of the eye.[7] Dull ocular pain exacerbated by light (photophobia) is most often present. Depending on the extent of involvement, there may be a decrease in visual acuity. The eye usually exhibits a ciliary flush (redness surrounding the sclera adjacent to the cornea), or generalized conjunctival

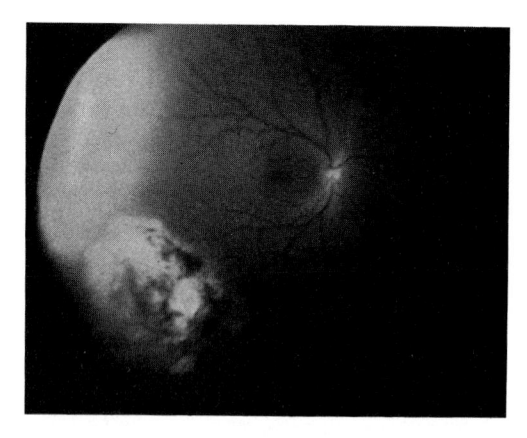

FIGURE 4–13. Retinitis. A focal inflammatory lesion within the retina. Since it does not involve the central retina, no visual symptoms may be present.

hyperemia may be present. The correct treatment depends on the etiology, which may be idiopathic, systemic, autoimmune, or infectious. The treatment must be directed toward the specific etiology and, unless biomicroscopy is performed, the condition may be confused with other ocular inflammations. Steroids should not be administered by themselves or in combination with antibiotics unless a specific diagnosis has been confirmed. Steroid-induced breakdown of the ocular defenses may be quite detrimental and may allow certain organisms to damage the eye irreparably.

Optic Nerve

Inflammation of the optic nerve may be primary or secondary to orbital disease. Primary inflammatory disease of the optic nerve is associated with a profound loss of visual acuity and the presence of an afferent pupillary defect (Marcus Gunn's phenomenon).[17] Swelling of the optic nerve is usually seen in anterior optic neuritis[18] and is associated with minimal pain symptoms. In retrobulbar optic neuritis, pain can be elicited by quick lateral eye movements. Although there is an association between optic neuritis and multiple sclerosis,[19] this association is weak and there is no benefit in telling the patient of this relationship. Some patients have contemplated suicide after being given the impression that they may develop multiple sclerosis in the future.

Tenon's Capsule

The connective tissue layer deep to the conjunctiva and superficial to the anterior sclera is Tenon's capsule.[20] This tissue may become primarily inflamed, as in autoimmune disease, or it may be secondarily involved in inflammations of the sclera or of the conjunctiva. When patients with primary tenonitis are examined in natural sunlight, there tends to be a blue hue to the inflamed tissues. This inflammation is steroid responsive.

Sclera

The connective tissue coat of the eye may itself become inflamed, usually on an autoimmune basis.[20, 21] These patients complain of a dull, penetrating pain deep within the eye. If the inflammation is involving the anterior portion of the globe, localized redness may be seen. If the posterior aspect of the sclera is involved, localized signs may not be apparent. Ultrasonography reveals a thickened sclera with surrounding edema in these cases. This disease is particularly steroid responsive.

Orbital Disease

Diseases of the soft tissues that surround the eye may also cause head pain.[17, 21, 22, 23] Depending on the extent of involvement, ocular signs may not be easily recognized. Within the orbit, the muscles, connective tissues, blood vessels, and individual nerves may become inflamed. The pain associated with orbital inflammatory disease is exacerbated by retropulsion of the globe which helps in localizing the source of head pain. To determine the extent of orbital involvement and to aid in the diagnosis, ultrasonography and/or a CT scan are indicated. Infection, thyroid disease (Fig. 4–14), tumor, and idiopathic inflammation can all be etiologic. If there is limitation of eye movement associated with signs of active infection, with or without proptosis, post-septal orbital cellulitis should be suspected and a CT scan is essential. Immediate systemic broad spectrum antibiotics should be started to impede the spread through the orbital walls to intracranial structures.

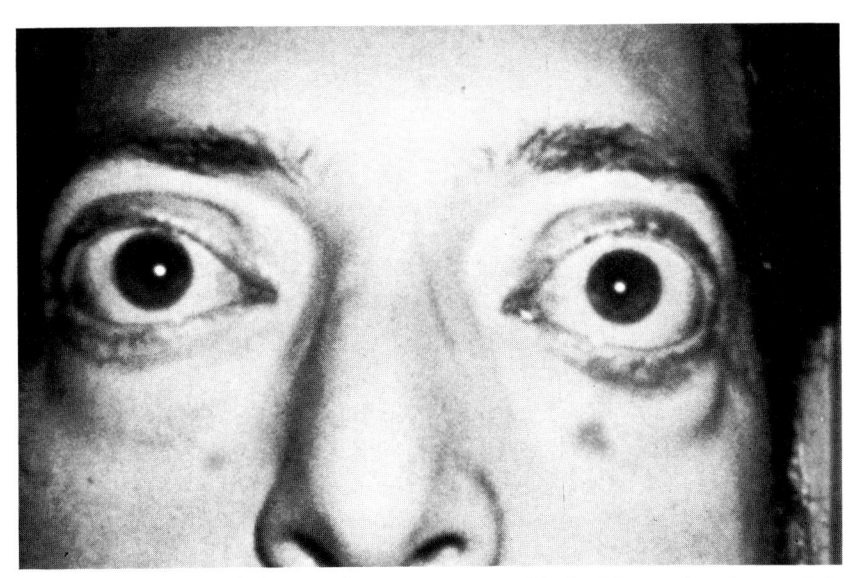

FIGURE 4–14. Thyroid disease. There is protrusion of both globes with widening of the orbital fissures. Ocular motility is also abnormal.

In all cases of retrobulbar pain, speed in making the correct diagnosis can be vital in maintaining ocular function.

Temporal arteritis usually occurs in individuals over the age of 60.[17, 24, 25] These patients present with head pain with or without loss of vision. An elevated sedimentation rate is usually present. Treatment, usually with high-dose steroids, is indicated to prevent visual loss. If visual loss has occurred in one eye, steroids are needed to prevent visual loss in the other eye. A biopsy of the temporal artery is indicated to document the diagnosis.

Inflammatory processes involving the sinus may also give rise to periocular pain and a secondary orbital cellulitis. Rapid diagnosis and appropriate treatment are required to reduce the likelihood of visual impairment.

Primary Nonocular Conditions Causing Secondary Ocular Symptoms

Migraine

Migraine headache is a specific disorder that should not be confused with other causes of head pain. Since it is vascular in origin, its symptom complex is predictable and is related to the various stages of vascular activity. Symptoms may be isolated to the eye or may involve the eye and head or the head alone. There is usually a prodrome that the patient learns to recognize. These symptoms are due to vasoconstriction in the cortical area responsible for vision. Ocular symptoms include an awareness that the vision is being gradually obscured in one eye, and then, moments later, vision gradually returns in reverse sequence. The part of the vision that is first to go is first to return. The diminution in vision may begin at the periphery and contract with scintillating light at the border, or it may seem as if a window shade were being drawn down, eventually covering the vision. The aura may last for seconds, minutes, or rarely hours. Once the blood vessels have dilated, the ocular symptoms subside, and the classic headache may occur. The headache, which may be located near the eye, temples, or hemicranially, may be quite unbearable, minimal, or absent. Light sensitivity may develop, and the patient may prefer a dark room.

Ophthalmoplegic Migraine

This is a pediatric disease that is also of vascular origin. Unlike ocular migraine, the headache occurs first and is followed by ocular muscle paresis, which usually lasts 12 to 24 hours, but these deviations may last for weeks. Since the nerve palsy occurs after the onset of pain, it is thought to occur in the vasodilation stage.

Summary and Conclusion

The nonophthalmologist can confidently perform the basic eye examination and may be able to correlate these findings with other manifestations of disease. It is essential to realize that complaints of head and facial pain may arise from the eye and that pain located behind the eye may be the result of intracranial tumor, central nervous system inflammation, meningitis, or circulatory decompensation. The importance of a thorough medical, family, and social history cannot be overemphasized. If the conditions mentioned in this chapter do not fully explain the patient's symptoms or signs, a full neurologic examination is warranted. Finally, it is necessary to realize that an ophthalmologist must be consulted for less straightforward ocular conditions.

References

1. Rubin, M. Optics for Clinicians. Gainesville, FL, Triad Publishing Company, 1974.
2. Milder, B., and Rubin, M. The Fine Art of Prescribing Glasses. Gainesville, FL, Triad Scientific Publishers, 1978.
3. Pau, H. Differential Diagnosis of Eye Diseases. Philadelphia, W.B. Saunders Co., 1978.
4. Lanchner, A. J. Headache in ophthalmic practice. CBL Ges Ophthalmol 60:289, 1953.
5. Parks, M. M. Alignment. In Clinical Ophthalmology. Vol. 1. Philadelphia, Harper & Row, 1987, Chap. 6.
6. Pavan-Langston, D. (ed.) Ocular viral disease. Int Ophthalmol Clin 15(4):141–150, 1975.
7. Aronson, F. B., and Elliott, J. H. Ocular Inflammation. St. Louis, C.V. Mosby, 1972.
8. Tunis, F. W., and Tatert, M. J. Acute retrobulbar neuritis complicating herpes zoster ophthalmicus. Ann Ophthalmol 19(12):453–460, 1987.
9. Sandor, E. V., Millman, A., Croxson, T. S., et al. Herpes zoster ophthalmicus in patients at risk for the acquired immune deficiency syndrome (AIDS). Am J Ophthalmol 101(2):153–155, 1986.
10. Thygeson, P. Complications of staphylococcic blepharitis. Am J Ophthalmol 68:446–449, 1969.
11. Frueh, B. R., and Schoengarth, L. D. Evaluation and treatment of the patient with ectropion. Ophthalmology 89:1049–1054, 1982.
12. Dortzbach, R. K., and McGetrick, J. J. Involutional entropion of the lower eyelid. In Advances in Ophthalmic, Plastic and Reconstructive Surgery. New York, Pergamon Press, 1983.
13. Abbot, R. L., and Abrams, M. A. Bacterial corneal ulcers. In Duane, T. D., and Jaeger, E. A. (eds.). Clinical Ophthalmology, Vol. 4. Philadelphia, Harper & Row, 1986.
14. Ritch, R., and Shields, M.B. (eds.). The Secondary Glaucomas. St. Louis, C.V. Mosby Co., 1982.
15. Kolker, A. E., and Hetherington, J. (eds.). Becker–Schaffer's Diagnosis and Therapy of the Glaucomas. 5th ed. St. Louis, C.V. Mosby Co., 1983.

16. Godfrey, W. A. Acute anterior uveitis. In Duane, T. D., and Jaeger, E. A. (eds.). Clinical Ophthalmology. Vol. 4. Philadelphia, Harper & Row, 1987, Chap. 40.
17. Walsh, T. J. Neuro-Ophthalmology: Clinical Signs and Symptoms. Philadelphia, Lea & Febiger, 1985.
18. Glaser, J. S. Tropical Diagnosis: Prechiasmal visual pathways. In Duane, T. D., and Jaeger, E. A. (eds.). Clinical Ophthalmology. Vol 2. Philadelphia, Harper & Row, 1978, Chap. 5.
19. Kurtzke, J. F. Optic neuritis or multiple sclerosis. Arch Neurol 42(7):704–710, 1985.
20. Watson, P. Diseases of the sclera and episclera. In Duane, T. D., and Jaeger, E. A. (eds.). Clinical Ophthalmology. Vol 4. Philadelphia, Harper & Row, 1987, Chap. 23.
21. Jakobec, S. A., and Jones, I. S. Orbital inflammations. In Duane, T. D., and Jaeger, E. A. (eds.). Clinical Ophthalmology. Vol 2. Philadelphia, Harper & Row, 1987, Chap. 35.
22. Fortson, J. K., Shapshay, S. M., Weiter, J. J., et al. Otolaryngologic manifestations of orbital pseudotumors. Otolaryngol Head Neck Surg 88(4):342–348, 1980.
23. Verma, N., and Singh, J. Bilateral idiopathic inflammatory pseudotumor of the orbit. Ann Ophthalmol 16(11):1076–1080, 1984.
24. Jay, W. M., et al. Bilateral sixth nerve pareses with temporal arteritis and diabetes. J Clin Neuro-Ophthalmol 6(2):91–95, 1986.
25. Clarke, A. E., and Victor, W. H. An unusual presentation of temporal arteritis. Ann Ophthalmol 19(9):343–346, 1987.
26. Hedges, T. R. The diagnosis and management of headache. Sem Ophthalmol 2(3):173–182, 1987.
27. Heyck, H. Headache and Facial Pain. Chicago, Yearbook, 1981, pp. 134–181, 232–235.

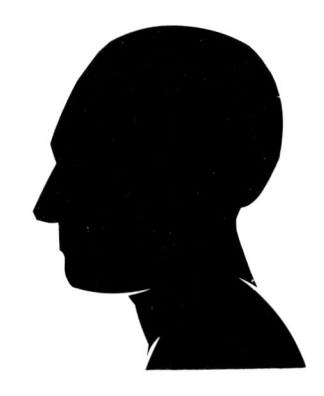

Chapter 5
Rhinologic Causes of Facial Pain

Charles P. Kimmelman

As the central structure of the face, it is not surprising that the nose is frequently the site of nociceptive stimuli of varied origins. This organ is richly endowed with nerves, blood vessels, and glands and is frequently affected by infections, neoplasms, inflammatory processes, and trauma, including the surgeon's knife. In fact, national expenditures for relief of nasal and paranasal sinus pain total in the billions of dollars annually. We have only to think of the common complaint of "sinus headache" to grasp the magnitude of the malady.

The following discussion organizes nasal pain into an etiopathologic classification. The methods of diagnosis are reviewed. Finally, the treatment of pain in each class is outlined. This approach offers the clinician a rational means of dealing with facial pain of rhinosinal origin.

Neuroanatomy

The nose develops from the region of the midface supplied by the field of the maxillary and ophthalmic divisions of the trigeminal nerve. The maxillary sensory nerve cell bodies reside in the gasserian ganglion on top of the petrous apex and send their peripheral processes through the foramen rotundum into the pterygopalatine fossa. Within the fossa the nerve takes an abrupt bend laterally to create a so-called bayonet course. The nerve continues anteriorly as the infraorbital nerve. Within the fossa, the maxillary nerve sends medial branches through the sphenopalatine foramen as the lateral posterior superior nerve, the medial posterior superior nerve, and the palatine nerves. The medial posterior superior branches pass over the roof of the nose to supply the posterior nasal septum. The lateral posterior superior nasal nerve provides sensation to the middle and superior turbinates. The posterior inferior nasal nerve supplies the inferior turbinate and is a branch of the anterior palatine nerve.[1]

The nasociliary branch of the ophthalmic division of the trigeminal nerve sends two branches medially from the orbit, the anterior and posterior ethmoid nerves. These supply the most anterior portions of the nasal septum and lateral nasal wall. The external nose is supplied by the external nasal branch of the anterior ethmoid nerve, which exits from the nose between the nasal bone and the upper lateral cartilage. The superior dorsum is supplied by the infratrochlear branch of the nasociliary nerve. The skin of the lateral dorsum is served by the infraorbital nerve.[1]

The mucous membrane of the frontal sinus is supplied by the supraorbital, supratrochlear, and anterior ethmoid branches of the ophthalmic nerve. The lateral posterior superior nasal branches of the maxillary division of the trigeminal nerve also play a role. The anterior ethmoid air cells are supplied by the anterior ethmoid nerve, and the posterior ethmoid air cells and the sphenoid sinus are supplied by the posterior ethmoid nerve and lateral and medial posterior superior nasal nerves.[2] The mucous membrane of the maxillary sinus is supplied by branches of the lateral posterior superior nasal nerve and the superior dental plexus, which is formed from the interdigitation of branches of all three superior alveolar nerves. The latter are branches of the maxillary division of the trigeminal nerve[1] (Fig. 5–1).

The autonomic nerve supply to the nose is accomplished predominantly through the pterygopalatine ganglion. The latter contains secretomotor parasympathetic nerve cell bodies and sends postganglionic peripheral fibers to the nasal blood vessels and glands by way of the branches of the nasal nerves.

Knowledge of the sensory innervation allows the clinician to interpret patterns of pain referral from the nose and sinuses. Frontal sinus pain may be sensed over the involved sinus, the temporal region, or the occiput. Ethmoid pain is perceived in the medial orbital region, the eye, the vertex, and the parietal region. Sphenoid pain may radiate to the temporal region, the vertex, the occiput, the postauricular region, and the canine tooth. This pattern of radiation can be explained by the fact that intracranial structures (blood vessels, dura) are also innervated by branches of the trigeminal nerve. Maxillary sinus pain is perceived over the involved sinus and extending into the posterior maxillary teeth. It is more difficult to explain the occasional radiation of ethmoid pain to the upper cervical region and sphenoid pain to the shoulder.[3] This pattern may be due to overlap of the nucleus and spinal tract of the trigeminal nerve with the dorsal horn of the

Rhinologic Causes of Facial Pain

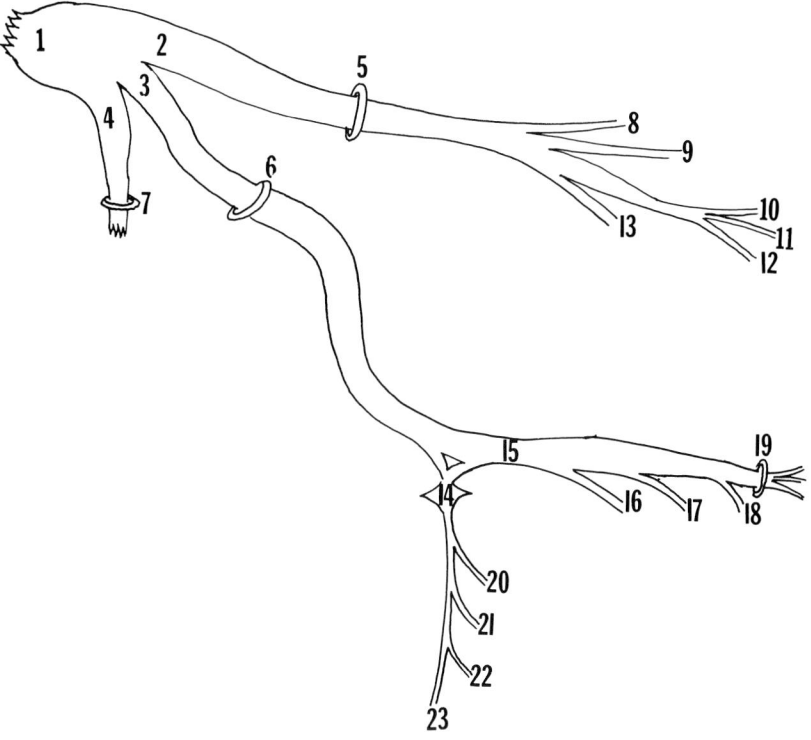

FIGURE 5–1. Schematic illustration of the sensory nerve supply of the nose and paranasal sinuses. (1) Trigeminal ganglion, (2) ophthalmic nerve, (3) maxillary nerve, (4) mandibular nerve, (5) superior orbital fissure, (6) foramen rotundum, (7) foramen ovale, (8) supraorbital nerve, (9) supratrochlear nerve, (10) infratrochlear nerve, (11) anterior ethmoid nerve, (12) external nasal nerve, (13) posterior ethmoid nerve, (14) pterygopalatine ganglion, (15) infraorbital nerve, (16,17,18) posterior, middle, and anterior superior alveolar nerves, (19) infraorbital foramen, (20) medial posterosuperior nasal nerve, (21) lateral posterosuperior nasal nerve, (22) posteroinferior nasal nerve, (23) palatine nerve.

cervical spinal cord. It has also been suggested that pain sensations are carried through the sympathetic fibers to the thoracic levels of the spinal cord, where, after efferent stimulation of sympathetic neurons, pain receptors are stimulated at the corresponding thoracic levels.

Etiology of Nasal and Sinus Pain

There are numerous pathologic entities that may lead to nasal pain. These may be classified as inflammatory, neoplastic, developmental, traumatic, and idiopathic.

Inflammatory Lesions

Inflammatory lesions produce most cases of nasal pain. Acute bacterial rhinitis and sinusitis are usually due to pyogenic organisms such as *Streptococcus pneumoniae, Hemophilus influenzae,* and *Staphylococcus aureus.* Viral upper respiratory infections are a common antecedent cause (Fig. 5–2). Occlusion of the ostium of the sinus coupled with mucosal injury and impaired ciliary activity leads to stasis of secretions and bacterial proliferation. Purulent drainage from the sinus ostium is a common finding in this disease. The mucosa may undergo hyperplastic changes leading to development of polyps, which further impede ventilation and drainage. Pain and purulent rhinorrhea are common findings.

Granulomatous infections, such as tuberculosis and syphilis, are destructive but rarely painful unless secondary pyogenic infection supervenes. Fungal rhinosinusitis is usually found in immunocompromised hosts, such as patients with the acquired immune deficiency syndrome (AIDS). *Aspergillus* and *Mucor* species invade the nasal and sinus mucosa and cause a gangrenous necrosis of bone and soft tissue. If left unchecked, the organisms invade the orbit and cranial cavity with fatal results. Occasionally a noninvasive form of *Aspergillus* causes local inflammation and pain in an immune competent patient.[4]

Rhinoscleroma (Fig. 5–3) is a granulomatous reaction to infection by *Klebsiella rhinoscleromatis.* The infection is acquired by residents of areas where the organism is endemic, such as Central and South America and

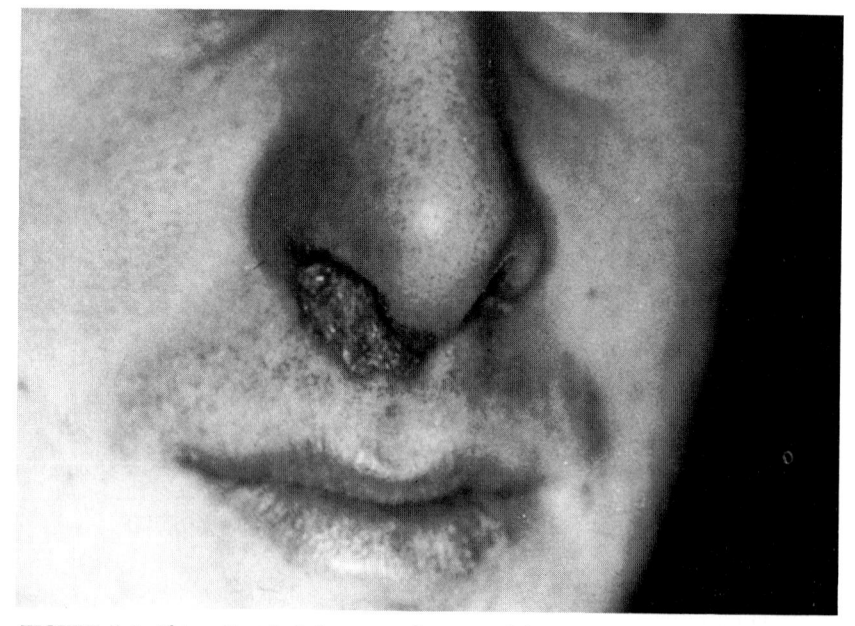

FIGURE 5–2. This patient had the acquired immunodeficiency syndrome and developed a granular, crusting, painful lesion of the nasal vestibule that extended onto the upper lip. The lesion was due to herpes simplex virus, activated by the loss of immune competence.

Rhinologic Causes of Facial Pain

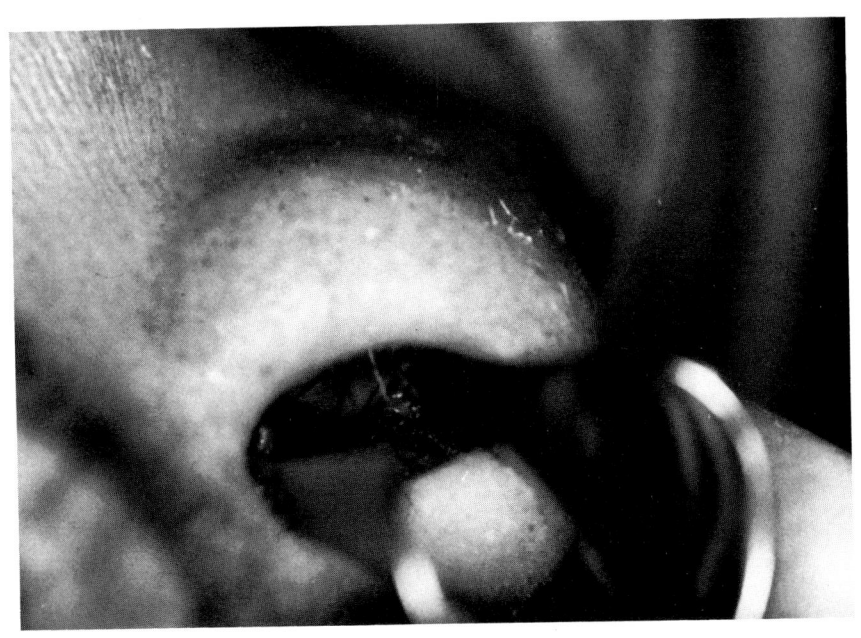

FIGURE 5–3. Right nasal vestibule in a patient with rhinoscleroma. There is a granular crusting lesion that was mildly painful and bled at a light touch.

eastern Europe. There is severe destruction of the nasal mucosa with secondary bacterial infection.[5]

Allergic rhinitis is a common cause of nasal inflammation. Submucosal mast cells and basophils degranulate when the immunoglobulin E on their surface comes in contact with specific antigen. The release of inflammatory mediators, such as histamine and leukotrienes, produces vascular congestion, edema, and glandular hypersecretion. The patient may complain of chronic discomfort due to nasal obstruction. Secondary bacterial infection may also cause pain. Persistent edema leads to polyp formation, which further obstructs the sinus ostia and can lead to chronic sinusitis.

Rhinitis medicamentosa is a nasal inflammation resulting from the abuse of topical sympathomimetic amine nasal sprays. The nasal mucosa shows a severe degree of inflammation and edema; often there is total nasal obstruction. An important cause of rhinitis medicamentosa is cocaine abuse. The ischemia caused by the intense vasoconstrictive effect of cocaine can lead to tissue necrosis and destruction. In the most severe cases there can be total destruction of the nasal septum with extensive nasal crusting.

The endocrine alterations that occur in pregnancy and hypothyroidism may lead to mucosal congestion and discomfort. Certain antihypertensive medications, such as reserpine, may also engender nasal obstruction.

Foreign bodies lead to nasal pain, discharge, and obstruction. These are most common in children and range from substances as innocuous as food to highly corrosive alkaline batteries (Fig. 5–4). Unilateral nasal pain and discharge in a child should lead to suspicion of an intranasal foreign body.

Wegener's granulomatosis deserves mention because of its life-threat-

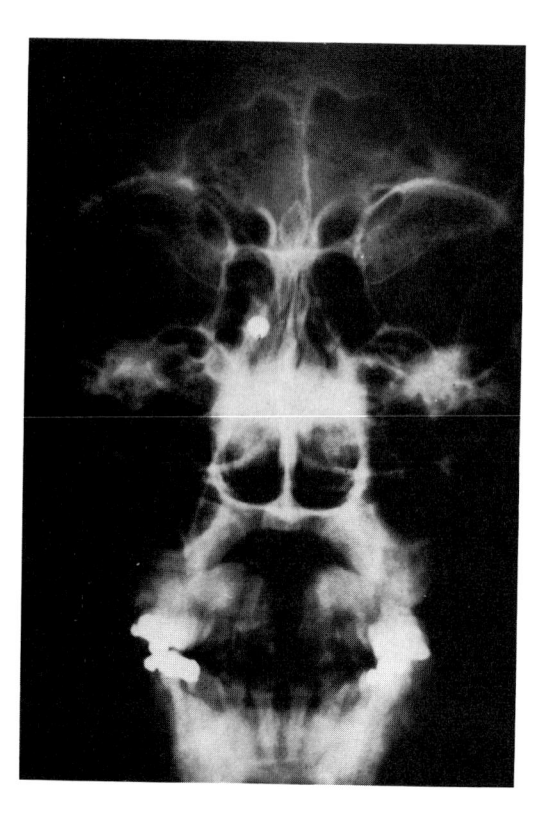

FIGURE 5–4. Plain x-ray (Caldwell projection) of a patient with a foreign body (bullet) of the superior portion of the right nasal cavity.

ening nature. It is a systemic vasculitis that preferentially affects the respiratory tract and kidneys. Sites of involvement usually include the nose and paranasal sinuses, larynx, and pulmonary parenchyma. The sinonasal complaints are often the first symptoms brought to the attention of a physician. There is a necrotizing ulceration of the nasal mucosa with mucopurulent exudate and severe crusting. The destruction often undermines the structural support provided by the nasal septum and leads to a saddle nose deformity (Fig. 5–5). Secondary infectious sinusitis or primary mucosal involvement with the vasculitis is common.[6]

Sarcoidosis gives rise to thick tenacious casts in the nasal cavity owing to alteration of epithelial mucociliary activity. There is destruction of the mucosa by noncaseating granulomas, probably triggered by an as yet unidentified antigen. Pain may result from secondary infection or sinusitis. Neuralgia may be the result of granulomatous involvement of nerves.

Sjögren's syndrome is an autoimmune condition involving destruction of salivary tissue that causes symptoms primarily in the head and neck. The nose becomes extremely dry and crusted. Secondary bacterial infection of the nasal fossa and sinusitis may result from inadequate mucociliary clearance.

Ulcerating mucosal disorders, such as pemphigus and Stevens-Johnson

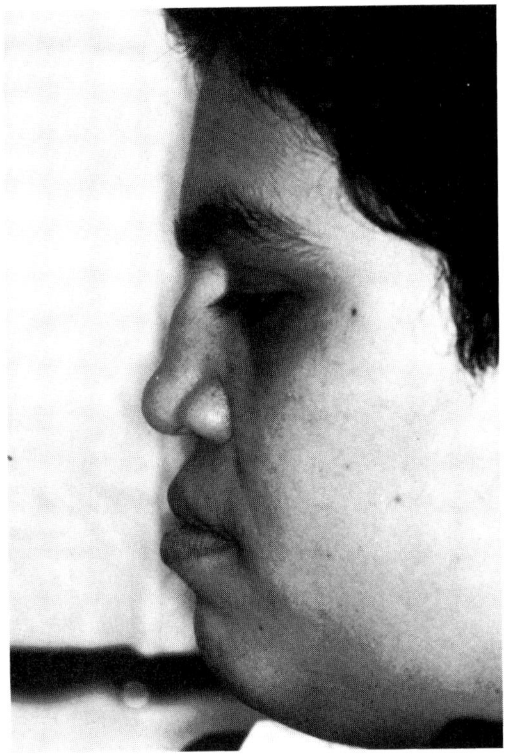

FIGURE 5-5. Patient with Wegener's granulomatosis and saddle-nose deformity caused by collapse of the structural framework of the nasal dorsum.

syndrome, often involve the nasal mucosa and give rise to nasal pain. The nasal involvement is usually only part of the clinical picture; oral and cutaneous involvement is more readily observed.

Necrotizing sialometaplasia is a benign, ulcerating condition that grossly resembles a neoplasm. It may occasionally involve the nasal cavity and cause nasal pain. It is a self-limited condition and resolves without treatment.[5]

Neoplasms

Most nasal neoplasms begin in the skin of the nasal dorsum in the alar region (Fig. 5-6). These areas are unshielded from actinic exposure, and basal cell carcinomas may develop there in lightly pigmented individuals. Squamous cell carcinoma is less frequent and may also occur in the region of the columella and nasal vestibule. Cancer of the nasal dorsum may prove very difficult to eradicate once the embryonic fusion planes of the face are invaded.[7] Pain develops with perineural invasion of the adjacent sensory nerves, but this usually occurs only with extensive disease. Melanomas occasionally are seen on the nasal dorsum, but these are rarely painful.

Neoplasms of the nasal and sinus mucosa are much less common than

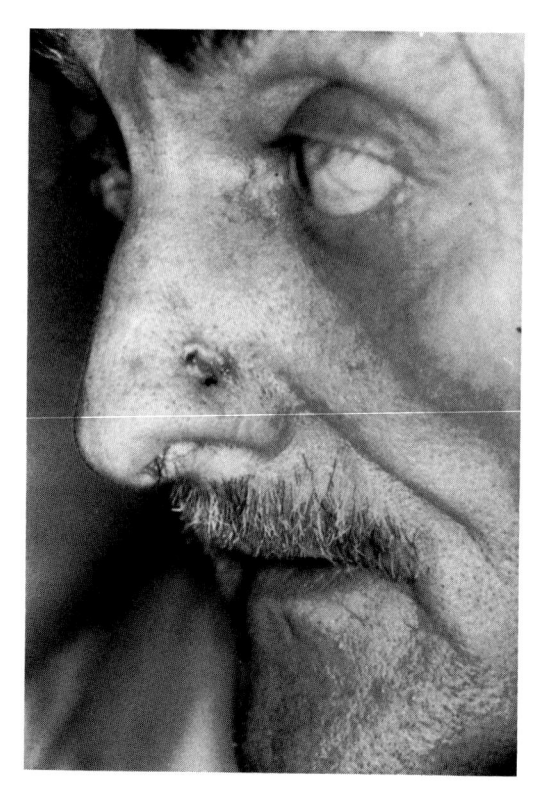

FIGURE 5–6. Small basal cell carcinoma of the left nasal ala.

those of the skin overlying the nasal dorsum. They tend to be asymptomatic until they attain a large size. The usual presenting symptoms are nasal obstruction, epistaxis, rhinorrhea, and pain. Since nasal neoplasms usually occur in older individuals, any elderly patient with nasal pain must be carefully evaluated for neoplasia.

Papillomas are the most common nasal neoplasms. They usually occur in the vestibule or lateral nasal wall. The latter type have the histologic picture of infolding papillary projections with microcysts—hence they are termed inverted papillomas. These lesions usually cause pain through secondary sinusitis due to ostial obstruction. In about 5 percent of cases there may be an associated squamous cell carcinoma.

Other benign tumors that may involve the nasal mucosa are minor salivary gland lesions, such as pleomorphic adenoma or papillary cystadenoma. Neurogenic tumors, including schwannomas and neurofibromas, are also occasionally seen and may be painful. Osteomas tend to develop at the frontoethmoid suture line. They are rarely painful themselves, but they cause secondary frontal or ethmoid sinusitis and pain.

Malignant intranasal neoplasms are very rare. Squamous cell carcinoma is the most common type. It usually originates in the maxillary sinus. Once again, it usually reaches a large size and extent before it is discovered. Nickel exposure is a risk factor.[6] Adenocarcinomas arising in nasal and paranasal sinus glandular tissue are also recognized. These seem to be more common in furniture makers and other workers handling wood products.[5] Neural invasion or mucosal ulceration leads to pain. Other, less common tumors are metastases from distant primary lesions (notably the prostate, lung, and breast), mucosal melanoma, esthesioneuroblastoma, and sarcomas (osteogenic sarcoma, rhabdomyosarcoma). Sarcomas are more common in children than nasal epithelial malignancies. Patients with AIDS may develop Kaposi's sarcoma or lymphoma of the nose.

Congenital and Developmental Lesions

Congenital disorders of mucociliary transport would be expected to predispose to sinusitis. These disorders include ciliary dysmotility syndromes, such as Kartagener's syndrome. Nasal polyposis, obstruction, and sinusitis are fairly common in cystic fibrosis.

Developmental cysts may enlarge and lead to sinus ostial obstruction. Odontogenic cysts and related lesions may thus present with nasal or sinus pain. Nasolabial and globulomaxillary cysts may become infected and cause pain (Fig. 5–7). Similarly, fibro-osseous lesions of the midface, such as fibrous dysplasia, may cause nasal and sinus pain from osteal occlusion.

Trauma

Blunt or penetrating trauma is an obvious cause of nasal and facial pain. The long-term, traumatically induced intranasal deformity may also lead to

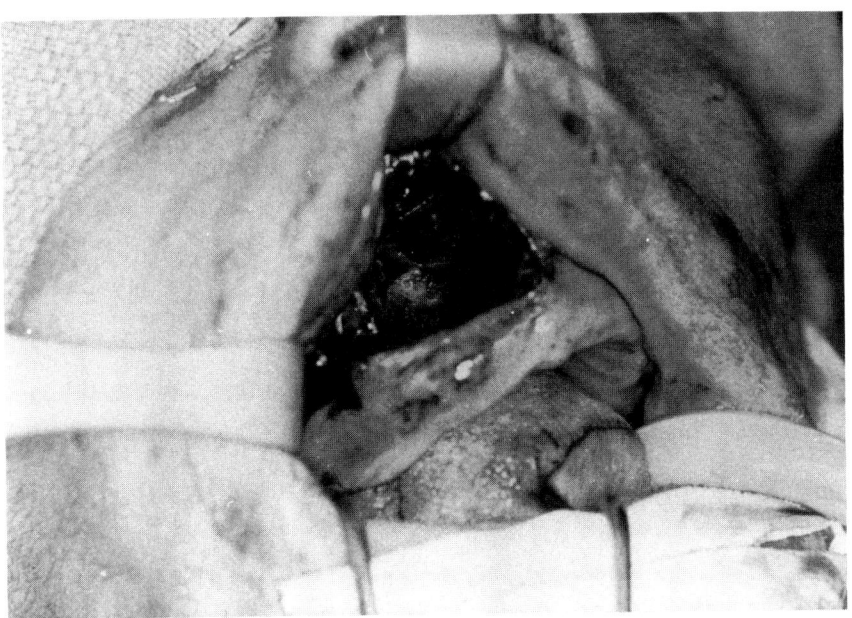

FIGURE 5–7. Intraoperative photograph of excision of a right nasolabial cyst. An incision of the gingivobuccal sulcus has been made, and the floor of the nose has been exposed to reveal the cyst.

nasal pain. For example, septal deflection can lead to sinusitis owing to impaired ostial ventilation. Some authorities state that contact between the deformed septum and lateral nasal wall may be a source of nasal pain.[8] Post-traumatic neuromas may lead to a neuralgic type of pain. Prolonged postoperative discomfort is not unusual following sinus surgery, especially when it involves the maxillary sinus (Caldwell-Luc procedure). This discomfort is probably due to injury secondary to intraoperative retraction of the infraorbital nerve. Patients undergoing osteoplastic frontal sinus surgery will have frontal tenderness for several months or longer (Fig. 5-8). Surgery of the pterygopalatine fossa, such as transantral ligation of the internal maxillary artery, commonly leads to postoperative neuralgia. Septal and rhinoplastic surgery rarely results in prolonged pain.

Neurologic Lesions

Sluder's syndrome, or sphenopalatine neuralgia, is postulated to arise from reflex parasympathetic hyperactivity and mucosal congestion.[8] The neural pathways are thought to be the nasal and palatal branches of the sphenopalatine ganglion, the greater superficial petrosal nerve, the connection within the medulla with the reticulospinal tract and through those, the segmental autonomic nerves in the lower cervical segments of the cord that supply the vasomotor innervation of the arteries of the regions involved.

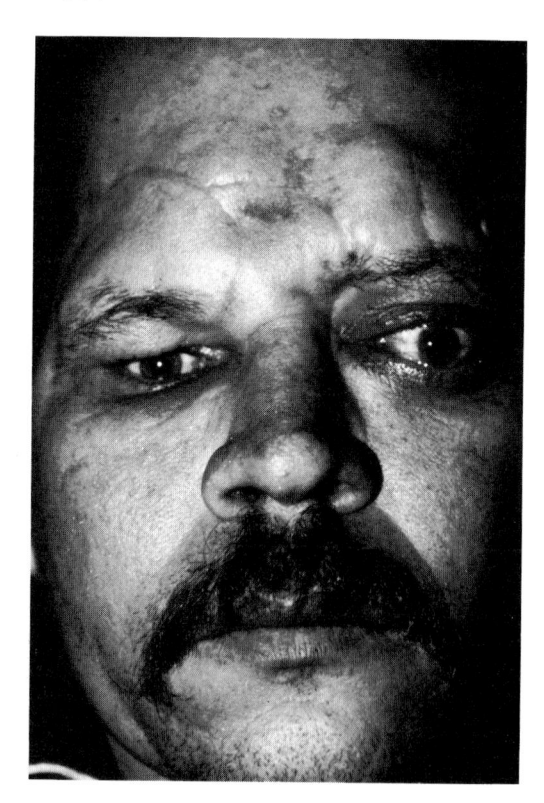

FIGURE 5-8. This patient sustained massive frontal trauma 20 years earlier and developed a chronic pain syndrome in the frontal region. A right frontal mucocele was a secondary development from an injury to the nasofrontal duct. This is revealed by bulging of the right supraorbital area and downward and outward displacement of the globe.

Migrate and trigeminal neuralgia may occasionally be the cause of nasal pain. For further information on these two conditions see Chapter 2.

Idiopathic Lesions

Atrophic rhinitis results in shrinking of the nasal mucosa with reduction of the ability to humidify and prepare the inspired air. Although the airways are widely patent, the patient complains bitterly of nasal obstruction and discomfort. The exact cause is unknown, but in some cases, *Klebsiella ozoenae* may be cultured. In other instances, overaggressive surgery, such as total inferior turbinectomy, may be a cause.

Vasomotor rhinitis is a term used to describe recurrent episodes of nasal obstruction and discharge that are precipitated by emotional stress, environmental incidents, or other activities that increase parasympathetic activity. The underlying cause is assumed to be an imbalance of sympathetic versus parasympathetic activity. Normally, the sympathetic tone predominates, but when parasympathetic tone is heightened, there is nasal congestion and hypersecretion. The sense of obstruction may lead patients to complain of nasal discomfort.[10]

Evaluation of the Patient

The historical aspects of the patient's complaint are exceedingly important in arriving at a diagnosis of the cause of nasal pain. The examiner should note any recent nasal or facial trauma. The presence of rhinorrhea, fever, nasal obstruction, or epistaxis should be ascertained. The patient should be questioned about the duration of pain, its quality, precipitating factors (foods, activity), and the use of intranasal drugs and medications. The patient should be questioned about the effect of position on the pain. Recent travel history or geographic region of birth is important because it may indicate exposure to pathogens. This is especially true of fungal infections and rhinoscleroma. Cranial nerve symptoms such as headache, altered visual acuity, diplopia, tearing, facial hypesthesia, dysphagia, or dysphonia are important; they may indicate extension of the disease process outside of the confines of the nasal or sinus mucosa. Previous nasal surgery or exposure to radiation is also noteworthy.

The physical examination should encompass the entire head and neck including the ears (to ascertain the presence of middle ear effusion), the face, the pharynx and larynx (with particular attention to the nasopharynx), the oral cavity and dentition, and the neck. The intranasal examination should be performed with and without topical vasoconstriction. The examiner should note the status of the nasal mucosa and the presence of any mass, ulceration, pigmentation, discharge, granulation, or bleeding. The use of telescopes and fiberscopes is necessary to obtain complete visualization. Orbital examination should be performed to determine any displace-

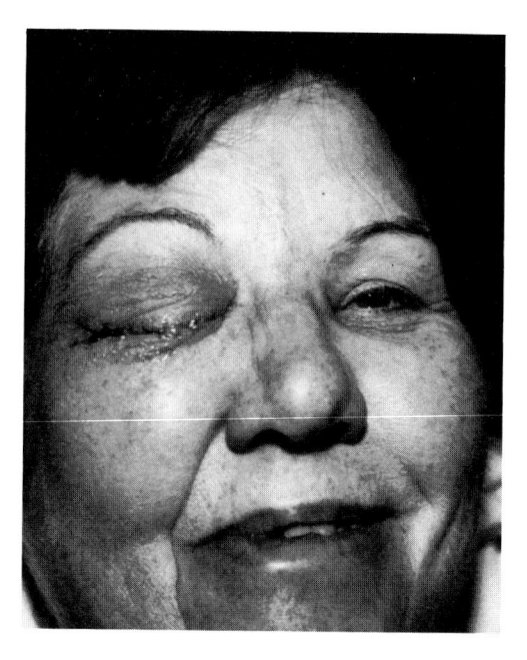

FIGURE 5-9. Severe edema and proptosis of the right eye in orbital cellulitis secondary to frontal and ethmoid sinusitis.

ment of the globe, disturbance of extraocular motion, a mass within the orbit, epiphora, papilledema, or optic atrophy (Fig. 5–9). Trigger points for pain, if any, should be identified.

The radiographic examination includes plain films of the paranasal sinuses and computed tomography (CT) of the nose and paranasal sinuses with axial and coronal cuts and contrast enhancement. If CT is performed, plain x-rays may be eliminated. The radiologist and requesting practitioner should pay special attention to the status of the nasal and sinus mucosa and bone. Thickening of the mucosa may be due to tumor (Fig. 5–10) or inflammation (Fig. 5–11); bone destruction is usually secondary to neoplasia (Fig. 5–12),

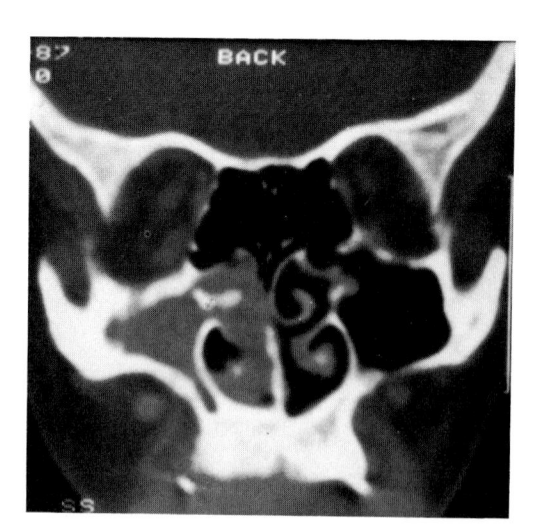

FIGURE 5-10. Coronal computed tomogram of the nose and paranasal sinuses demonstrating a mass of the right nasal cavity extending into the right maxillary sinus with minimal bone destruction. This was an inverted papilloma of the right lateral nasal wall.

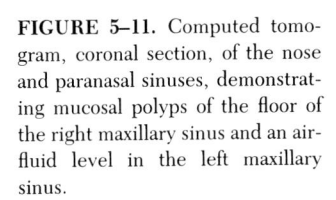

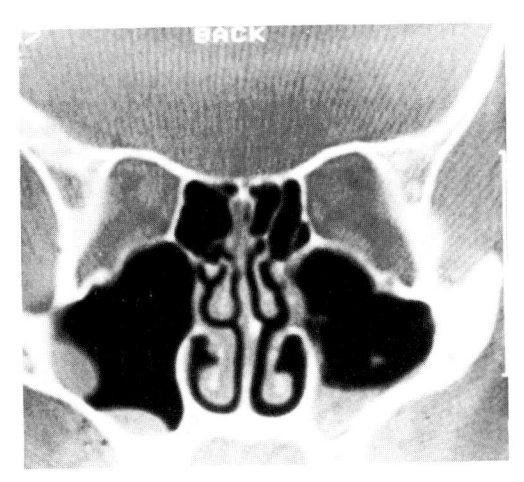

Rhinologic Causes of Facial Pain

FIGURE 5–11. Computed tomogram, coronal section, of the nose and paranasal sinuses, demonstrating mucosal polyps of the floor of the right maxillary sinus and an air-fluid level in the left maxillary sinus.

although cocaine abuse and Wegener's granulomatosis can cause this as well. Orbital and intracranial invasion can be delineated by CT. Sphenoid disease is very difficult to ascertain without CT.

Magnetic resonance imaging (MRI) is a new modality that is rapidly assuming importance in head and neck imaging. Although bone is not visualized, MRI allows very good delineation of soft tissue changes. The brain is especially well seen, and small lesions, such as those due to multiple sclerosis, are evident. At present it complements but does not replace CT, since the bony confines of the nose and sinuses are not seen on MRI.

Other radiographic studies that may be required are chest x-rays or CT if the pulmonary changes of sarcoidosis or Wegener's granulomatosis are being considered. Contrast cine-esophagography is indicated in pharyngo-esophageal disease, as might occur with neoplasia or rhinoscleroma. Angiography is utilized in searching for a cause of hemorrhage or vascular occlusion.

Other studies include culture of nasal discharge for aerobic bacteria, anaerobic bacteria, mycobacteria on Ziehl-Neelsen stain, and fungi. Syphilitic gummas should be examined with dark-field microscopy. A tissue

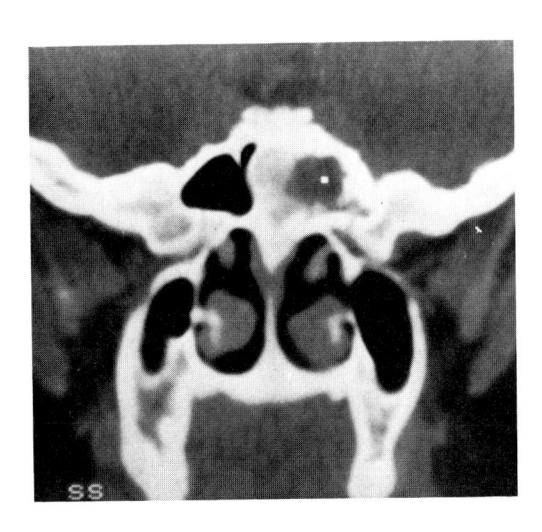

FIGURE 5–12. Coronal computed tomogram of the paranasal sinuses with attention to the sphenoid bone. There is a combined sclerotic and lytic lesion of the left sphenoid sinus. Exploration of the sinus revealed fibrous dysplasia.

biopsy specimen for histologic examination and culture may also be indicated. Special immunohistologic stains may be required in cases of pemphigus or tumor. Blood studies including a complete blood count with differential may reveal leukemia. The serum calcium level may be elevated in sarcoidosis. A serologic test for syphilis is also important.

Treatment

Treatment options for rhinologic sources of pain vary with the etiology. This fact emphasizes the need for a definitive diagnosis of nasal pain.

Infectious processes can be treated with the appropriate antimicrobial agent. Fungal infections in the immunocompetent individual usually respond to aeration of the affected sinus and surgical debridément. In immunocompromised patients, pharmacologic therapy as well as aggressive surgical intervention is usually required, although the prognosis is grim unless the immunocompromised state is improved. Both acute and chronic bacterial sinusitis usually respond well to systemic antibiotics based on the most likely pathogens. Intranasal culture is notoriously unreliable. When life-threatening complications develop or are impending, specimens obtained directly from an infected sinus are crucial. Irrigation and lavage of a chronically infected maxillary sinus may be of value if medical therapy fails.

Frontal sinusitis can be particularly serious because of the possibility of intracranial complication. Because the posterior wall of the sinus has a large interface with the dura overlying the frontal lobes, the extension of bacterial infections by way of a septic thrombophlebitis is a distinct possibility (Fig. 5–13). Such an extension can lead to meningitis, brain abscess, epidural abscess, subdural empyema, or cavernous sinus thrombosis. For this reason acute frontal sinusitis often requires aggressive management with intravenous antibiotics and topical application of vasoconstrictors to the middle meatus of the ipsilateral side of the nose. If clinical improvement is not noted within 24 to 48 hours, frontal sinusotomy should be considered.

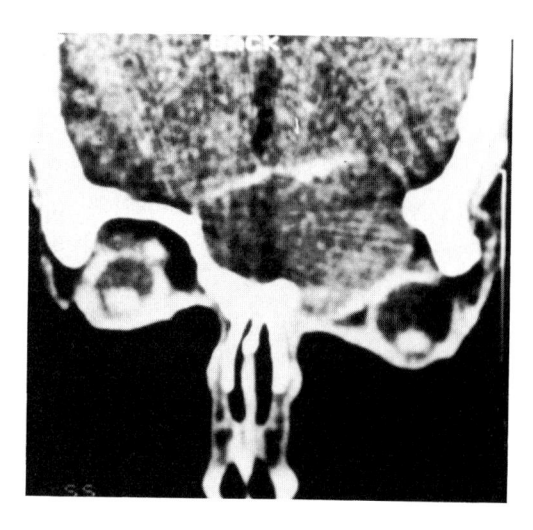

FIGURE 5–13. Computed tomogram, coronal section, of the anterior skull and orbits. There is intracranial extension of a left frontal sinus mucocele with destruction of the bone of the posterior table of the sinus so that the dura is in contact with the mucocele. There is downward and outward displacement of the left globe.

When medical therapy for chronic sinusitis fails to alleviate symptoms, surgical treatment of the affected sinus or sinuses is appropriate. This may be performed either externally or transnasally. The goal is to remove irreversibly altered mucous membrane and bone while achieving ventilation and drainage of the sinus contents. Chronic frontal sinusitis is usually dealt with in a different manner. Because attempts to create a large opening between the nasal cavity and the frontal sinus lumen often result in stenosis of the communication, frontal sinus obliteration is preferred by many surgeons. The diseased epithelium is completely removed from the sinus wall, and the lumen is obliterated with fat harvested from abdominal subcutaneous tissue.

Rhinitis medicamentosa usually responds well to abstinence from the offending nasal spray or drops coupled with a topical corticosteroid spray for 2 weeks.

Allergic rhinitis is treated conservatively with antihistamines, systemic decongestants, and topical corticosteroid spray. Cromalyn sodium spray, which prevents mediator release from mast cells and basophils, may also be of value. Immunotherapy using injections of increasing dosage of antigen is also used when specific allergens can be identified.

Wegener's granulomatosis can be a life-threatening disorder if not diagnosed. The disease activity can be held in check by chronic administration of systemic corticosteroids and cyclophosphamide. Most cases resolve spontaneously after several years, and the drugs can then be stopped.

Sarcoidosis involving the nose requires frequent debridément and antibiotic treatment if secondary infection supervenes. Topical corticosteroid spray can be of value.

The dry mucosa of Sjögren's syndrome may benefit from topical saline nasal drops and room humidification.

Nasal neoplasms are usually treated surgically. Inverted papillomas usually require a medial maxillectomy approach to completely eradicate the disease. Malignancies of the nasal dorsum may be excised locally and reconstructed with local tissue advancement or facial flaps. Mucosal malignancies often require extensive resection of the bony skeleton of the midface, and on occasion require sacrifice of the orbital contents or floor of the anterior cranial fossa. Most intranasal malignancies are also treated with postoperative radiation therapy.

Nasal cysts are treated surgically. Fibrous dysplasia is also approached surgically if it is symptomatic.

Pain developing after nasal trauma can be extremely frustrating. If there is displacement of the skeletal framework, reduction of the fracture or fractures is indicated. If bony healing has already taken place (usually after 4 to 6 weeks), osteotomy may be required to reposition the displaced structures. Nasal discomfort associated with a severely deformed nasal septum may respond to septoplasty, with the admonition to the patient that the procedure may not be curative.

Sluder's syndrome is said to respond to topical cocaine application to the region of the sphenopalatine foramen (mucosa of the lateral wall of the nose just posterior to the terminus of the middle turbinate). Sphenopalatine ganglioneurectomy may also be considered.[10] Other neuralgias may be effectively treated with phenytoin or carbamazepine.

Atrophic rhinitis is particularly frustrating to treat. This condition may occur after overly aggressive nasal surgery, such as total inferior turbinectomy. In these instances, prevention is the key to treatment. Treatment options include identification of any bacterial pathogens and appropriate antimicrobial therapy. Surgical procedures to narrow the nasal lumen with submucosal bone chips or surgical closure of the anterior nares are infrequently utilized. Prevention of intranasal drying with topical saline and emollients is also useful.

Summary

Nasal and paranasal sinus pain may be of varied origin. It constitutes a large segment of facial pain syndromes. Many patients are already convinced before seeing a physician that their facial or head pain is of sinonasal origin. A thorough understanding of the various pathologic processes that give rise to pain in this region is essential in making the diagnosis and initiating the appropriate treatment.

References

1. Schaeffer, J. P. Morris' Human Anatomy, 10th ed. Philadelphia, Blakeston Co., 1942, pp. 1380–1381.
2. Moss-Salentign, L. Anatomy and embryology. In Blitzer, A., Lawson, W., and Friedman, W. H. (eds.). Surgery of the Paranasal Sinuses. Philadelphia, W. B. Saunders Co., 1985, pp. 18–20.
3. English, G. M. Sinusitis. In English, G. M. (ed.). Otolaryngology, Vol. 2. Philadelphia, Harper & Row, 1987, Chap. 21, p. 9.
4. Stevens, M. H. Primary fungal infections of the paranasal sinuses. Am J Otolaryngol 2:348–357, 1981.
5. Hyams, V. J. Pathology of the nose and paranasal sinuses. In English, G. M. (ed.). Otolaryngology, Vol. 2. Philadelphia, Harper & Row, 1987, Chap. 8, pp. 17–18.
6. Batsakis, J. G. and Sciubba, J. J. Pathology. In Blitzer, A., Lawson, W., and Friedman, W. H. (eds.). Surgery of the Paranasal Sinuses. Philadelphia, W. B. Saunders Co., 1985, p. 79.
7. Granstrom, G., Aldenbory, F. and Jeppsson, P. Influence of embryonal fusion lines for recurrence of basal cell carcinoma of the head and neck. Otolaryngol Head Neck Surg 95:76–82, 1986.
8. Hinderer, K. H. Fundamentals of Anatomy and Surgery of the Nose. Birmingham, Ala, Aesculapius, 1971, p 39.
9. Sluder, G. Etiology, diagnosis, prognosis and treatment of sphenopalatine ganglion neuralgia. JAMA 61:1201–1206, 1913.
10. Kimmelman, C. P., and Ali, G. H. A. Vasomotor rhinitis. Otolaryngol Clin North Am 19:65–71, 1986.
11. Cepero, R., Miller, R. H., and Bressler, K. L. Long-term results of sphenopalatine ganglioneurectomy for facial pain. Am J Otolaryngol 8:171–174, 1987.

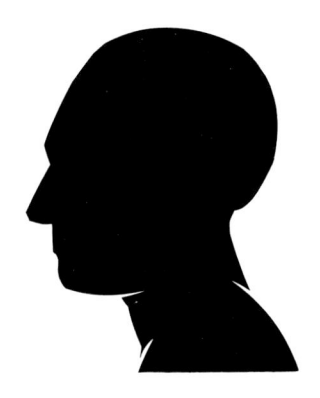

Chapter 6
Intraoral Pain

Barry C. Cooper

Patients frequently complain of oral or facial pain caused by defects in their teeth or the tissues that support the teeth. The patient may be able to localize the source of pain to a specific tooth or teeth or may feel discomfort originating in a generalized area of the oral cavity. Sometimes the pain radiates from a dental structure to adjacent areas. At other times, patients complain of diffuse pain or discomfort in the cheek, side of the jaw, angle of the mandible, ear, or throat. Such diffuse pain may make isolation of the etiologic agent and diagnosis difficult or impossible.[1] The physician may be called upon to make a primary diagnosis or may be asked to rule out pathology in the nondental tissues of the face in cases of diffuse facial pain. If the pain is clearly localized in the dental apparatus, the dentist is the health care practitioner usually called upon by the patient to make a diagnosis and render treatment. In this chapter a description of the various causes of intraoral pain will be presented. For the medical reader, the chapter will provide a brief overview of intraoral pain and a description of the causes, clinical signs, history, and treatment of various pathologic conditions that affect the dentition and surrounding oral tissues.

The information in this chapter, together with that found in Chapter 8, provides the basis for making a differential diagnosis between facial pain of dental origin, pain associated with the functioning of the mandible, and pain originating in other structures in the head and neck that is discussed in other chapters in this book.

Craniomandibular disorders can result in abnormalities of the teeth and their supporting structures. The reverse is also true in that diseases that result in loss of tooth structure or changes in tooth position can affect the functioning of the mandible and its associated muscles and temporomandibular joints.

More complete knowledge of the functional interrelationships between the various structures in the head and neck will lead to a better understanding of the causes of pain in this area.

Causes of intraoral pain include dental and nondental (soft and hard tissue) problems.

Dental Problems

Symptoms

Symptoms associated with dental intraoral disease include sensitivity to temperature (hot or cold), percussion (biting), and chemicals (sweets) as well as spontaneous pain. The pain can be felt in a single tooth, in multiple teeth, or in a diffuse area emanating from the teeth or including the teeth.[2]

Patients may report pain in both maxillary and mandibular teeth, especially when the source of dental pain is in the most posterior teeth. Pain from erupting mandibular molars may produce areas of discomfort adjacent to the teeth, such as the throat, side of the face, or ear. Careful examination of these areas may be necessary to rule out primary pathology or coincident pathology. It should be pointed out that cardiac pain sometimes produces pain in the mandible.[3]

When a single tooth is the cause of pain, the patient can usually localize the tooth, although in the early stages of pulpal inflammation this is not always possible.[4] The various stages of pulpal disease present with different symptoms. The dental pulp contains nerve fibers and a complete circulatory system. Mechanical, chemical, or thermal trauma and infection elicit an inflammatory response, which causes pain in the tooth. Pain is the only sensation that can be transmitted by pulpal nerve fibers.

Periodontal or gingival abnormalities often present as diffuse pain in a quadrant of the mouth or in multiple quadrants rather than as pain in a specific tooth.

Causes

Dental problems that may cause intraoral pain include caries (tooth decay), pulpal and periapical pathology, periodontal disease, impacted teeth, dental cysts, erupting or exfoliating teeth, retained roots, impacted food, faulty dental restorations, fractured teeth, traumatic occlusion, neoplastic processes, and postoperative pain.[5]

Despite the widespread use of fluoride in recent years, dental caries continues to be a major source of dental pain in the middle-aged and elderly populations as well as in some younger individuals.[6,8] Dental caries has been largely controlled in younger individuals who have been exposed to its benefits during the years of tooth formation,[9,10] although notable exceptions include children with a genetic or developmental predisposition to caries and those who have been exposed to excessive cariogenic agents throughout their childhood.[11, 12] Caries beneath existing dental restorations is frequently a source of dental pain.[13]

Fractures of the teeth or breakage of dental restorations within the teeth may also cause pain. Mechanical, chemical, and thermal trauma may likewise cause dental pain. The reaction of the vital pulp tissues to any trauma is inflammation.[14] That inflammatory response hyperactivates the normal sensitivities of the pulp. The tooth will at first be sensitive to mechanical and thermal stimuli, both hot and cold. Prolonged or excessive inflammation within the tooth's rigid pulp canal of the root may result in strangulation of the pulpal tissues. With pulpal necrosis, extreme sensitivity to heat and pressure, which is sometimes relieved by the application of cold, is observed. This reaction reflects the accumulation of liquids and gases beneath the root of the tooth in a bony confinement. It is a pathognomonic sign of pulp death. Sustained hyperemia in the dental pulp may be reversible or irreversible. In the reversible stage, pain caused by hyperemia is associated with stimulus and is not spontaneous. In the irreversible stage, pain may be spontaneous.

Teeth may become nonvital with or without bacterial involvement. Trauma that does not cause breakage of the tooth's integrity may result in pulp hyperemia, which can, if sufficiently intense or prolonged, result in pulp death. The specific symptoms, changes in symptom patterns, and history of circumstances accompanying the onset of symptoms are of great importance in making a diagnosis.

Periodontal pain may be either isolated around a single tooth or widespread. It is caused by inflammation in the tissues surrounding the teeth. That inflammation is caused by accumulation of foreign matter including food, bacterial plaque, and calculus (calcified plaque).[15] Food debris not removed, together with the normal oral bacterial flora, moisture, and warmth, create a perfect environment for bacterial replication, resulting in a periodontal inflammation and infection.[16] With swelling, the area of infection is often isolated, and a periodontal abscess results.[17] If it proceeds apically, it may destroy the nerve supply of the tooth or teeth, and a periapical abscess results with devitalization of the tooth or teeth.[18-22] The teeth involved become exceedingly sensitive to even the slightest touch and may feel elongated as they are extruded from their bony sockets. Mobility of the teeth is also often observed as teeth are raised out of their sockets by the accumulated liquid or gases beneath.[23] This is often accompanied by facial swelling.

Dental treatment may also result in pulpal hyperemia. The injection of local anesthetics in the tissues around the teeth may cause localized sensitivity. Actual dental procedures involving use of a dental drill,[24] chemical agents, and restorative materials[25] can sensitize teeth. If not excessive, the pulpal reaction is usually reversible. Changes in occlusal relationships following dental restorative procedures due to modifications in the dental anatomy may result in pulpal irritation and hypersensitivity, with dental pain and irritation of the periodontal supporting tissues.[26]

Occlusal changes created by restorative dentistry may also precipitate craniomandibular disorders.[27] This subject is discussed in Chapter 8.

Impacted teeth are prevented from erupting fully into the oral cavity by contact with an adjacent tooth or, in the case of the mandibular third molars (wisdom teeth), insufficient room distal to the tooth in the mouth for complete eruption. In some cases the most posterior portion of the crown of such a tooth is covered with the soft tissue that covers the ascending ramus. The erupting or unerupted tooth can cause pressure within the alveolar bone and soft tissue, producing intraoral pain.[28] A partially erupted tooth causes inflammation in the gingiva as it breaks through the soft tissue. This is also frequently accompanied by local inflammation in the tissue due to food impaction and a substantial bacterial presence. This condition is known as pericoronitis.[29] Exfoliating deciduous (primary) teeth can be a source of oral pain.[28] In the initial stages of primary tooth loss, there is movement of the tooth as it comes into contact with its antagonist in the opposite arch. In the later stages, when the tooth is almost lost, even the tongue can move the tooth, since it no longer has root substance to retain it firmly in bone. Finally, it is only held by the gingiva, from which it gradually detaches. The undersurface of the exfoliating tooth may be extremely sharp as a result of the dissolution of the root structure. It is this sharp edge of the tooth separating from its gingival attachment that causes the pain reported by children losing a primary tooth.

History

A thorough patient history often offers a clue to the cause of dental pain. It is important to note the onset of the pain relative to recent trauma to the teeth or face, whether pain is subtle or overt, and its relation to recent dental procedures. The history should include the factor(s) that precipitates the pain, the nature (severity, quality) and duration of the pain, and what ameliorates or exacerbates the pain.[30]

Trauma to teeth can result from a severe blow to the face, as in accidents involving direct facial contact.[31] Indirectly, the teeth may be traumatized by a cervical whiplash injury resulting from automobile accidents. In this case the head is abruptly thrust backward and then forward, with the mandible likewise being jolted.[32] This combination of whiplash and jawlash will be discussed further in the section dealing with temporomandibular joint dysfunction in Chapter 8. In the abrupt jarring of the head and jaw, the mandibular and maxillary teeth may be instantly forced into traumatic contact. Subtle traumatic insults to the teeth may also initiate hyperemia in the pulp, producing pain.[26, 27] Such insults may arise from an unintentional bang of a coffee cup against the anterior teeth or an unguarded bite against a fork. They may also result from the chronic trauma present in a patient who frequently clenches or grinds the teeth while asleep or awake, a condition called *bruxism*. Premature points of contact between the upper and lower teeth in entering the dental occlusal position (prematurities) may likewise cause pulpal irritation and dental pain. Both bruxism and occlusal prematurities may also cause muscle hyperactivity, as discussed in Chapter 8.

Dental procedures can traumatize teeth. Teeth being restored can be pulpally irritated by the debridément of decay with a drill or hand instruments.[24] The pulp of the tooth may be irritated or even invaded in this essential process. The pulp may also be invaded by the decay process itself. Teeth that are antagonistic to a newly restored tooth or the restored tooth itself may be traumatized if the occlusion or bite is excessive vertically or produces lateral interferences during normal functional contacts between upper and lower teeth. If teeth that have been recently restored or those adjacent or antagonist to recently restored teeth are painful, traumatic occlusion should be considered as well as pulpal involvement from the caries or restorative procedures.

If teeth are thermally sensitive to both hot and cold, pulpal vitality should be expected.[33] If there is a history of hot and cold sensitivity, with a current heat sensitivity that is relieved by cold, the pulpal tissues are probably necrotic. Liquids and gases expand with heat and contract with cold; hence pain is precipitated by the application of heat and is ameliorated by cold. If teeth become painful during eating, suspect either a broken dental restoration, a fractured tooth, or food impaction as the cause of the pain.[34]

A history of pain in the posterior portion of the mandibular dental arch in a patient aged approximately 18 to 25, with repeated episodes possibly accompanied by discomfort in the angle of the mandible and throat, should suggest third molar eruption or impaction.

A history of frequent episodes of pain (often posture-dependent) in or above healthy maxillary posterior teeth in a patient with a history of sinus problems should suggest maxillary sinusitis.[35] The maxillary sinus lies immediately above the bicuspid and molar roots and often drapes around these roots.[36] The history is important here for the examining physician, who must determine whether to treat the patient, refer him to an otolaryngologist or dentist, or have sinus radiographs taken.[37] The history is also important to a dentist, who may be the primary examiner and after both clinical and radiographic examination, may have found no evidence of tooth pathology or defective dental restoration.[38]

Teeth that are sensitive to sweets or artificial sweeteners most often have defective restorations. It should be noted that a superficial layer of carious dentin and enamel can act as an insulator to thermal sensitivity in a vital tooth. In contrast, a decay-free restored tooth with an incomplete peripheral seal of the restoration will react painfully to sweets and to thermal stimulation. Thermal and chemical stimuli are transmitted through the dentinal tubules to the pulp tissue.

Clinical Examination

Although a detailed clinical examination for dental pathology in the oral cavity lies within the realm of the dentist and oral surgeon, examination of this area should be a part of every evaluation of pain when an intraoral disease is suspected.[39] The examining physician should be familiar with the normal anatomy of the dentition. In looking for abnormalities, similar teeth on both sides of the dental arch should be observed. Missing portions of teeth should be visible, as should overt decay. Decay (caries) appears either as a dark substance within the tooth or a chalky surface.[8] Missing restorations or large portions of restorations may also be obvious. Fractures in teeth will not be obvious unless they permit movement of significant portions of a tooth or teeth on digital examination.[34] Fractures may also be visualized utilizing transillumination. The ability to produce visible movement of teeth by the examiner signifies an abnormality in, around, or beneath a tooth.[23] Soft tissue examination around the teeth is valuable in this regard and will be discussed shortly.

Further Diagnostic Measures

Evaluation of dental abnormalities does not stop with the clinical examination.[5] Dental radiographs are performed routinely, but many other tests play a role in assessing the status of the dental apparatus. Dental radiographs show caries,[13] the status of dental restorations, loss of bone support around the teeth, periapical pathology if it has existed long enough to have produced hypocalcification of the periapical bone,[40] cystic lesions, fractures in teeth if the plane is not parallel to the film, and impactions or retained root fragments. Dental radiographs are two-dimensional and as such do not fully demonstrate all of the tooth's form.

Electrical testing of pulp vitality is utilized to compare a symptomatic tooth with its neighbors.[33] A relative measurement of reactivity to electrical stimuli is made as an adjunct to the diagnosis of pulp hyperacruity or nonvitality. Vitality testing may not be valid in the post-trauma setting. Thermal testing is also utilized to diagnose the status of the dental pulp. Hot materials are applied to individual teeth, as are chilled substances, such as ice or ethyl chloride on a cotton roll. Asymptomatic teeth are always stimulated as controls. Healthy teeth are sensitive to thermal stimuli, both hot and cold. The sensitivity is mild and momentary, usually lasting only as long as the thermal stimulus is applied. Severe sensitivity and sensitivity that lingers long after the stimulus is removed are signs of pulp hypersensitivity.

Percussion of sensitive teeth with a rigid instrument, such as the end of the handle of a dental mirror, is utilized to localize which tooth is the painful one and to determine whether a tooth is indeed the cause of the pain. Pain on percussion indicates that the pulpal inflammation has proceeded into the periapical tissues.[41, 42] Palpation along the gingiva in the region of the root of the suspected tooth may elicit pain due to either periapical or a periodontal pathologic lesion.

Biting can be used to localize tooth sensitivity as well. A soft wooden block or cotton roll is placed between a maxillary and a mandibular tooth, and the patient is instructed to bite together firmly. Pain is an indication of pulpal disease. Pain on release of biting pressure often indicates a fracture.[34] Once again, similar biting on neighboring asymptomatic teeth is utilized as a control, since their reaction will be less painful.

Finally, exploratory examination into a tooth may be necessary to determine the status of the dental pulp if other noninvasive diagnostic means are inconclusive. Even radiographic examination of teeth sometimes fails to show caries beneath large restorations, which, in the case of metallic fillings and crowns, block the x-ray beam. The danger here is that in the process of removing and excavating an old restoration a vital pulp may be uncovered and injured. That excavation may be harmful to the pulp if it initiates an inflammatory reaction.[24] As stated before, the inflammatory response may cause pulp strangulation and lead to necrosis. Therefore, great care must be exercised in performing exploratory excavation of carious lesions in the teeth and exploratory removal of old restorations. Sometimes the presence of extensive metal restorations on or in teeth limits the value of radiographic analysis. Likewise, extensive restorations make explorative procedures difficult and sometimes costly because restorations must be disturbed or destroyed in the process. Obviously, invasive procedures are the last diagnostic modalities to be employed.

Treatment

The most conservative treatment for a tooth that has been traumatized without damage to the hard tooth structure is rest. If occlusion against an antagonist tooth aggravates the sensitive tooth, judicious removal of tooth structure is performed to eliminate the occlusal contact temporarily. Natural eruption of the tooth will follow, and occlusion will naturally be restored in a matter of days if the amount of enamel removed was minimal.

If a tooth or teeth have been loosened by a traumatic injury or have been moved out of place, they are carefully set manually in their proper place in the dental arch, their position is verified by having the patient occlude the upper and lower teeth, and the teeth are stabilized by splinting to adjacent firm teeth.[43] This procedure can be done with various materials. The recent advances in bonding to tooth structure enable the dentist to join teeth together securely and for long periods of time. This process enables teeth to become secured in bone. Occlusion or biting contacts are relieved as described above.[40]

A severely traumatized tooth is a tooth that has been forcibly evulsed from the alveolar bone.[45] If the tooth is reimplanted quickly and stabilized by fixation to adjacent teeth, it has a good chance of remaining functional in the future.[46] The tooth must be maintained in a moist environment and must be gently cleaned without much debridément prior to reimplantation. It may become devitalized soon after the trauma or in the future, and therefore endodonture (root canal therapy) should be instituted within 2 weeks. Patients must be made aware of this possibility as well as the more serious possibility of failure of reimplantation and resorption of root structure.

Fractured teeth can be restored if the fracture does not extend below the margin of the attached gingiva (just below the junction of the enamel-covered coronal portion of the tooth and the root). The fractured portion can be removed and the remainder of the tooth restored. Fractures that extend below that junction prohibit successful restoration, since gingival attachment is essential to long-term periodontal health of the tooth.[47] Without such an attachment, future local irritation of the periodontal attachment apparatus may lead to loss of attachment essential to the longevity of the tooth in the alveolar bone. If the fracture extends to the pulpal tissue or if the trauma that produced the fracture severely irritates the pulp, the pulp may undergo necrosis. Successful endodontic therapy requires perfect isolation of the pulp chamber from the oral environment as well as from the periodontal environment.[48]

A vertical fracture down the root makes endodontic treatment impossible and extraction necessary. A fracture of a coronal tooth that does not extend below the gingival epithelial attachment can be successfully restored even if the entire coronal portion of the tooth is lost. Removal of the pulp tissue may be necessary if the pulp has been injured and becomes devitalized. Removal of a vital pulp may be necessary for proper restoration. Techniques for restorative dentistry utilizing reinforcing screws, cast gold, or preformed posts and bonding together with traditional restoration using crowns, inlays, and onlays permit major portions of teeth to be restored successfully, re-establishing normal function and esthetic appearance.

Teeth that have become painful due to decay or defective restorations are also restored as described above. After carious material or old defective restorations are removed, suitable sedative materials are placed to calm an aggravated pulp and insulate the pulp from thermal stimulation. A variety of materials are currently utilized.[25, 50] They include some that have eugenol as an anodyne, others with calcium hydroxide, which stimulates dentinoblastic activity in the pulp to create additional insulation, and the newest glass ionomer cements, which permit bonding of composite restorative materials for maximum sealing between restoration and tooth. This material also releases fluoride into the tooth, which reduces sensitivity.

Treatment for the dentition in which a tooth or teeth cannot be restored and must be extracted involves the use of either removable or fixed (attached) restorations.[49] Removable dentures are either complete or partial. Complete dentures replace all of the functioning teeth within a dental arch. Removable partial dentures replace only those teeth that are missing. Fixed bridges are of many types. Most attach to at least two stationary objects, referred to as *abutments*, which may be natural teeth or metallic objects implanted into the alveolar bone. When natural teeth are utilized as abutments, they are attached to the artificial replacement teeth by crowning or covering the abutment completely or partially or merely by being bonded to the replacement teeth.

If impacted teeth are the cause of dental pain, they can be extracted. Some impacted teeth are surgically exposed and then orthodontically brought into the dental arch.[29] Sometimes the impacted tooth cannot be extracted because it is inaccessible. In that case, an adjacent tooth may be sacrificed and the impacted one allowed to erupt normally. This eruption may be aided by orthodontic treatment.

Periodontally caused dental pain is treated first by debridément of the unhealthy material and soft tissue within the periodontal space surrounding the tooth or teeth.[51] This material includes food debris, plaque, calculus, and necrotic tissue. Sometimes surgery must be performed to change the bony and soft tissue architecture of the tissues that surround and support the teeth to establish healthy maintainable tissues.

If periapical disease is the cause of dental pain, it must be resolved.[41] Endodontic therapy has a high success rate in resolving periapical disease.[52] If the periapical area has become cystic or if endodontic treatment is impossible because of inaccessibility or calcification of the pulp canals, surgical intervention may be necessary.[53, 54] An apicoectomy, involving removal of the tip of the root, can sometimes be performed to remove the cyst or debride the periapical area. Extraction of the affected tooth is another means by which the diseased root canal system can be removed.

Surgical intervention may also be necessary if a retained root from a previous extraction or exfoliation of a deciduous tooth becomes an active cause of pathology within the alveolar bone.[29, 55] Although not common, foreign substances within the alveolar bone can be a cause of pain. Pieces of restorative material (e.g., amalgam),[56] portions of endodontic instruments, and objects implanted in the gingiva[57] and alveolar bone that have been introduced into the mouth by the patient may ultimately cause irritation and possibly infection with pain as the presenting symptom.[51] These objects must be surgically removed.

Foreign substances, the most common of which are food and calculus, when present in the gingival tissues may be a cause of pain in the oral cavity. The treatment is obviously removal of the substance. Proper oral hygiene measures by the patient should prevent reoccurrence. Pericoronitis found in the mandibular molar area associated with erupting teeth is treated first by removing the foreign substances under the operculum and by utilizing warm saline washes every 2 to 3 hours until the discomfort is relieved; oral antibiotics are used if infection is suspected. If the pericoronitis is repeated frequently, and the tooth that is erupting is the third molar, extraction is often done, especially if the tooth has no restorative value. If the second molar is present and is in no imminent danger of being lost, the third molar has no restorative value, since it would not be required as a posterior abutment for a removable or fixed restorative appliance.

Prognosis

The prognosis for painful teeth is good if the teeth are firmly supported by the alveolar bone and surrounded by healthy periodontium. Pulpal tissues traumatized by mechanical, chemical, or thermal irritants have a questionable prognosis depending on the severity of the inflammatory response within the hard tooth pulpal canal.[14] If the pulp becomes necrotic, endodontic therapy is usually performed and has a very high degree of success.[52] Sometimes surgical intervention in debriding the periapical area is combined with endodontic treatment.[54] With the variety of sophisticated restorative techniques and materials now available, severely broken-down teeth can be restored to proper function and esthetic appearance.[50] The prognosis for teeth with severely compromised bony and periodontal support is quite guarded.[23] Teeth that are traumatically evulsed have a guarded prognosis even with prompt and effective reimplantation and stabilization techniques.[43] Finally, a tooth that is fractured vertically on its long axis has a hopeless prognosis and must be extracted.[33, 47]

Soft and Hard Tissue Diseases

This section will not include a discussion of the bony supporting structure or the gingiva and periodontium surrounding the teeth because they have been discussed above. It will include the palate, tongue, floor of the mouth, and inner mucosa of the oral cavity as well as the maxilla and mandible.[58] Discussion of the mandible will not include the posterosuperior termination of the mandible, the condyle, which is covered in Chapter 8.

Symptoms

Diseases of the soft and hard tissues of the oral cavity may present symptoms of pain, burning,[59] numbness, chemical sensitivity, thermal sensitivity, and fullness or swelling and pressure.[1, 30, 60, 61]

Causes

Discomfort in the soft and hard tissues may be caused by trauma within the oral cavity. Trauma may be a major insult involving a significant foreign body entering the mouth as in a gunshot wound. It may also be a minor common injury, in which a food substance, pencil, or other small object penetrates or traumatizes the oral mocusa on the inner cheek, floor of the mouth, or palate.[51, 57] Hard and soft tissue pain may also accompany abnormalities in the tissues of the oral cavity.[62] These abnormalities include inflammatory, infective, neoplastic, endocrine, connective tissue, developmental, and nutritional disorders.[63, 64]

Infectious processes within the soft tissues may include aphthous ulcers, herpetic or syphilitic lesions, major aphthous stomatitis, and acute necrotizing ulcerative gingivitis (ANUG or Vincent's infection).[55, 62]

History

A careful history must be taken. It should include inquiries about conditions accompanying the onset of symptoms. An attempt to isolate the etiologic agent or agents should be made based on this information.[60] Changes in the symptoms as well as exacerbating and ameliorating agents should be noted.[1] A general health history should also be elicited because there are numerous systemic conditions that manifest in the oral cavity.[65–68]

Clinical Examination

A clinical examination of the oral cavity should be performed in an orderly manner and repeated in the same sequence for all patients to ensure thoroughness. The examination should begin with an extraoral inspection and palpation of the entire head and neck complex.[69]

A visual and manual examination of the cheeks should be performed, looking for indications of inflammation, swelling, induration, ulceration, and any lesions that alter or interrupt the normal continuity and constitution of the buccal mucosa and the muscles and parotid glands that lie beneath.[70] The cheeks are followed from one side of the mouth upward to the deepest fold where the buccal mucosa reflects and becomes the gingiva and downward to the lower gingiva. After viewing that side of the mouth, the upper lip is raised to allow examination of the vermilion border, the inner aspect of the lip, the labiogingival fold, and the gingiva. The same maneuver is done with the lower lip. The opposite side of the mouth is viewed in a similar manner. Close attention should be paid to bilateral symmetry.

The palate is now examined, again observing unusual alterations in the normal color, texture, and architecture of this region.[71] Examination can proceed as far into the oropharynx as one's skills and optic instruments permit. A more detailed description of this area can be found in Chapter 7.

The tongue and floor of the mouth are examined by grasping the tip of the tongue with a dry gauze pad and moving the tongue out of the mouth and toward one corner of the mouth and then the other to obtain a good view of the lateral borders of the tongue. The floor of the mouth should be carefully viewed as well. These areas are common locations for neoplastic lesions, which should not be confused with traumatic injuries, which are frequently found here as well. The gingival tissues on the outer and inner aspects of the dental arches should be observed for swelling and indications of infection and foreign objects. It is at this time that the teeth are examined as described earlier in this chapter. Teeth out of normal position in the dental arch in a patient complaining of pain in that area should alert the examiner. The possibilities of an infective process beneath the tooth in the gingiva should be investigated. An erupting tooth below the tooth being moved may also be considered. The history and age of the patient are important. A developmental cyst or neoplastic lesion may also forcibly displace a tooth or teeth from its normal position in the alveolar bone.[63]

Further Diagnostic Measures

If infection is considered in the periodontal (around the tooth) or periapical (above or below the root ends) area, a dental radiograph should be taken.[5]

This can be a routine periapical radiograph or a panoramic x-ray of the entire dentition. If more extensive bony pathology is considered, more complex imaging modalities should be employed. Such modalities include computed axial tomography (CT scan) and magnetic resonance imaging (MRI). Other single-plane radiographic imaging modalities are also employed, although the CT scan and MRI are considered the most efficacious.

Bacterial cultures are utilized when infection is suspected.[72] Incisional or exisional biopsy is performed if soft tissue and possibly hard tissue pathologic lesions that are not infective are being considered. Exploratory surgery may be employed to assist in making a diagnosis if all noninvasive techniques fail to make a diagnosis and pain continues.

It is important to note here that sometimes patients report areas of pain in the oral cavity either in the teeth or the soft or hard tissues for which no physical cause is discernible in the mouth.[1, 60, 61, 73, 74] No invasive procedure should be undertaken until *all* conservative diagnostic means have been employed.[75, 76] Sometimes consultation with other health care providers is necessary.[39] Various physical and psychological disorders may produce the perception of pain in the oral tissues when its causes do not lie in the oral cavity.[30, 64, 77, 78] Recall the admonition of Hippocrates: "above all else, do no harm."

Treatment

Treatment for the various pathologic conditions of the soft and hard tissues is as diverse as the conditions themselves. If localized irritants are the cause of an inflammatory or infective tissue response, the etiologic agent is removed and appropriate antibiotics are prescribed, together with palliative measures.[79] These measures include saline rinses, application of topical anesthetics, and oral analgesics. Some infections require surgical excision.[16, 17]

In the case of periapical disease, endodontic treatment is initially performed through the tooth's root canal. If that therapy does not eliminate the infection beneath the root, surgical entry is made through the alveolar bone, and the root tip is removed by apicoectomy; this is followed by placement of an amalgam restoration at the end of the root after the area of infection has been debrided.[53]

Periodontal surgery is sometimes necessary to remove hyperemic or hypertrophic gingival tissue and recontour alveolar bone to establish healthy, hygienic periodontal tissues.

Cystic lesions within the maxilla and mandible may be developmental. They are removed surgically if they are expanding and exerting pressure on teeth. Cysts occur around developing and impacted teeth such as third molars. They also occur in developmental suture lines between the maxillary central incisors and between the maxillary cuspids and lateral incisors.[80, 81]

Inflammatory soft tissue lesions such as pemphigus vulgaris are treated with systemic or local medications.[82–84] Neoplastic lesions within the soft and hard tissues may be treated surgically or by chemotherapy and radiation.

Traumatic injury to the maxilla and mandible involving fracture of the bone requires intervention including fixation to reduce the fracture and stabilize the segments.[31, 45]

Prognosis

The prognosis for pathology in the soft and hard tissues of the oral cavity is as diverse as the variety of pathologic conditions found there. Surgical intervention for the treatment of periodontal pathologic lesions may or may not produce long-term control, depending on the severity of loss of the supportive bone and the quality of oral hygiene maintained by the patient. Treatment of periapical pathology by endodontic therapy with or without surgical entry into the apical area (apicoectomy) has an excellent prognosis.[54] Reduction of fractures in the maxilla and mandible likewise has a favorable prognosis.

Pharmacologic management of chronic inflammatory lesions in the oral cavity has a variable prognosis. Sometimes control is achieved with comfort rather than elimination of disease. The treatment of pemphigus vulgaris with corticosteroids is an example of this. Treatment of neoplastic disease has a variable prognosis depending on the type of neoplasm, its severity, and the reaction of the patient to therapy.[85]

References

1. Kreisberg, M. K. Atypical odontalgia: Differential diagnosis and treatment. J Am Dent Assoc 104:852, 1982.
2. Glick, D. H. Locating referred pulpal pains. Oral Surg 15:613, 1962.
3. Matson, M. S. Pain in orofacial region associated with coronary insufficiency. Oral Surg 16:284, 1963.
4. Mitchell, D., and Tarpley, R. Painful pulpitis. Oral Surg 13:1360, 1960.
5. Wood, N. K., and Goaz, P. W. Differential Diagnosis of Oral Lesions, 2nd ed. St. Louis, C.V. Mosby Co., 1980.
6. Barnes, D. E. Epidemiology of dental disease. J Clin Periodontol 4:80–92, 1977.
7. Mandel, I. D. Dental caries. Am Sci 67:680–688, 1979.
8. Newbrun, E. Cariology, 2nd ed. Baltimore, Williams & Wilkins, 1982.
9. Carlos J. P. The prevention of dental caries, ten years later. J Am Dent Assoc 104:193–197, 1982.
10. Heifetz, S. B., Horowitz, H. S., and Driscoll, W. S. Effects of school water fluoridation on dental caries: Results in Seagrove, N.C. after eight years. J Am Dent Assoc 97:193–196, 1978.
11. Dreizen, S. The role of diet in dental decay. Nutr News 29:1–2, 1966.
12. Mansbridge, J. N. Heredity and dental caries. J Dent Res 38:337–347, 1959.
13. Hensen, B. F. Clinical and roentgenologic caries detection. Dentomaxillofacial Radiol 9(1):34–36, 1980.

14. Bernick, S. Vascular and nerve changes associated with the healing of the human pulp. Oral Surg 33:983, 1972.
15. Dawes, C., Jenkins, G. N., and Tenge, C. H. The nomenclature of the integument of the enamel surface of teeth. Br Dent J 115:65, 1963.
16. Kannangara, D. W., Thadepelli, H., and McQuiter, J. L. Bacteriology and treatment of dental infections. Oral Surg 50:103, 1980.
17. Chow, A. W., et al. Oral-facial odontogenic infections. Ann Intern Med 88:392, 1978.
18. Seltzer, S., Bender, I. B., and Zionty, M. The interrelationship of pulp and periodontal disease. Oral Surg 16:1474, 1963.
19. Bender, I. B., and Seltzer, S. The effect of periodontal disease on the pulp. Oral Surg 33:458, 1972.
20. Blair, H. A. Relationships between endodontics and periodontics. J Periodontol 43:209, 1972.
21. Mazur, B., and Massler, M. Influence of periodontal disease on the dental pulp. Oral Surg 17:592, 1964.
22. Sinai, I. H., and Soltanoff, W. The transmission of pathologic changes between the pulp and the periodontal structures. Oral Surg 36:558, 1973.
23. Morris, M. L. Diagnosis, prognosis and treatment of the loose tooth. Oral Surg 6:957–964, 1963.
24. Langeland, K., and Langeland, L. K. Pulp reactions to cavity and crown preparation. Aust Dent J 15:261, 1970.
25. Spangbert, L., Engstrom, B., and Langeland, K. Biologic effects of dental materials. Oral Surg 36:856, 1973.
26. Dotto, C. A., Carranza, F. A., Jr., Cabrini, R. L., et al. Vascular changes in experimental trauma from occlusion. J Periodontol 38:183, 1967.
27. Landay, M. A., and Seltzer, S. The effects of excessive occlusal force on the pulp. Oral Surg 32:623, 1971.
28. Tanner, H. A., and Kitchen, R. N. An effective treatment for pain in the eruption of primary and permanent teeth. J Dent Child 31:289–292, 1964.
29. Kruger, G. Textbook of Oral and Maxillofacial Surgery, 5th ed. St. Louis, C.V. Mosby, 1979.
30. Sicher, H. Problems of pain in dentistry. Oral Surg 7:149, 1954.
31. Rowe, N. L., and Killey, H. C. Fractures of the Facial Skeleton, 2nd ed. London, E. & S. Livingstone, 1956.
32. Kinnie, B. H. From the outside looking in. Presented to the American Academy of Dental Radiology, October 19, 1984.
33. Bhaskar, S. N., and Rappaport, H. M. Dental vitality tests and pulp status. J Am Dent Assoc 86:409, 1973.
34. Cameron, C. Cracked tooth syndrome; additional findings. J Am Dent Assoc 93:971, 1976.
35. Evans, F. O., Jr., et al. Sinusitis of the maxillary antrum. N Engl J Med 293:735, 1975.
36. Killey, H. C. and Kay, L. A. The Maxillary Sinus and Its Dental Implications. Bristol, John Wright, 1975.
37. Ryan, R. E., Jr., and Kern, E. B. Rhinologic causes of facial pain and headache. Headache 18:44, 1978.
38. Lyon, H. E. Reliability of panoramic radiography in the diagnosis of maxillary sinus pathosis. Oral Surg 35:124–128, 1973.
39. Robertson, S., Goodell, H., and Wolff, H. G. The teeth as a source of headache and other pain. Arch Neurol Psychiatr 57:277, 1947.

40. Andran, C. M. Bone destruction not demonstrable by radiograph. Br J Radiol 24:107, 1951.
41. Bhaskar, S. N. Periapical lesions—types, incidence and clinical features. Oral Surg 21:657, 1966.
42. Blechman, H. Infections of pulp and periapical tissues. In Nolte, W. A. (ed.). Oral Microbiology, 3rd ed. St. Louis, C.V. Mosby, 1977.
43. Andreasen, J. O. Traumatic Injuries of the Teeth. St. Louis, C.V. Mosby, 1972.
44. Andreasen, J. O. Etiology and pathogenesis of traumatic dental injuries. A clinical study of 1298 cases. Scand J Dent Res 78:329–342, 1970.
45. Edgerton, M. T. Emergency care of maxillofacial injuries. In Zuidema, G. D., Rutherford, R. B., and Ballinger, W. F. II (eds.). The Management of Trauma, 3rd ed. Philadelphia, W.B. Saunders Co., 1979.
46. Braham, R. L., Roberts, M. W., and Morris, M. E. Management of dental trauma in children and adolescents. J Trauma 17:857–865, 1977.
47. Clyde J. S. Transverse-oblique fractures of the crown with extension below the epithelial attachment. Br Dent J 120:402–406, 1968.
48. Grossman, L. I. Endodontic Practice, 9th ed. Philadelphia, Lea & Febiger, 1978.
49. Henderson, D., and Steffel, V. L. McCracken's Removable Prosthodontics, 5th ed. St. Louis, C.V. Mosby, 1977.
50. Baum, L., Phillips, R. W., and Lund, M. R.: Textbook of Operative Dentistry, 2nd ed. Philadelphia, W.B. Saunders Co., 1985.
51. Cataldo, E., and Santis, H. Response of the oral tissue to exogenous foreign materials. J Periodontol 45:93, 1974.
52. Bender, I. B., Seltzer, S., and Soltanoff, W. Endodontic success—a reappraisal of criteria. Oral Surg 22:780, 1966.
53. Freedland, J. B. Conservative reduction of large periapical lesions. Oral Surg 29:455, 1970.
54. Luebke, R. G., Glick, D. H., and Ingle, J. I. Indications and contraindications for endodontic surgery. Oral Surg 18:97, 1964.
55. Shafer, W. G., Hine, M. K., and Levey, B. M. A Textbook of Oral Pathology, 4th ed. Philadelphia, W.B. Saunders Co., 1983.
56. Bryan, A. W. Some common defects in operative restorations contributing to the injury of the supporting structures. J Am Dent Assoc 14:1486, 1927.
57. Orban, B. Discoloration of the oral mucous membrane by metallic foreign bodies. J Periodontol 17:55, 1946.
58. Schoenberg, B., et al. Chronic idiopathic orolingual pain. NY State J Med 71(8):1832–1837, 1981.
59. Gruskka, M. Burning mouth: A review and update. Ont Dent 60(4):56–61, 1983.
60. Roberts, A. M., and Person, P. Etiology and treatment of idiopathic trigeminal and atypical facial neuralgias. Oral Surg 48:298, 1979.
61. Marbach, J. J., et al. Incidence of phantom tooth pain: An atypical facial neuralgia. Oral Surg 53:190, 1982.
62. Mitchell, D. F., Standish, S.M. and Fast, T. B. Oral Diagnosis/Oral Medicine, 3rd ed. Philadelphia, Lea & Febiger, 1978.
63. Gorlin, R. J., et al. Odontogenic tumors. Cancer 14:73, 1961.
64. Bell, W. E. Orofacial Pains, Classification, Diagnosis, Management. Chicago, Year Book, 1985.
65. Trapnell, D. H., and Bowerman, J. L. E. Dental manifestation of systemic disease. London, Butterworth, 1973.

66. Cutress, T. W. Periodontal disease and oral hygiene in trisomy 21. Arch Oral Biol 16:1345–1355, 1971.
67. Benveniste, R., Bixler, D., and Conneally, P. M. Periodontal disease in diabetics. J Periodontol 38:271–279, 1967.
68. Segelman, A. E., and Doku, H. C. Treatment of the oral complications of leukemia. J Oral Surg 35:469, 1977.
69. Robertson, M. S., and Snape, L. The malignant gland in the neck as a presenting sign in head and neck cancer. N Z Med J 92:303, 1980.
70. Fu, K. K., et al. Carcinoma of the major and minor salivary glands. Cancer 40:2882, 1977.
71. Saunders, W. H. Nicotine stomatitis of the palate. Ann Otol Rhinol Laryngol 67:618, 1958.
72. Bender, I. B., Seltzer, S., and Turkenkopf, S. To culture or not to culture? Oral Surg 18:527, 1964.
73. Denaley, J. F. Atypical facial pain as a defense against psychosis. Am J Psychol 133:1151, 1976.
74. Brooke, R. Atypical odontalgia. Oral Surg 49(3):196–199, 1980.
75. Feinman, C. Psychogenic facial pain: Presentation and treatment. J Psychosom Res 27(5):403–410, 1983.
76. American Psychiatric Association. Diagnostic and Statistical Manual of Mental Disorders, 3rd ed. Washington, D.C., American Psychiatric Association, 1987.
77. Thompson, J. Diagnosis of head pain. An Ideographic approach to assessment and classification. Headache 22(9):221–232, 1982.
78. Seltzer, S. Pain Control in Dentistry. Philadelphia, J. B. Lippincott, 1978.
79. Roed-Peterson, B. Nasolabial cysts: A presentation of five patients and review of the literature. Br J Oral Surg 7:8, 1963.
80. Stafne, E. C., et al. Median anterior maxillary cysts. J Am Dent Assoc 23:801, 1936.
81. Shklar, G. The oral lesions of pemphigus vulgaris. Oral Surg 23:629, 1967.
82. Laskaris, G. Oral pemphigus vulgaris: An immunofluorescent study of fifty-eight cases. Oral Surg 51:626, 1981.
83. Lozada, F., Silverman, S., and Cram, D. Pemphigus vulgaris. A study of six cases treated with levanisole and prednisone. Oral Surg 54:161, 1982.
84. Ackerman, L. V., Del Regato, J. A., and Spjut, H. J. Cancer: Diagnosis, Treatment and Prognosis, 5th ed. St. Louis, C.V. Mosby, 1977.

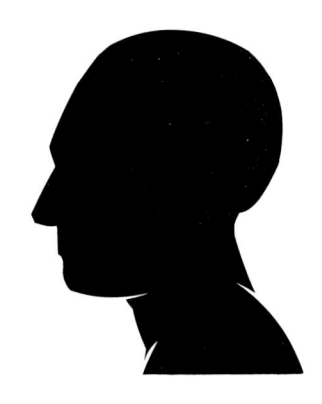

Chapter 7
Oropharyngeal, Laryngeal, and Neck Pain

Robert L. Pincus

Perhaps no other complaint stimulates a patient more readily to seek medical care than pain. Pain is a sensation of discomfort, distress, or agony resulting from the stimulation of specialized nerve endings. Head and neck pain is particularly alarming to most patients because the food and air passages are frequently involved with the symptom.

Pain is a complex psychobiologic phenomenon that has both physical and emotional components. Individuals vary widely in their perceptions of and reactions to pain. The intensity and duration of pain is not proportional to the severity of disease. Only 50 percent of patients with deep lacerations complain of pain in the emergency room,[1] whereas patients with tic douloureux have severe lancinating pain. Inflammatory lymphadenitis may be quite painful, whereas metastatic lymph nodes are not. Pain in the head and neck is frequently heterotopic or referred as well as homotopic or local. In order to understand these complaints, the physician must understand the neural pathways in the head and neck.

A careful, detailed history and thorough examination with a knowledge of head and neck anatomy and pathophysiology and pain syndromes are essential to diagnose and treat the patient in pain appropriately. The characteristics of the pain in terms of onset, duration, intensity, and trigger point, if any, should be noted. The patient should be asked how the pain affects him or her. The patient's perception of the cause of the pain should be sought. The patient should be asked if friends or relatives have had similar complaints. Any addictive, habituating, or abusive habit should be noted. Medications taken and relief afforded should be charted. Additionally, the examiner should seek out clues of cancer or acquired immune deficiency phobia. Young children present a special problem because an accurate history may be difficult or impossible to obtain.

In examining the patient with head and neck pain, the physician should first assess the general medical condition of the patient as well as the patient's level of anxiety. Cranial nerves I through XII should be carefully evaluated. Sensory distribution to the face should be tested in each of the branches of the trigeminal nerve. The distribution of the mandibular branch is the most common trigger point in trigeminal neuralgia.[2] The autonomic nervous system of the head and neck should also be evaluated. Evidence of normal lacrimation and salivation suggests that the parasympathetic system related to cranial nerves VII and IX is intact. A Horner's syndrome (ptosis, miosis, and anhydrosis) would indicate a dysfunction of the cervical sympathetic system.

A complete evaluation of the patient's oral mucosa with bimanual palpation and visual inspection should be done. The color and condition of the gingivae and teeth should be noted. The buccal mucosa should be examined for changes in color, evidence of trauma, and the condition of the parotid duct orifices opposite the upper second molar. The mucosa of the tongue should be evaluated for masses. A tongue depressor is used to manipulate the tongue to allow complete examination of the undersurface and sides of the tongue. Tongue mobility, both on protrusion and side-to-side motion, should be noted. The hard and soft palate should be evaluated for lesions, symmetry, and motion on phonation. The oropharynx, including the tonsillar fossae and the posterior pharyngeal walls, can be examined by gentle downward pressure on the tongue. The mucosa of the floor of the mouth should be examined, paying attention to the orifices of the submandibular ducts, just lateral to the frenulum. The floor of the mouth, tongue, and submandibular glands should be palpated bimanually (Fig. 7–1).

The patient's hypopharynx and larynx can be examined indirectly with a mirror as well as directly with a fiberoptic nasopharyngoscope. The neck should be palpated for masses, spasm, and areas of tenderness. The sternocleidomastoid muscle should be gently retracted laterally so that the underlying venous system and lymphatics can be evaluated. The carotid arteries should be auscultated and palpated individually. External examination of the laryngeal structures involves palpation of the hyoid bone and the thyroid and cricoid cartilages. The size, consistency, and symmetry of the thyroid gland should be noted. The examination should be tailored so that the area of pain is examined last. Imaging should be done as indicated by the complaint.

Oral and Oropharyngeal Pain

The glossopharyngeal nerve supplies sensation to almost the entire pharynx, from the level of the eustachian tube down (Fig. 7–2). A branch of the glossopharyngeal nerve, the tympanic branch of cranial nerve IX or Jacob-

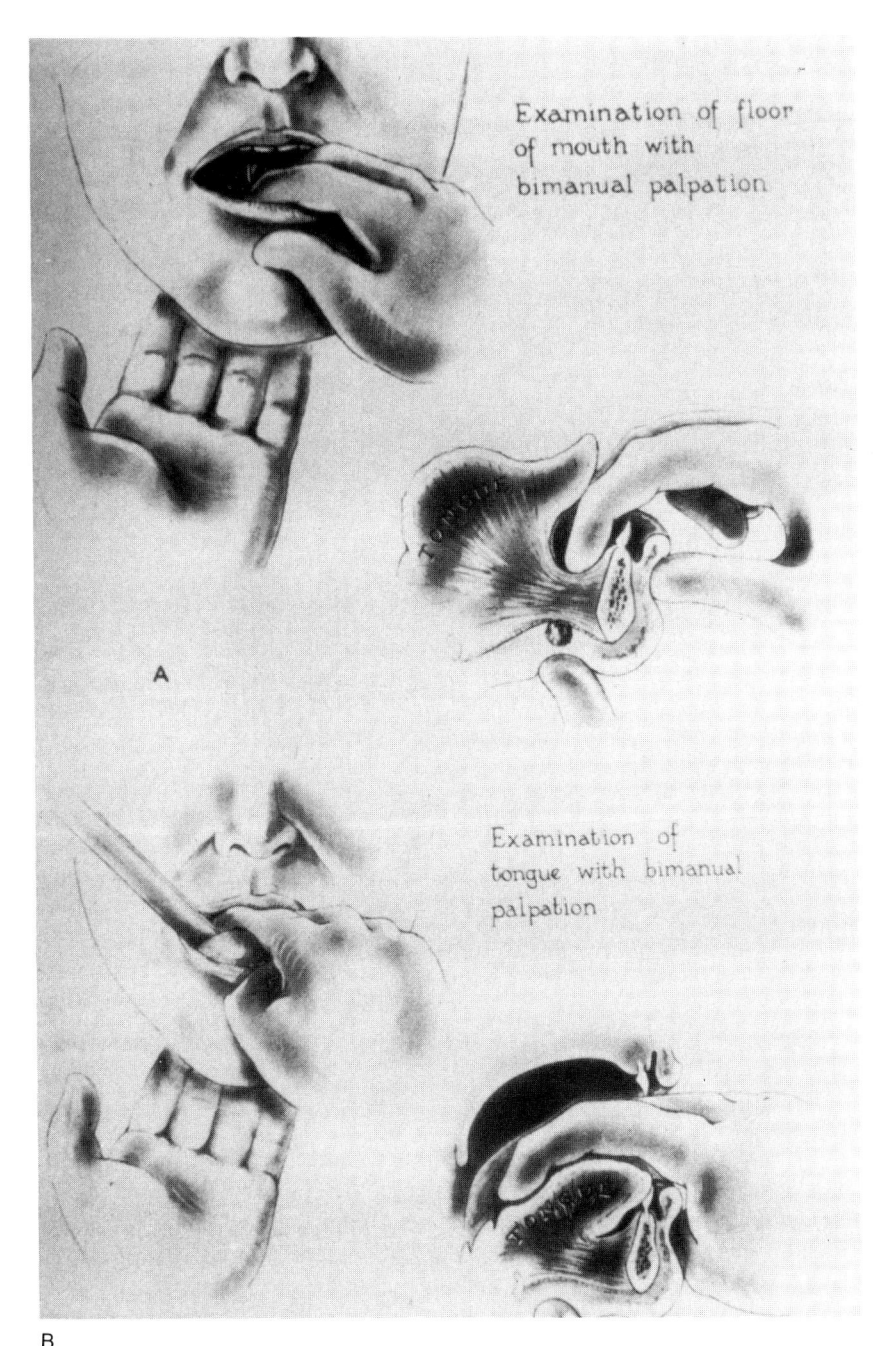

FIGURE 7–1. *A*, Bimanual palpation of the floor of the mouth. *B*, Bimanual palpation of the tongue. (From Paparella, M. M., and Shumrick, D. A. [eds.]. Otolaryngology. Vol. 3. Head and Neck. Philadelphia, W. B. Saunders Co., 1973.)

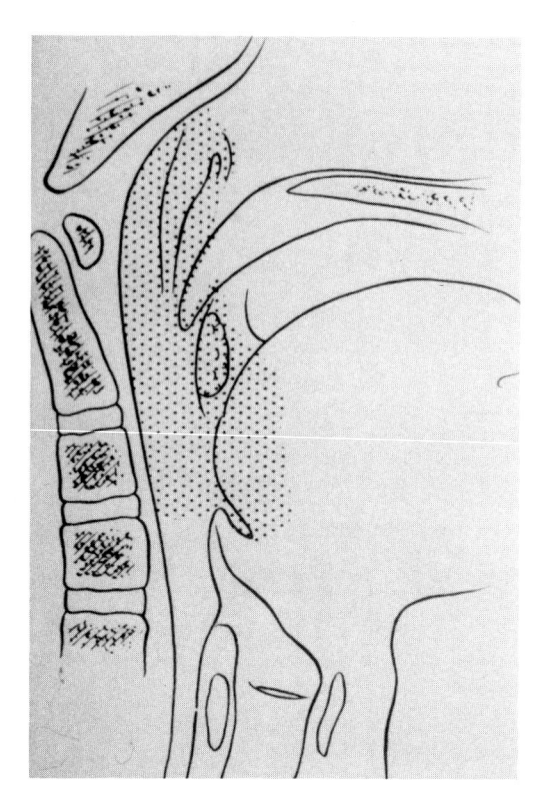

FIGURE 7–2. Area of sensation supplied by glossopharyngeal nerve. (From Hollinshead, W. H. Anatomy for Surgeons. Vol. 1. Head and Neck. New York, Harper & Row, 1968.)

son's nerve, supplies the middle ear mucosa and a small area of the external meatus and ear. It is responsible for referred otalgia with pharyngeal inflammation. Above the opening of the eustachian tube a limited upper part of the nasopharynx is supplied by maxillary nerve fibers that reach it through the pharyngeal branch of the pterygopalatine ganglion. The lower pharynx has sensory innervation supplied by the superior laryngeal branch of the vagus nerve.[3]

Neuralgia

Glossopharyngeal neuralgia is 70 to 100 times less common than trigeminal neuralgia. There is no sexual predominance. Glossopharyngeal neuralgia is unusual in patients under 20 years of age. Left-sided symptoms are more common than right, and in 2 percent of patients the neuralgia is bilateral.[4] Patients usually describe sharp, knifelike paroxysmal pain. It may last seconds or minutes and is rare at night. A dull ache may persist between attacks. Attacks are usually induced by swallowing, yawning, coughing, or chewing or even by particular tastes.[5] Pain usually starts in the tonsil or the base of tongue but may spread to or begin in the ear. The glossopharyngeal nerve usually pierces the dura separately from the vagus at the jugular foramen and can be lysed independently.

Postherpetic Neuralgia

Postherpetic neuralgia occurs in specific dermatomes. Cranial nerve involvement is second most frequent after the thoracic dermatomes.[6] Cranial nerve involvement tends to be severe and may involve the glossopharyngeal distribution. Pain occurs with a vesicular eruption over single or adjacent dermatomes served by segmental or cranial nerve branches. Biopsy shows multinucleated giant epithelial cells with intranuclear inclusions. These can be differentiated from varicella and herpes simplex by fluorescent antibody staining. Postherpetic neuralgia is often difficult to manage but usually diminishes over a period of months or years.

Pharyngitis

Pharyngitis is one of the most common illnesses and is probably the most common cause of head and neck pain. The areas affected by a "sore throat" usually are the soft palate, tonsils, adenoids, and oropharyngeal mucosa. Pharyngitis may be bacterial, viral, fungal, or noninfectious in etiology. Extension of infections into the deep spaces adjacent to the pharynx may cause fascial space infections or abscesses. The most commonly involved spaces are the peritonsillar, parapharyngeal, and retropharyngeal spaces.

Pharyngitis usually presents with a sore throat, often with dysphagia, fever, and malaise. It may occur in epidemics. The pharynx is usually uniformly affected and erythematous. Regional lymph tissue and lymph nodes may be enlarged and tender. Purulent debris may accumulate on the tonsils or pharyngeal wall. There may be a membranous exudate or ulceration.

BACTERIAL PHARYNGITIS

Acute streptococcal pharyngitis has received most of the emphasis since the work done in the early 1950s showing that acute rheumatic fever could be prevented by treating pharyngitis with penicillin.[7, 8] Prior to the use of penicillin, there were 200,000 to 250,000 new cases of acute rheumatic fever annually.[9] This incidence has fallen to 0.49 per 100,000 in middle-class areas but not quite as low in areas of endemic poverty.[10]

Clinical differentiation of streptococcal pharyngitis from viral pharyngitis is not reliable, although cultures in children may be correctly predicted in 75 percent of cases.[10] Pharyngeal swab culture is the most common diagnostic test. However, 20 percent of asymptomatic children are carriers of group A beta-hemolytic *Streptococcus*, and 10 percent of patients with proven streptococcal pharyngitis have false-negative cultures.[11] A fourfold increase in the antistreptolysin O antibody titer is evidence of invasive infection. Enzyme-linked immunosorbent assays (ELISA) are available for rapid antigen identification. The treatment of choice is either penicillin G, 200,000 to 250,000 units orally four times a day for 10 days, or benzathine penicillin G, 600,000 to 1.2 million units intramuscularly once a day.

However, today only 15 to 20 percent of cases of acute pharyngitis are caused by beta-hemolytic *Streptococcus*.

Diphtheria is caused by *Corynebacterium diphtheriae*. There are still 200 to 300 cases annually in the United States. Release of a toxin causes local inflammation, exudate formation, and cellular necrosis. A membrane, composed of fibrin exudate and sloughing epithelium, appears. A bleeding ulcerative base is found deep to the membrane. Death may result from airway obstruction or from the effect of the diphtheroid toxin on the conduction system of the heart and peripheral nervous system.[12] Neutralization of the unbound toxin is the therapeutic goal.

Oropharyngeal gonorrhea has been found in up to 20 percent of homosexual men and 10 percent of women examined at venereal disease clinics. Two-thirds of those with positive cultures were asymptomatic.[13] The clinical picture is nonspecific. The diagnosis is made by culture on a Thayer-Martin plate and only if the physician has a high index of suspicion.

Vincent's angina is caused by anaerobic bacilli and spirochetes. Although more common in the gingiva, where it presents as "trench mouth," it may present on the tonsil with a distinctive, necrotic tonsillar ulceration covered by a dirty gray membrane. Vincent's angina is a disease of young adults and teenagers. There may be malaise, low-grade fever, and unilateral adenopathy. Although the lesion may look similar to a carcinoma, crystal violet staining of the exudate will show *Fusobacteria* and spirochetes. Treatment includes a 7- to 10-day course of penicillin and improved oral hygiene. Luetic pharyngitis should be ruled out. Primary syphilitic lesions, however, are usually painless.

Other bacterial organisms may cause pharyngitis less frequently. Among these are *Staphylococcus aureus*, *Haemophilus influenzae*, and *Bacteroides melaninogenicus*. *Bacteroides melaninogenicus* is a common oral anaerobe that is present frequently on the tonsil and in core aspirates of chronically infected tonsils. Its role as a pathogen, however, is uncertain.

VIRAL PHARYNGITIS
Most pharyngitis is viral, the common cold alone accounting for about one-third of all sore throats. Most cases are due to rhinovirus or coronavirus, and pharyngeal involvement is usually not severe. Symptoms are mild, and the illness is self-limited.

Adenovirus causes about 10 percent of cases of pharyngitis. It usually occurs in childhood but may be epidemic in groups living in close quarters, such as military recruits. Adenovirus pharyngitis typically presents with throat pain, fever, chills, hoarseness, cough, malaise, and myalgias. Pharyngoconjunctival fever, which includes fever, sore throat, and conjunctivitis, may be due to adenovirus.[14]

Herpetic gingivostomatitis may present with vesicular lesions on the palate, pharyngeal walls, and tonsils as well as the labial mucocutaneous border, buccal mucosa, and gingiva. Primary infection usually occurs in infants, and recurrent lesions are common in adults. Over 80 percent of adults have antibodies to herpesvirus.[10] The lesions begin as 2- to 3-mm vesicles with larger red bases. These later ulcerate and are painful. Systemic symptoms are present with the primary infection but are uncommon in recurrent lesions. Acyclovir may be useful in treatment.

Herpangina, a viral infection due chiefly to group A coxsackievirus infection, presents with a characteristic clinical picture. It is epidemic, usually occurring in late summer in children. Herpangina is characterized by multiple, discrete, 1- to 2-mm vesicles on the palate, tonsillar pillars, and uvula. There is a sudden onset of high fever and sore throat. Abdominal pain, vomiting, and diarrhea may occur. In older children and adults group A coxsackievirus may cause acute lymphonodular pharyngitis, with sore throat, fever, malaise, and headache. There will be raised, yellow-white, submucosal nodules on the pharyngeal wall without ulceration. Treatment is symptomatic.

Infectious mononucleosis is an acute pharyngitis due to the Epstein-Barr virus (EBV), a member of the herpes group of viruses. It is typified by fever, pharyngeal exudate and edema, cervical adenopathy, hepatosplenomegaly, and an increase in the white blood cell count with over 10 percent atypical lymphocytes. Clinical manifestations may vary from a mild sore throat to diffuse lymphoreticular hyperplasia, high fever, airway obstruction, jaundice, splenic rupture, and aseptic meningitis. Fatalities are rare.

Infectious mononucleosis is a disease of older children and young adults. It is spread by way of the saliva, and oropharyngeal shedding of the virus may continue for months after the illness. Approximately 50 percent of college students have EBV antibodies, and there is an incidence of infection of about 12 percent per year in the remaining students.[10] Diagnosis is made by the clinical picture, examination of the peripheral blood smear, and serologic tests for the heterophil antibody and for EBV antibodies. Treatment is symptomatic.

Other viral infections may result in pharyngitis as part of their clinical pictures. Among these are influenza, parainfluenza, rabies, measles, and varicella.

FUNGAL PHARYNGITIS

Candidiasis may involve the pharynx, especially in the immunocompromised patient. *Candida* usually appears as adherent white plaques on the pharyngeal mucosa and is frequently accompanied by severe pharyngeal pain. *Candida* is identified by microscopic examination of pharyngeal scrapings and can be grown on Sabouraud's agar. The incidence of pharyngeal fungal infections can be expected to rise with the increasing incidence of acquired immune deficiency syndrome (AIDS).

NONINFECTIOUS PHARYNGITIS

The pharynx may be irritated from noninfectious causes. Symptoms and physical findings may be similar to those characteristic of a mild viral pharyngitis. Among the causes are smoker's pharynx and mouth breathing due to nasal obstruction. Reflux esophagitis may also be severe enough at times to cause pharyngeal symptoms.

Recurrent aphthous ulcers, or "canker sores," are seen frequently, especially in younger patients. The etiology is unknown. Minor aphthae are most common.[15] These present as small ulcerations, less than 1 cm in diameter, with a central pseudomembrane and peripheral erythema. Major ulcers (Fig. 7–3) may be 2 to 3 cm in diameter. Lesions are painful, and frequently new lesions appear as the old lesions heal. Aphthous ulcers should be differentiated from herpetic and other viral lesions. Aphthous ulcerations rarely affect the hard palate and gingiva and rarely cause systemic symptoms. Viral cultures are negative, and pathologic specimens show no evidence of viral effect. Treatment is frequently unsatisfactory. Topical and systemic steroids have been used.

Space Infections

The peritonsillar, parapharyngeal, and retropharyngeal spaces may be involved by direct or lymphatic spread from pharyngeal infections. Space infections may develop into abscesses and require drainage. Pain is often a major symptom in these patients owing to irritative muscle spasm caused by the infections. Retropharyngeal space infections typically present with refusal to take food, pain, neck rigidity, dysphagia, odynophagia, low-grade temperature elevation, and adenopathy. Physical examination shows a bulging posterior pharynx just to the side of the midline. Lateral soft tissue x-rays show a widening of the soft tissue shadow (Fig. 7–4). Treatment includes securing the airway, if necessary, and early drainage.

The parapharyngeal space becomes involved most often owing to spread from tonsillitis, pharyngitis, or peritonsillar infection. The patient presents with fever and dysphagia and develops trismus due to irritation of the internal pterygoid muscle. The lateral pharyngeal wall and tonsil are displaced medially, and the tail of the parotid is displaced laterally. Treatment includes use of antibiotics and early drainage.

The peritonsillar space is more frequently involved. Infection may spread

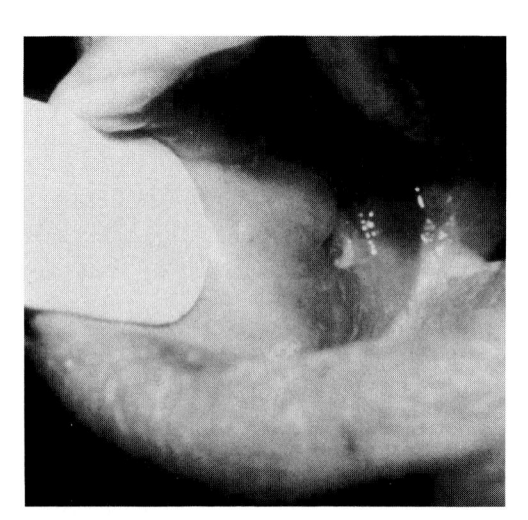

FIGURE 7–3. Major aphthous ulcer of the buccal mucosa.

Oropharyngeal, Laryngeal, and Neck Pain

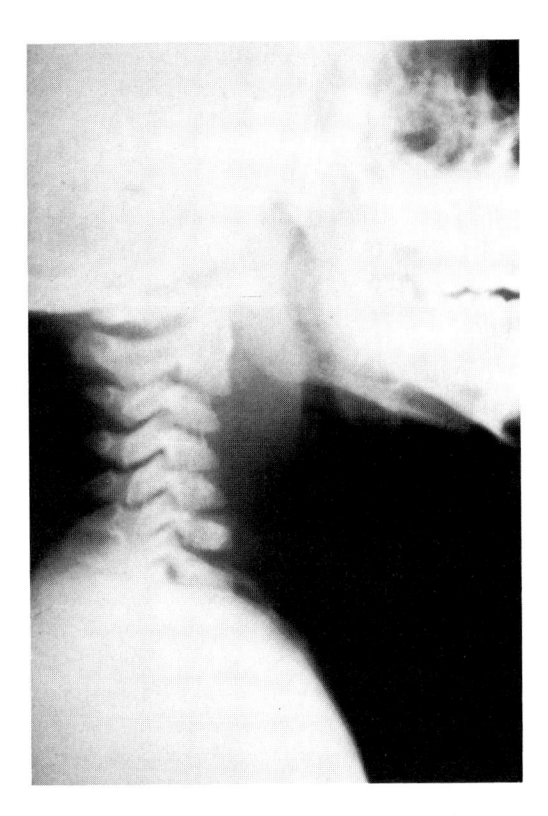

FIGURE 7–4. Widened posterior pharyngeal soft tissue shadow with abscess of the retropharyngeal space.

from the tonsils to the potential space about the tonsil. Patients usually present with sore throats that persist and worsen in spite of treatment. Pain increases and becomes more localized. Systemic signs may become more prominent, and trismus may develop owing to spasm of the internal pterygoid muscle. Physical examination shows a bulging of the tonsil and uvula, almost always unilaterally. If cellulitis is present without abscess formation, treatment is accomplished with antibiotics. Abscesses require drainage or repeated aspiration.

Other Causes of Oropharyngeal Pain

Pemphigus and benign mucous membrane pemphigoid both involve the oral and oropharyngeal mucosa. Pemphigus appears to be due to an autoimmune response to an intercellular substance of the epidermis and mucosa. Half of patients with pemphigus have oral and oropharyngeal mucosal involvement, which often presents 1 to 2 years before the onset of cutaneous lesions.[16] Bullae erode and leave sloughed areas with friable edges. The lesions are quite painful. Smears from the base of a bulla stained with Giemsa stain demonstrate acantholysis, the loss of intercellular bridges. Immunofluorescent studies identify immunoglobulin directed against the intercellular spaces of the epithelium. Treatment includes the use of steroids and often cytotoxic therapy. Prior to the use of steroids pemphigus was universally fatal owing to dehydration and superinfection.

Benign mucous membrane pemphigoid is probably an autoimmune disease as well. Lesions occur most often in the oral cavity, usually as blisters with a surrounding area of erythema. These lesions then ulcerate. The buccal mucosa, gingiva, and palate are involved most often.[17] These lesions are frequently painless. Biopsies show subepithelial clefting. There are linear deposits of IgG and C3 in the basement membrane zone on immunofluorescence. Topical and systemic steroids as well as dapsone have been used for therapy.

Erythema multiforme may resemble pemphigus and pemphigoid. It usually presents in young patients, however, and most commonly affects the lips, buccal mucosa, and tongue when the oral cavity is involved.

Oropharyngeal pain may be due to local trauma, such as eating hot or coarse foods or local injury from a foreign body or caustic ingestion. Children may suffer palatal and oropharyngeal lacerations from falling while holding an object in their teeth. There is usually an irregular ulcer with a raised erythematous border. Pain and local tenderness are the major symptoms. If uncomplicated, healing usually occurs in 1 to 2 weeks. Possible complications include space infections, and some practitioners recommend prophylactic antibiotics. Biopsies should be taken if the lesion persists.

Foreign bodies frequently become lodged in the base of the tongue. Typically, a fish or chicken bone may lodge in the tonsil or lingual lymph tissue, presenting as a sharp sticking pain on swallowing. These objects can be seen on a mirror examination and require removal. General anesthesia is rarely required.

The styloid process is lateral to the tonsillar fossa within the parapharyngeal space. Eagle pointed out that in 4 percent of patients the styloid process is elongated and may impinge on either the internal or the external carotid artery or the tonsillar region.[18] Although most elongated styloid processes are asymptomatic, they may produce pharyngeal pain, sometimes with extension to the ear. Babbitt reported a case of spontaneous styloid fracture causing oropharyngeal pain.[19] Diagnosis of Eagle's syndrome is accomplished by bimanual palpation of the tonsillar fossa.

Neoplastic Causes of Oropharyngeal Pain

Most benign neoplasms of the oropharynx are not painful. Ninety percent of oropharyngeal malignancies are squamous cell carcinomas. These occur predominantly in males, smokers, and drinkers. Most carcinomas are painless when small and cause symptoms only when large, often due to deep muscular invasion or invasion of the sensory nerves. Chronic sore throat may be the only early symptom. Dysphagia, ear pain, and trismus are uncommon early. Lesions may be overlooked without bimanual palpation of the area. Between 40 and 75 percent of these patients will have metastatic disease at the time of presentation.[20] Diagnostic evaluation includes indirect examination, direct examination, and bimanual palpation. The extent of the lesion should be drawn on a standard template and be made part of the patient's permanent record. General anesthesia should be used for direct laryngoscopy, cervical esophagoscopy, and often bronchoscopy to evaluate the lesion and to look for second primaries.

Both Hodgkin's and non-Hodgkin's lymphomas occur in the oropharynx and constitute 16 percent of malignancies of the tonsil.[21] They may occur as solitary foci of involvement or as part of generalized disease. Oropharyngeal lymphomas generally present with a unilateral tonsillar enlargement. They are usually painless.

Minor salivary glands are scattered throughout the oropharynx. More than half of minor salivary gland tumors are malignant. Adenoid cystic carcinoma comprises about 35 percent of minor salivary gland carcinomas.[22] These tend to show perineural spread and frequently cause local pain with destruction of sensory nerves. Although survival is often prolonged, the cure rate for adenoid cystic carcinoma is small.

Hypopharyngeal Pain

Sensation in the hypopharynx is supplied by the glossopharyngeal and superior laryngeal nerves. Hypopharyngeal pain is frequently due to a dysfunction of the upper esophageal sphincter, particularly the cricopharyngeus. The cricopharyngeus muscle is actually part of the inferior constrictor muscle of the pharynx and a circumferential part of the upper esophageal sphincter. In patients with significant gastric reflux, the cricopharyngeus may go into spasm or develop incoordination of relaxation during swallowing. On swallowing, elevation of intrapharyngeal pressure proximal to the upper esophageal sphincter may result in a pulsion hypopharyngeal diverticulum.

Hypopharyngeal diverticula, or Zencker's diverticula, are most common in the sixth through ninth decades. Dysphagia is the major symptom.[23] With growth of the diverticulum, undigested food may remain trapped in the pouch and cause odor, delayed regurgitation of partially digested food, and a choking sensation. There may be laryngeal irritation, aspiration, and pneumonia. Local distention causes pain and fullness. Diagnosis is made on the basis of barium swallow or cervical esophogram. Esophagoscopy is dangerous in these patients because perforation may occur through the thin-walled diverticulum. Cricopharyngeal spasm without hernia formation can be shown as a shelf on ciné esophogram. Manometric examination shows spasm of the upper esophageal sphincter or delayed relaxation with swallowing. Most authors recommend myotomy as part of the therapy for hypopharyngeal diverticula combined with excision or diverticulopexy. Dohlman's technique uses endoscopic diathermy.[24]

Foreign bodies frequently come to rest just above the cricopharyngeus or are pushed into the esophageal wall by the upper sphincter's contraction and wedge just below the cricopharyngeus. Usually the patient can give a good history of the ingestion of the foreign body and point to the spot where the object has come to rest. In children this is more difficult. Smaller coins may lodge at the upper esophageal sphincter for weeks, causing persistent dysphagia and sore throat until a radiograph is taken or a complication ensues. Diagnosis is made radiographically or on mirror or fiberoptic examination (Fig. 7–5). Since fishbones rarely show on plain films, indirect signs such as thickening of the posterior pharyngeal shadow must be used for diagnosis. Foreign bodies should be removed under direct visualization.

Caustic ingestion may involve the hypopharynx, especially at the level of the upper esophageal sphincter, with or without intraoral injuries. History, including the agent ingested, and physical examination are essential. Acids when ingested cause a coagulation necrosis, which limits their penetration. Alkalis cause a liquefaction necrosis, tend to dissolve tissue, and penetrate more deeply. Household bleach usually causes first-degree burns only, and complications are unusual.[25]

Neoplasms

Benign neoplasms of the pharynx are unusual. About 95 percent of hypopharyngeal carcinomas are squamous cell carcinomas.[26] The hypopharyngeal areas involved are the piriform sinus, the pharyngeal wall, and the postcricoid region. Patients with hypopharyngeal carcinomas generally present with persistent, progressive soreness or pain. There may be the

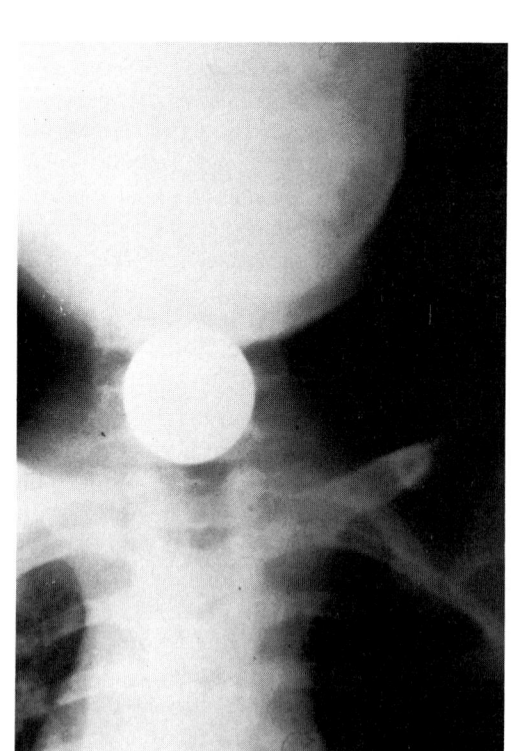

FIGURE 7–5. Coin at upper esophageal sphincter in child.

feeling of fullness or a lump in the throat, and otalgia is often present. Later symptoms include dysphagia, weight loss, blood-tinged sputum, foul odor, aspiration, and weight loss. Lesions are generally discovered late. Because of the abundance of lymphatics and blood vessels in the hypopharynx, more than half the patients present with metastases (Fig. 7–6). Diagnosis is made on indirect laryngoscopy. Treatment usually includes surgery with postoperative radiotherapy; however, cure rates are poor.

Infections

The hypopharynx is often involved in esophageal candidiasis. This is seen as white plaques on the oral and pharyngeal mucosa. Involvement of the hypopharynx can be readily seen on mirror examination. Barium swallows show the typical cobblestoning of the esophagus with esophageal involvement (Fig. 7–7). Symptoms include pain, dysphagia, and blood-tinged saliva. This is frequently seen in patients with AIDS and is the most common infection of the esophagus.

The hypopharynx may be involved in herpetic esophagitis in immunocompromised patients. It is often diagnosed when severe dysphagia thought to be due to candidal esophagitis does not respond to antifungal therapy.[27] Herpes esophagitis looks similar to candidal esophagitis radiographically, except that there may be focal ulcerations with viral esophagitis. Cytologic examination will show multinucleated cells containing intranuclear inclusion bodies.

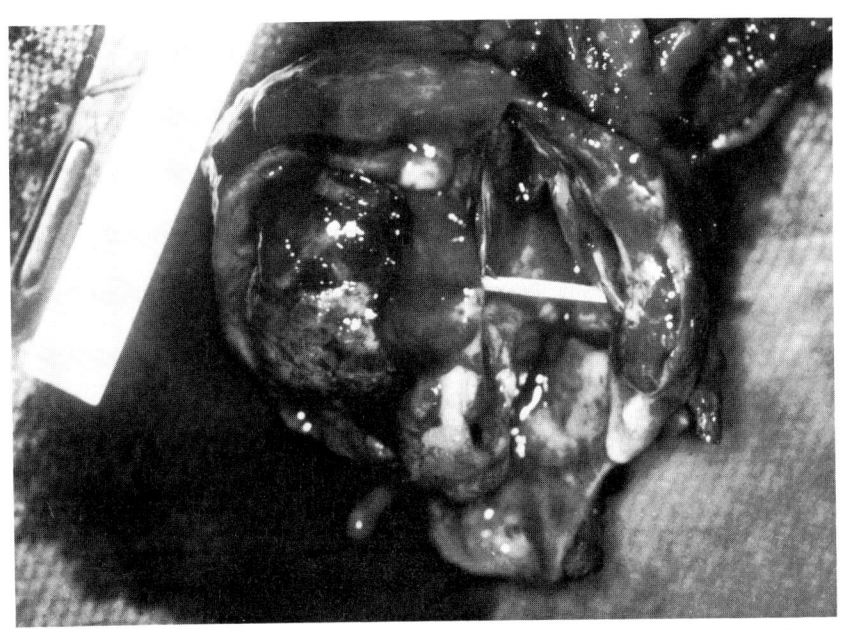

FIGURE 7–6. Large pyriform sinus carcinoma in 34-year-old woman. Patient presented with neck metastasis.

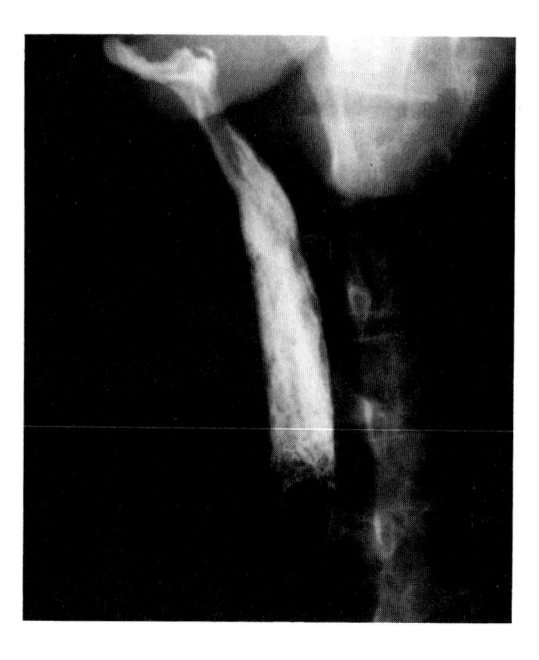

FIGURE 7–7. Cobblestone appearance of esophageal mucosa with esophageal candidiasis in patient with AIDS.

Laryngeal Pain

Innervation

Sensory nerve fibers to the supraglottic larynx are derived from the internal branch of the superior laryngeal nerve. Subglottically, sensation is supplied through the recurrent laryngeal nerve. A small area of anterior subglottic mucosa and the cricothyroid joints are supplied by the external division of the superior laryngeal nerve.[28] Chemoreceptors and thermoreceptors appear to be limited to the anterior supraglottis and the epiglottis.[29]

Trauma

Blunt and penetrating trauma to the larynx can cause pain. The most frequent cause of blunt laryngeal trauma remains automobile accidents, usually due to steering wheel or dashboard contact. Strangulation injuries also can cause blunt laryngeal trauma. Sharp trauma is most often due to knife wounds, gunshot injuries, or broken glass (Fig. 7–8).

Patients with laryngeal trauma typically present with dysphagia, odynophagia, vocal changes, dyspnea, and hemoptysis. In sharp traumatic injuries, entry and exit wounds should be searched for. In blunt trauma, examination may show soft tissue crepitus and blunting of the thyroid eminence. The vascular, respiratory, digestive, and neurologic systems must be evaluated.[30] Surgical exploration should be done in patients with major vascular compromises. Fiberoptic endoscopy is of major use in evaluating the airway for mucosal lacerations, edema, hematoma, and fractures of the cartilaginous structures of the larynx. CT scanning has

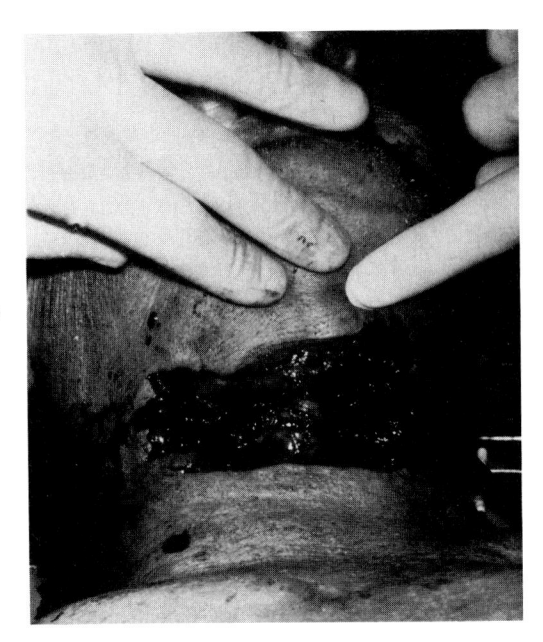

FIGURE 7-8. Self-inflicted knife wound with autolaryngotomy.

replaced many alternative imaging studies of the neck in these patients. An esophagogram may be done if digestive tract injury is also suspected. Maintenance of an adequate airway with early surgical repair of those injuries requiring it offers the best chance for maintaining a functioning glottis.

Neuralgia

Post-traumatic pain may persist in patients with fractures of the hyoid bone and laryngeal cartilages. If there is no mucosal disruption and the fractures do not need reduction, patients should be treated with warm soaks and analgesics. Post-traumatic pain may last for months.

Laryngeal Inflammation

Inflammation, either infectious or noninfectious, may affect the larynx and the cricoarytenoid joints and cause pain. Acute, nonspecific laryngitis is probably the most common laryngeal disorder. Symptoms include hoarseness, and often pain or discomfort accompanies attempts at phonation. Patients frequently complain of a dry, nonproductive cough. Acute laryngitis may be infectious or due to noninfectious causes such as vocal abuse, chemical irritants, or trauma. Treatment includes voice rest, removal of any known irritant, and possibly antibiotics.

Acute laryngitis from other causes may also be accompanied by pain. Laryngeal tuberculosis, although now quite uncommon, is still seen in urban areas where tuberculosis remains endemic. It usually occurs only in advanced cases of pulmonary tuberculosis and is due to contamination of the laryngeal mucosa with infected sputum. Symptoms include cough, odynophagia, weight loss, fever, and night sweats. Treatment consists of antituberculosis chemotherapy.

Syphilis and leprosy may affect the larynx with signs that appear similar to tuberculosis. They may cause discomfort when they are advanced enough to cause perichondritis, chondritis, or chondronecrosis. Patients may have otalgia, hoarseness, and hemoptysis.

Rhinoscleroma is a chronic granulomatous infection caused by *Klebsiella rhinoscleromatis*. Laryngeal involvement is present in 15 percent of patients[31] and may be the sole area of clinical infection (Fig. 7–9). Mikulicz's cells, foamy histiocytes, are seen on biopsy, often surrounded by areas of fibrosis. Diagnosis is made on the basis of a biopsy, and treatment includes oral tetracycline.

Mycotic infections may involve the larynx, most probably secondary to pulmonary disease. These lesions should be considered in the differential diagnosis of any nontuberculous granuloma of the larynx. Tissue should be sent for fungal smears, cultures, and biopsy.

Herpetic infection of the larynx produces recurrent severe pain due to involvement of the superior laryngeal nerve or glossopharyngeal nerve. Vesicles occur early, followed by shallow ulcerations and erythema. Treatment is symptomatic; however, the infection frequently recurs.

The cricoarytenoid joint is a true synovial joint and is subject to all of

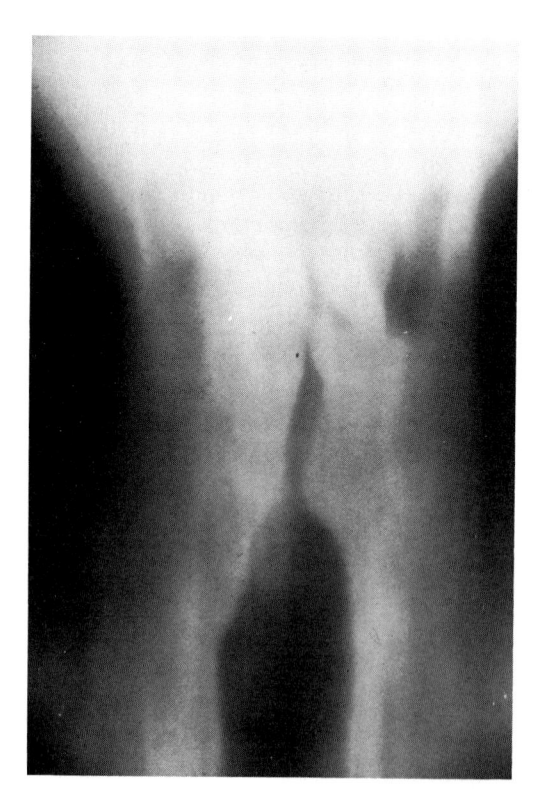

FIGURE 7–9. Laryngeal stenosis presenting as "recurrent asthma" in patient with isolated laryngeal rhinoscleroma.

the afflictions of true synovial joints, including rheumatoid arthritis, osteoarthritis, and infectious arthritides. Montgomery and Lofgren classified cricoarytenoid arthritides by their etiologies as either:

1. Part of a generalized arthritis (usually rheumatoid)
2. Direct extension from an acute infection in the larynx or hypopharynx
3. Traumatic
   a. External trauma
   b. Internal trauma (endoscopy, intubation)
4. Immobilization of the cricoarytenoid joint (long-standing paralysis of the intrinsic laryngeal musculature)

Although most of their patients had generalized rheumatoid arthritis, others had laryngeal arthritis associated with gout, Reiter's syndrome, or systemic lupus erythematosus.[32]

Grossman found rheumatoid changes in the cricoarytenoid joints in 5 of 11 patients with rheumatoid arthritis on biopsy.[33] Patients present with hoarseness, referred otalgia, odynophagia, and a feeling of fullness in the throat. The vocal cords may look normal or slightly thickened. Frequently erythema and fullness exist over the arytenoid. Diagnosis is made by palpating the joint and finding limited motion at endoscopy. Bilateral cricoarytenoid involvement may present with airway obstruction.

A laryngocele is a herniation of the mucosa of the ventricle and saccule of the larynx. It is believed that increased intraluminal pressure forces these sacs to expand upward. When the laryngeal opening is blocked these sacs may become secondarily infected laryngopyoceles, which may present with tender swellings in the neck. Treatment includes diagnosis on radiographs and endoscopy to be certain that there is no malignancy. Excision is generally performed through an external approach after the acute infection has resolved.

Most vocal cord nodules are painless, although the patient may describe a fullness and discomfort as he or she strains to speak. Intubation granulomas, however, frequently are painful. They are more common in women and are due to direct trauma to the perichondrium of the vocal process of the arytenoid. If the lesions persist, they should be surgically removed when mature.

Laryngeal Carcinomas

Glottic carcinomas generally present with hoarseness and are therefore found earlier than supraglottic or subglottic lesions. Pain is unlikely to be a presenting complaint in these patients. In patients with supraglottic or subglottic carcinomas, hoarseness may be a late symptom. These patients are more likely to present with pain, often referred to the ipsilateral ear, sore throat, dysphagia, and later airway obstruction. Diagnosis is made by direct laryngoscopy and biopsy.

Neck Pain

The cervical plexus supplies sensation to the muscles and skin of the anterior neck. It is formed by the union of the ventral rami of the second, third, and fourth cervical nerves. There may also be a contribution from the first cervical nerve. The posterior neck is supplied by the dorsal roots of the same cervical nerves.[34]

Pain may persist after trauma or surgical damage to a cutaneous nerve. A neuroma so formed may require surgical excision.

Neck infections may present with pain. Lymphadenitis from any cause may present with pain, tenderness, guarding, and frequently systemic symptoms. Treatment includes finding the source of the infection and treating both the primary focus and the inflamed nodes with the appropriate antibiotic. When unsure of the pathogen, or if treatment is not successful, the lymph node should be aspirated for culture and sensitivity (Fig. 7–10).

Actinomycosis may cause a chronic suppurative cervical infection with the formation of nodular lesions that resemble inflamed cervical lymph nodes. Actinomycosis is usually due to dental infection and is not a true adenitis. Diagnosis is made by biopsy and culture. Treatment includes a prolonged course of penicillin (Fig. 7–11).

Secondary infections of congenital cysts may cause painful, tender neck masses. Second and third branchial cleft cysts appear along the anterior border of the sternocleidomastoid muscle. They are generally asymptomatic, presenting as nontender fluctuant masses. However, the cysts may become inflamed and tender and form abscesses when inflamed. Inflammatory

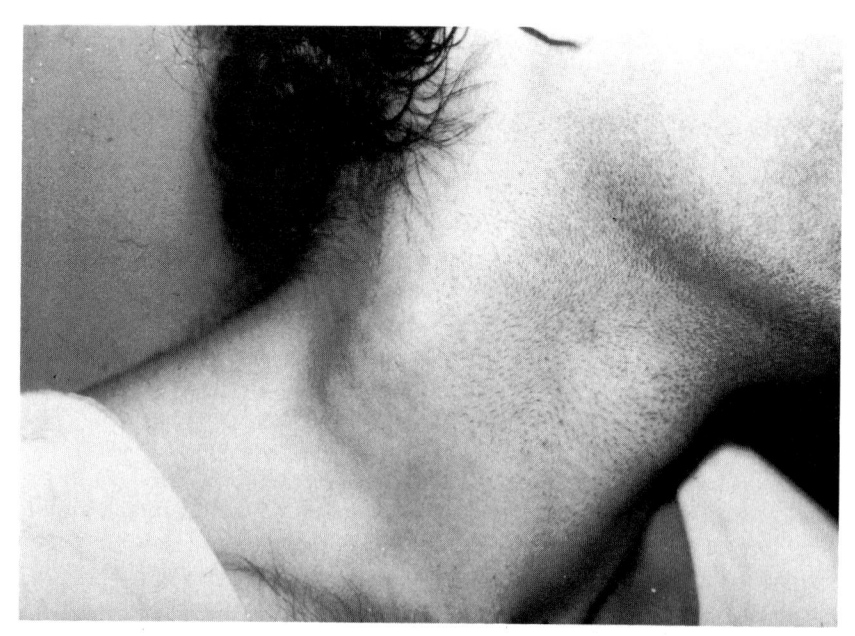

FIGURE 7–10. Scrofulous lymph node due to *Mycobacterium tuberculosis*.

Oropharyngeal, Laryngeal, and Neck Pain

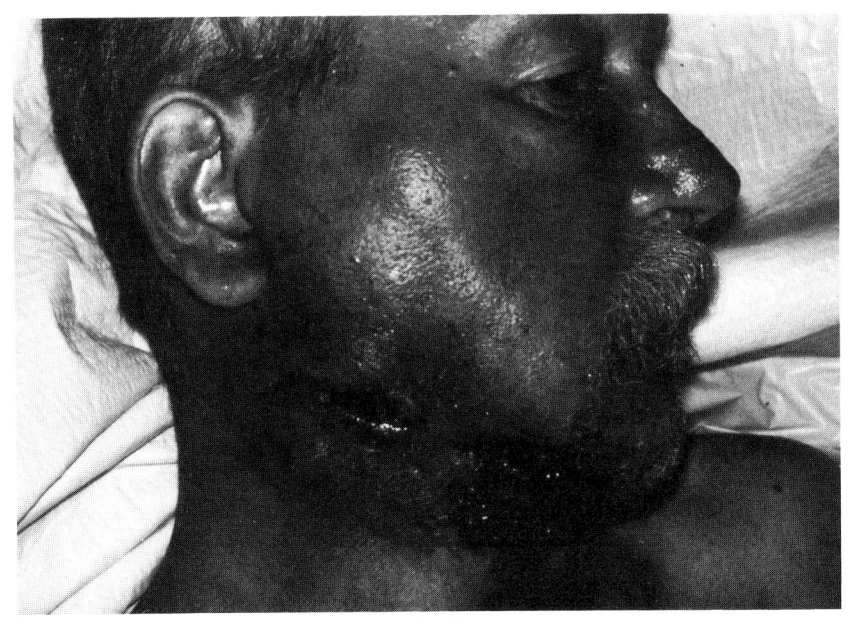

FIGURE 7–11. Fistulae due to actinomycosis.

episodes may occur frequently associated with upper respiratory tract infections. Branchial cleft cysts are removed surgically.

Lymphangiomas (cystic hygromas) are congenital malformations of the lymphatic channels. The neck is involved in 80 percent of patients with lymphangiomas.[35] These lesions present as soft, compressible, painless masses, usually within the first 2 years of life. With suprainfection, the masses may become painful and look like deep neck infections (Fig. 7–12).

Thyroglossal duct cysts are found in the midline and can occur anywhere from the foramen cecum to the thyroid gland. Cysts usually move up and down with the hyoid bone during deglutition. They result from persistence

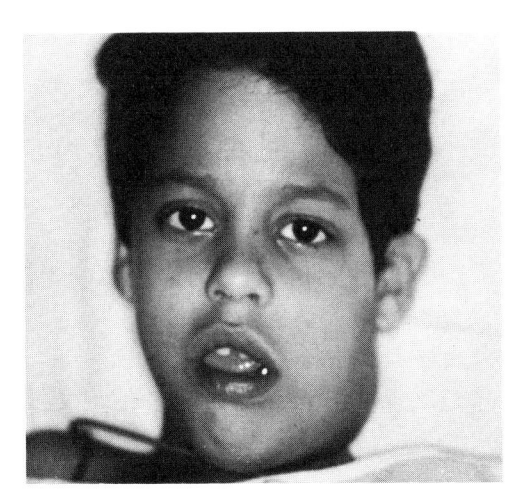

FIGURE 7–12. Infected lymphangioma presenting as parapharyngeal space infection.

of the thyroglossal duct. The cysts may be susceptible to frequent inflammations and abscess formation. When infected, the patient will have a tense, fluctuant, tender cyst in the midline or just off the midline of the neck. Treatment includes incision and drainage and later excision. Uninfected thyroglossal duct cysts should be removed after it is determined that the patient has other functioning thyroid tissue.

Most thyroid masses are painless unless there has been an acute enlargement due to recent bleeding into the nodule. However, thyroiditis is frequently accompanied by pain. Acute suppurative thyroiditis is rare and is due to bacterial infection of the thyroid gland. Infection may result from trauma, hematologic spread, or direct extension from a neck infection. Symptoms include malaise and severe pain that may extend to the ear. Diagnosis is made clinically and by needle aspiration.

Subacute thyroiditis is probably a viral disease. It is self-limited and lasts several weeks to several months. Malaise, fatigue, and an upper respiratory infection generally precede the development of neck pain that radiates to the ears. The thyroid gland is firm and tender. Diagnosis is based on the history and physical findings, an elevated sedimentation rate, and an initial elevation in triiodothyronine and thyroxine values. Symptomatic relief may be obtained with aspirin and steroids. Pain is not a prominent symptom of chronic thyroiditis.

Salivary glands may be a source of pain in the head and neck. Sudden distention of the gland caused by blockage will cause pressure and pain. Infection due to obstruction will also cause local pain, redness, and often toxicity. Purulent drainage may be seen from Stenson's (parotid) duct or Wharton's (submandibular) duct. Treatment includes hydration, antibiotics, and at times sialolithotomy. Chronic infections may require excision of the involved gland. Most tumors of the major salivary glands are painless unless they cause secondary obstruction. Adenoid cystic carcinomas are notorious, however, for perineural spread and may frequently present with pain and tenderness. Treatment is surgical excision. Although survival is prolonged, cures are unusual.

Neuromuscular pain and cervical spine pain are probably best dealt with by the neurologist or orthopedist. However, several syndromes of special interest seen in the neck will be mentioned here.

Grisel's syndrome is due to the subluxation of the atlantoaxial joint of the cervical vertebrae. The patient presents with pain and swelling in the superior neck and tilts his or her neck away from the affected side. The swelling may be easily confused with a tender lymph node. Treatment includes application of warmth, analgesics, and orthopedic evaluation.

Torticollis is a severe sustained contraction of the sternocleidomastoid muscle. It is usually unilateral and causes a tilting of the head and neck toward the involved side. It may be either congenital or acquired. In the congenital form, striated muscles are replaced by fibrous tissue. Acquired torticollis may result from trauma, inflammation, or a neuromuscular disorder (spasmodic torticollis) of either neurologic or psychological etiology.[36] There may be varying degrees of pain associated with torticollis.

Carotidynia is a painful carotid artery at its bifurcation. The etiology is unknown; however, it is important to be certain that there is no occlusive or neoplastic etiology. Additionally, the possibilities of true arteritis elsewhere in the head and neck should be investigated. Treatment consists of salicylates and warm soaks.

The thoracic outlet syndrome is caused by compression of the subclavian and axillary vessels. Symptoms include pain, paresthesias or numbness, and decreased circulation to the involved arm. The syndrome may be caused by compression from a cervical rib, a rudimentary first thoracic rib, subclavian artery aneurysm, neoplasm, or anterior scalene muscle compression. Treatment includes removal of the cause of compression.

References

1. Ty, T. C., Melzack, R., and Wall, P. D. Acute trauma. In Wall, P. D., and Melzack, R. (eds.). Textbook of Pain. New York, Churchill Livingstone, 1984, pp. 209–214.
2. Lisney, S. W. J. Current topics of interest in the physiology of trigeminal pain. J R Soc Med 76:292–296, 1983.
3. Hollinshead, W. H. The pharynx and larynx. In Hollinshead, W. H. (ed.). Anatomy for Surgeons: Head and Neck. Hagerstown, Md., Harper and Row, 1968, pp. 440–500.
4. Rushton, J. G., Stevens, J. C., and Miller, R. H. Glossopharyngeal neuralgia. Arch Neurol 38:201–205, 1981.
5. White, J. C., and Sweet, W. H. Pain and the Neurosurgeon. Springfield, Ill., Charles C Thomas, 1969.
6. Ragozzino, M. W., et al. A population-based study of herpes zoster and its sequelae. Medicine 61:310–316, 1982.
7. Denney, F. W., et al. Prevention of rheumatic fever. JAMA 143:151–153, 1950.
8. Wannamaker, L. W., et al. Prophylaxis of acute rheumatic fever by treatment of the preceding streptococcal infection with various amounts of depot penicillin. Am J Med 10:673–695, 1951.
9. Bisno, A. L. The rise and fall of rheumatic fever. JAMA 254:538–541, 1985.
10. Gates, G. A. Pharyngitis. In Johnson, J. T. (ed.). Antibiotic Therapy in Head and Neck Surgery. New York, Marcel Dekker, 1987, pp. 151–175.
11. Breese, B. B., and Disney, F. A. The accuracy of diagnosis of beta streptococcal infections on clinical grounds. J Pediatr 44:670–673, 1954.
12. Healey G. B. Pharyngitis. In Cummings, C. W., et al. (eds.). Otolaryngology—Head and Neck Surgery. St. Louis, C. V. Mosby, 1986, pp. 1185–1188.
13. Wiesner, P. J., et al. Clinical spectrum of pharyngeal gonococcal infection. N Engl J Med 288:181–185, 1973.
14. Jackson, G. G., and Muldoon, R. L. Viruses causing common respiratory infection in man. IV. Reoviruses and adenoviruses. J Infect Dis 128:811–866, 1973.
15. Antoon, J. W., and Miller, R. L. Aphthous ulcers—a review of the literature on etiology, pathogenesis, diagnosis and treatment. J Am Dent Assoc 101:803–808, 1980.
16. Blozis, G. B., and Allen, D. M. Oral mucosal lesions. In Cummings, C. W.,

et al. (eds.). Otolaryngology—Head and Neck Surgery. St. Louis, C. V. Mosby, 1986, pp. 1429–1448.
17. Laskaris, G., Sklavounou, A., and Stratigos, J. Bullous pemphigoid, cicatricial pemphigoid, and pemphigus vulgaris. Oral Surg 54:656–662, 1982.
18. Eagle, W. W. Elongated styloid process: Further observations and a new syndrome. Arch Otolaryngol 47:630–640, 1948.
19. Babbit, J. A. Fracture of the styloid process and its tonsil fossa complications, with report of a case. Ann Otol Rhinol Laryngol 42:789–798, 1933.
20. Conley, J. Concepts in Head and Neck Surgery. Stuttgart, G. Thieme Verlag, 1970.
21. Crawford, B. E., et al. Oral pathology. Otolaryngol Clin North Am 12:29–43, 1979.
22. Batsakis, J. G. Neoplasms of the minor and "lesser" major salivary glands. In Batsakis, J. G. (ed.). Tumors of the Head and Neck. Baltimore, Williams & Wilkins, 1979, pp. 76–99.
23. Doyle, P. J., and Stevens, H. E. Esophageal diverticula. In Cummings, C. W., et al. (eds.). Otolaryngology—Head and Neck Surgery. St. Louis, C. V. Mosby, 1986, pp. 2410–2416.
24. Dohlman, G., and Mattsson, L. The endoscopic operation for hypopharyngeal diverticula: A roentgencinematographic study. Arch Otolaryngol 71:744–752, 1960.
25. Tucker, J. A., and Yarington, C. T. The treatment of caustic ingestion. Otolaryngol Clin North Am 12:343–350, 1979.
26. Toomey, J. M. Cysts and tumors of the pharynx. In Paparella, M. M. and Shumrick, D. A. (eds.). Otolaryngology. Philadelphia, W. B. Saunders, 1980, pp. 2323–2342.
27. Donner, M. W., Saba, G. P., and Martinez, C. R. Diffuse diseases of the esophagus: A practical approach. Sem Roentgenol 16:198–213, 1981.
28. Suzuki, M., and Kirchner, J. A. Afferent nerve fibers in the external branch of the superior laryngeal nerve in the cat. Ann Otol Rhinol Laryngol 77:1059–1070, 1968.
29. Sasaki, C. T. Laryngeal physiology. In Bailey, B. J., and Biller, H. F. (eds.). Surgery of the Larynx. Philadelphia, W. B. Saunders Co., 1985, pp. 27–44.
30. May, M., Tucker, H. M., and Dillard, B. M. Penetrating wounds of the neck in civilians. Otolaryngol Clin North Am 9:361–391, 1976.
31. Acuna, R. T. Endoscopy of the air passages with special reference to scleroma. Ann Otol Rhinol Laryngol 82:765–769, 1973.
32. Montgomery, W. W., and Lofgren, R. H. Usual and unusual causes of laryngeal arthritis. Arch Otolaryngol 77:43–47, 1963.
33. Grossman, A., et al. Rheumatoid arthritis of the cricoarytenoid joint. Proc Canad Otol Soc 14:40–54, 1960.
34. Hollinshead, W. H. The pharynx and larynx. In Hollinshead, W. H. (ed.). Anatomy for Surgeons: Head and Neck. Hagerstown, Md., Harper and Row, 1968, pp. 440–500.
35. Lee, K. J., and Klein, T. R. Surgery of cysts and tumors of the neck. In Paparella, M. M., and Shumrick, D. A. (eds.). Otolaryngology. Philadelphia, W. B. Saunders, 1980, pp. 2987–2997.
36. Ramanurthy, S. Cervical pain. In Raj, P. P. (ed.). Practical Management of Pain. Chicago, Year Book, 1986, pp. 418–430.

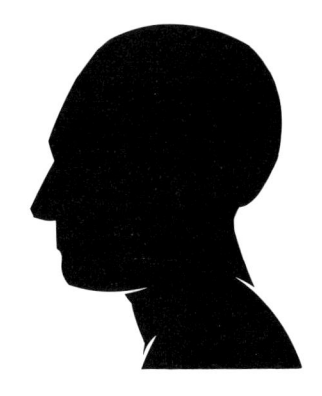

Chapter 8
Craniomandibular Disorders

Barry C. Cooper

Craniomandibular disorders can be defined as alterations in the morphology or function of the mandible with respect to both its articulation to the skull and the neuromuscular function associated directly or indirectly with that articulation. Craniomandibular disorders can be considered true medical diseases in that they cause a deviation or interruption in the normal structure or function of the stomatognathic system.[1]

Craniomandibular disorders can be classified for discussion into abnormalities within the temporomandibular joint (intrinsic disorders) and those occurring outside the joint (extrinsic disorders).[2] Extrinsic conditions may involve the mandible, skull, cervical vertebrae, and structures within the oral cavity as well as the muscles and connective tissues that support and move these structures.

Classifications of intrinsic and extrinsic disorders are often clinically difficult because each affects the other. This interaction may make the determination of a primary etiologic agent impossible, because examination of a patient may reveal the presence of both temporomandibular joint and musculoskeletal dysfunction.[3, 4]

In this chapter descriptions of both intrinsic and extrinsic diseases will be presented, including their clinical appearances, symptomatology, history, current diagnostic and therapeutic modalities, and prognosis. Because craniomandibular disorders affect the dental apparatus and are affected by changes in the dentition, references will be made to Chapter 6 (Intraoral Pain).

Extracapsular Disorders

Extracapsular disorders involve the musculoskeletal components of the entire craniomandibular system and the interrelationships between the neuromuscular system and the hard structures of the temporomandibular joints and dentition. Extracapsular craniomandibular disorders can be affected by and can affect the craniocervical system as well. These disorders are considered under the very nonspecific rubric of musculoskeletal dysfunction of the head and neck. Among these disorders is the myofacial pain dysfunction syndrome, which specifically applies to musculoskeletal disorders arising from an unhealthy functional relationship between the dental apparatus, the temporomandibular joints, and the neuromuscular system responsible for mandibular movement and posturing.

Intracapsular Disorders

Abnormalities within the temporomandibular joint (TMJ) include developmental and acquired aberrations. Developmental conditions include aplasia, hypoplasia, and hyperplasia of the mandibular condyle. Acquired abnormalities include traumatic injury, infection, inflammation, and neoplasm. Traumatic injury, inflammation, and subsequent degeneration are the most common acquired abnormalities within the temporomandibular joints.

Craniomandibular Disorders

Anatomy and Physiology of the Craniomandibular System

TEMPOROMANDIBULAR JOINT

To discuss diseases that affect the temporomandibular joint, it is necessary to describe the anatomy and physiology of this structure.[5,6] This section surveys the important anatomic and physiologic concepts relating to the joint (Figs. 8–1, 8–2).

The temporomandibular joints, left and right, are diarthrodial or synovial joints.[7] They are discontinuous articulations that permit movement between their component parts. The joints are surrounded by a fibrous capsule attached at the periphery of the articulating sufaces. The capsule's vascularization allows fluid interchange with the synovial fluid within the joint. The capsule is highly innervated and has numerous sensory receptors that are used for proprioceptive monitoring. The articular surfaces of the temporomandibular joint are composed not of hyaline cartilage, which is customarily found in synovial joints, but rather of nonvascularized and noninnervated, dense, fibrous connective tissue.

The condyle is the most superior posterior terminal projection of the mandible. It is an ovoid, cylindrical object, which is canted in such a way that its medial pole is situated more anterior and its lateral pole more superior. Each condyle fits into a concavity in the inferior surface of the petrous portion of the temporal bone. This concavity is called the *temporomandibular* or *glenoid fossa*. The fossa is lined with cartilage with the exception of the posterior wall that approximates the external auditory canal. The anterior portion of the fossa is called the *articular eminence*.

Craniomandibular Disorders

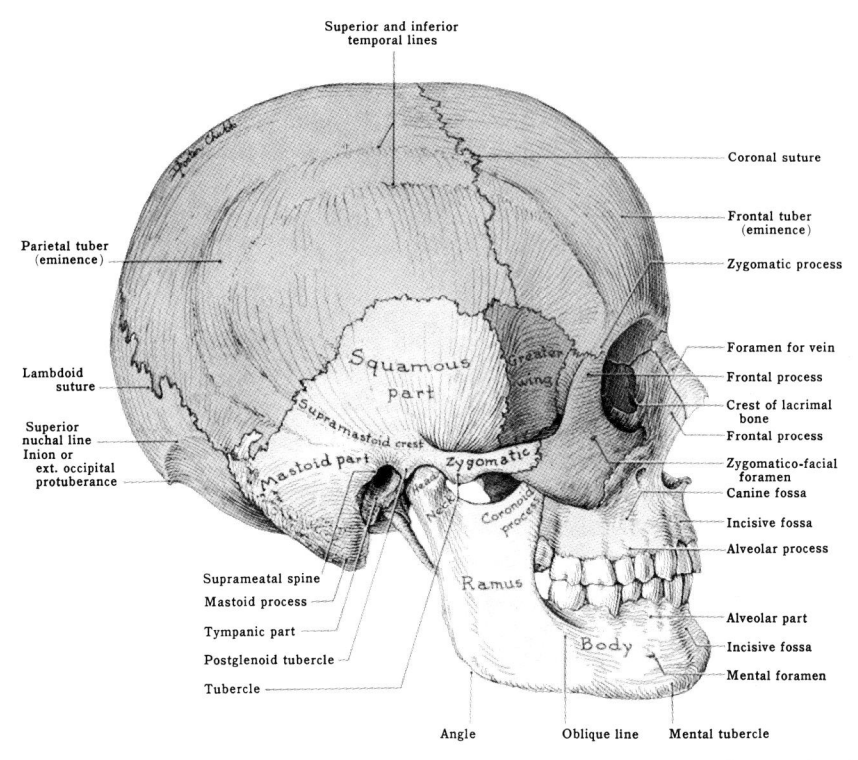

FIGURE 8–1. Lateral view of normal skull. (Note position of temporomandibular joint (TMJ) at posterior superior termination of mandible, anterior to external auditory meatus.) (From Anderson, J. (ed.). Grant's Atlas of Anatomy, 8th ed. Baltimore, The Williams & Wilkins Co., 1983.)

Interposed between the condyle and the fossa is a biconcave disk of fibrocartilage (dense fibrous connective tissue). The disk is attached medially and laterally to the joint capsule and condyle and posteriorly to the wall of the fossa by the retrodiskal tissue. This tissue is highly vascularized and innervated. Anteriorly, the disk attaches to the superior portion (belly) of the lateral pterygoid muscle.

All synovial joints are pressure-bearing joints. Normally, the articular surfaces of these joints are in contact at all times. In the case of the temporomandibular joints, the two bones are in contact with their respective approximating surfaces of the disk. Diarthrodial joint movement in general is limited by the articular surfaces, fibrous capsule, ligaments, and muscles. In the special case of the temporomandibular joints, the position and morphology of the articular disk also are limiting factors in mandibular movement, and hence in joint function. The interdigitation of the teeth also affects the positioning of the components of the temporomandibular joint.

The temporomandibular joints, left and right, are the most complex joints in the human body for two reasons. First, these joints are unique in permitting both rotational and translational movements owing to the dual articulation of the condyle within each joint. The condyle articulates with the inferior surface of the disk; the posterior portion of the articular eminence articulates with the superior surface of the disk. The temporomandibular joint is thus classified as a compound ginglimyoarthrodial joint, consisting of a ginglimyoid (hinge) joint and an arthrodial (sliding) joint.

Second, there are two joints (left and right), which are connected by a single bone (the mandible) and function simultaneously. Any movement of the mandible involves activity in both left and right joints. The movement in the two joints need not be the same in either direction or magnitude.

For example, in a horizontal rotation of the mandible toward the patient's right side, the left condyle rotates clockwise as it translates forward and

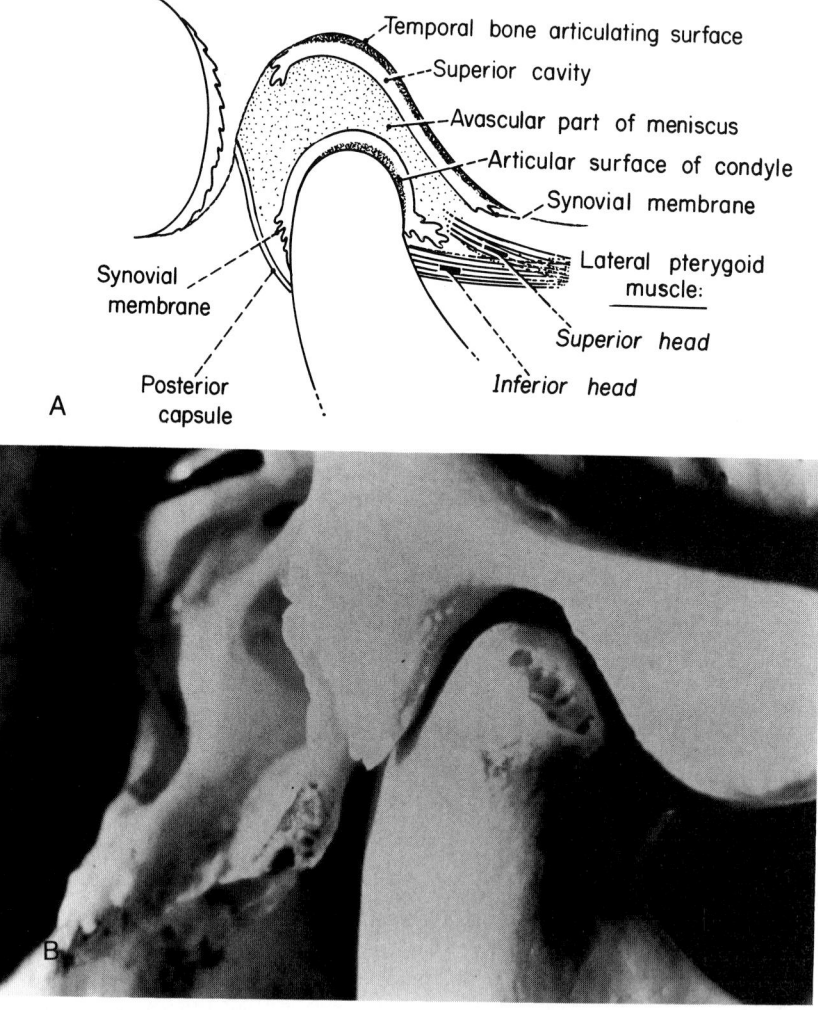

FIGURE 8–2. *A*, Schematic representation of the temporomandibular joint. *B*, Bony structures of the temporomandibular joint. (From Ramfjord, S., and Ash, M. M. (eds.). Occlusion, 3rd ed. Philadelphia, W. B. Saunders, Co., 1983.)

downward along the posterior surface of the articular eminence in its socket. The lateral pole of that condyle moves anteriorly and inferiorly, while its medial pole moves inferiorly and posteriorly. At the same time, in the right temporomandibular joint the condyle may not move bodily anteriorly or posteriorly, but merely rotates on its vertical axis with its lateral pole moving posteriorly and its medial pole moving anteriorly. This movement is opposite to the direction of motion of the poles of the left condyle. The disk is not stationary during this mandibular movement. It rotates about the head of the condyle with all mandibular movement in response to pulling force by the superior portion of the lateral pterygoid muscle, elastic resilience of the posterior attachment fibers, and mechanical compression between the condyle and the articular eminence. In normal healthy function all of these movements occur smoothly. This is obviously a complex mechanism: The variety of movements that can and must be made by the mandible in performing its functions of speech, expression, respiration, mastication, and deglutition of food and saliva require intricate coordination of function between the two joints and their components. This system is liable to trauma and dysfunction.

Development of the Temporomandibular Joint

There is an old maxim in medicine that states that form follows function. Moss described a functional matrix theory in which development responds to functional demands.[8,9] Joints have the capacity to undergo development and redevelopment, called *remodeling*, as an adaptational response to functional activity throughout life.

Phylogenetically, the temporomandibular joint is recent and is found only in mammals. It is not the same in humans as it is in other mammals because of both the vertical posture of humans and their dietary patterns. Some structures of the temporomandibular joint and ear are intimately related both developmentally and by common innervation. They are the tensor tympani muscle, the tensor veli palatini muscle, and the anterior malleolar ligament, known as Pinto's ligament.[10,11] The tensor tympani and the tensor veli palatini muscles are innervated by the mandibular division of the trigeminal nerve, which innervates most of the muscles responsible for mandibular function.

In the temporomandibular joints the shape of the condyle and articular eminence in the fetus is quite different from that in the newborn and developing child. In fetal life the swallowing reflex requires a purely rotational movement of the mandible. At that stage of development, the articular surfaces and the disk are vascularized and innervated. That situation changes after birth as compressive forces are applied to these tissues.

At birth the temporomandibular joint is in line with the occlusal plane of the dentition rather than above it as it is in the fully developed child. The articular eminence is flat, and the fossa behind it is shallow, a structure that is adequate for the hinge movement that existed before birth. With postpartum life, swallowing is accompanied by sucking and later chewing and speech, all of which require different movements of the mandible. The joint develops to accommodate these functions.

Remodeling is a process that occurs after development is completed. It is accomplished by selective addition and removal of tissues in response to mechanical and chemical stimuli. It is a normal physiologic, nonpathologic process that is a response to functional needs. It involves both hard and soft tissues. If the mechanical pressures or chemical irritants applied to the tissues exceed the remodeling capacity of the tissues, the delicate balance of adaptive response shifts toward pathology. This is known as degenerative joint disease. In its earliest stages it can be inflammatory, and in the later stages it involves destruction of hard and soft structures.

MUSCULOSKELETAL SYSTEM

The craniocervical skeletal system includes the skull, mandible, hyoid bone, laryngeal cartilages, and cervical vertebrae. The muscular system includes the masticatory muscles, facial muscles, and anterior, lateral, and posterior cervical muscles. The muscles primarily involved in mandibular function are collectively called the *muscles of mastication* and will be described in detail here.[12]

Although a more complete discussion of the cervical muscles can be found in Chapter 9, it is useful to discuss them here because they have functional interactions with the facial and masticatory muscles (Fig. 8–3).

Mandibular posture is affected both by the posture of the skull on the cervical spinal column and by the posture of the mandible itself in relation to the skull. The former is dictated to a large extent by the anterior, lateral,

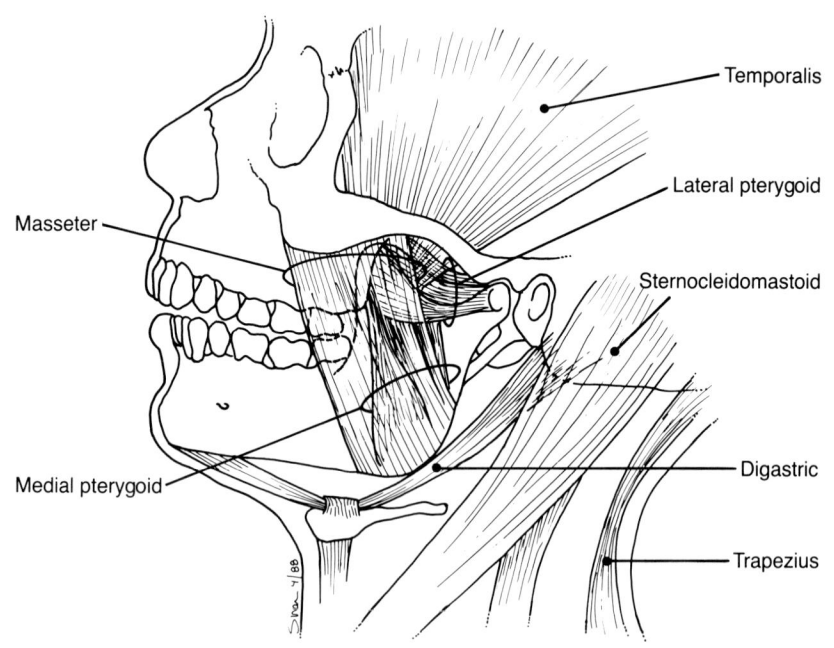

FIGURE 8–3. Mandibular masticatory and cervical muscles. (From Cooper, B. Myofacial pain dysfunction: Cause, clinical appearance and current therapy. Primary ENT 3(3):2–7, 1987. P.W. Communications Int. for Schering. Reproduced with permission.)

and posterior cervical muscles as well as by the trapezius and sternocleidomastoid muscles. The posture of the mandible itself—held at rest near the opposing maxillary arch—is accomplished by suspending the mandible in a dynamic sling of opposing muscle groups. The muscles are functionally grouped as either elevators or depressors.

The posturing and movement of the mandible cannot be considered solely in terms of activity in the masticatory musculature, independent of the entire craniocervical musculoskeletal system.[13] In fact, because the mandible moves during speech, respiration, deglutition, and mastication, its movement is part of coordinated reflex arcs and cerebral movement patterns that involve all of the craniocervical musculature.[14]

One can see a vivid example of this in the aged, in whom curvature of the cervical spinal column results in rounding of the shoulders and a forward, downward tilting of the head. As a compensatory mechanism for maintaining an adequate airway, the head is brought forward. Although this seemingly innocuous act by the posterior cervical muscles should have little effect of the mandible, the resulting head position puts increased tension of the suprahyoid muscles, pulling up on the hyoid bone and resulting in increased tension in the infrahyoid muscles to stabilize the hyoid bone.

In patients who have chronic nasal obstruction and are of necessity obviate mouth breathers, the mandible must be lowered in its resting postural position. The tongue, normally resting on the anterior palate, is dropped to the lower portion of the mouth, draping over the mandibular posterior teeth. The lips are parted, and the mouth is left open to provide an oral airway. This totally alters the normal resting posture of the mandible and all of the musculature of the stomatognathic system.

Mandibular Elevators and Depressors

The muscles of mastication are functionally grouped as mandibular elevators and mandibular depressors (Fig. 8–4). This grouping is an oversimplification, since smooth, fine, controlled movements of the mandible involve coordinated contraction and relaxation of antagonistic muscles bilaterally.[15]

The temporalis is a broad, fan-shaped, radiating muscle located on the lateral aspect of the skull. It arises from the entire temporal fossa and from the deep surface of the temporal fascia. The fibers of the temporalis muscle converge into a tendon, which passes deep to the zygomatic arch and inserts onto the mandible along the medial surface, apex, and anterior border of the coronoid process (the anterior superior terminal process of the mandible) as well as along the anterior border of the ramus of the mandible almost as far anteriorly as the most posterior molar. This muscle is a mandibular elevator. Its posterior fibers, nearly horizontal in position, act to retrude the mandible as it is elevated. The temporalis is innervated by the masseteric nerve from the mandibular division of the trigeminal nerve (cranial nerve V_3).

The masseter is a broad, thick muscle consisting of superficial and deep portions. The larger superficial portion originates on the inside of the zygomatic arch and the zygomatic process of the maxilla and inserts onto

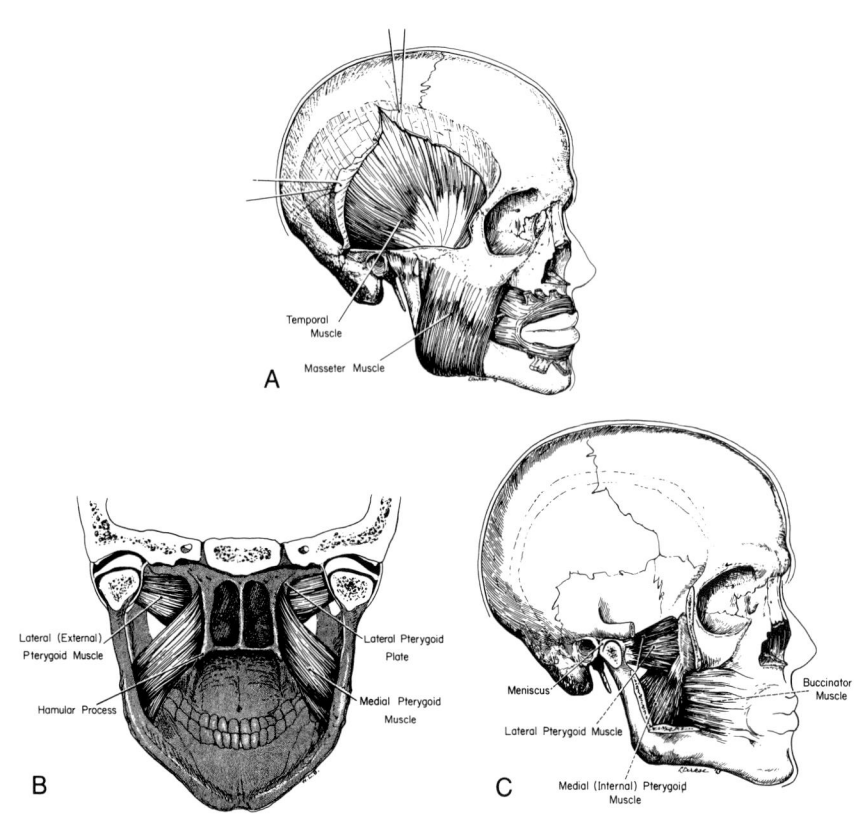

FIGURE 8–4. Masticatory muscles. *A*, Anatomic features of the temporalis and masseter muscles. *B*, Schematic representation of the medial and lateral pterygoid muscles (PA view). *C*, Medial and lateral pterygoid muscles, sagittal view. (From Ramfjord, S., and Ash, M. M. (eds.). Occlusion, 3rd ed. Philadelphia, W. B. Saunders Co., 1983.)

the angle and inferior surface of the ramus of the mandible. The deep portion of the masseter arises from the posterior third of the inferior border of the zygomatic process of the maxilla and the zygomatic arch and passes anteriorly, inserting into the superior half of the ramus and the lateral surface of the coronoid process. The masseter elevates the jaw. It is innervated by the masseteric nerve from the mandibular division of the trigeminal nerve (V_3).

The medial (internal) pterygoid is a thick, quadrilateral-shaped muscle located inside the ramus of the mandible in relatively the same position as the location of the masseter muscle outside the mandible. Together, the medial pterygoid and the masseter form a sling that supports the mandible. The medial pterygoid arises from the medial surface of the lateral pterygoid plate and the grooved surface of the pyramidal process of the palatine bone. It also has a second site of origin for a portion of the muscle, the lateral surface of the pyramidal process of the palatine and tuberosity of the maxilla. This second portion lies superficial to the lateral pterygoid muscle, whereas the main portion is located deep to the lateral pterygoid muscle.

The fibers of the medial pterygoid pass inferiorly, laterally, and posteriorly, inserting through a strong tendinous layer into the inferior posterior portion of the medial surface of the ramus and angle of the mandible. The medial surface of this muscle is closely related with the tensor veli palatini and the superior pharyngeal constrictor. The medial pterygoid muscle is a mandibular elevator that closes the mandible and is innervated by the medial pterygoid nerve, arising from the mandibular division of the trigeminal nerve (V_3).

The lateral (external) pterygoid is a short conical muscle, which runs almost horizontally between the infratemporal fossa and the condyle of the mandible (its most posterior, superior terminal projection). It has a superior and an inferior belly. The superior belly originates from the inferior part of the lateral surface of the great wing of the sphenoid and from the infratemporal crest. The inferior belly arises from the lateral surface of the lateral pterygoid plate. The fibers of the lateral pterygoid muscle run horizontally backward and laterally, with the inferior belly inserting into a depression in the anterior part of the neck of the mandibular condyle and the superior belly inserting into the anterior margin of the articular disk of the temporomandibular joint. The lateral pterygoid muscle acts to open the mouth by depressing and protruding the mandible and moving it laterally to the contralateral side. It is innervated by the lateral pterygoid nerve of the mandibular division of the trigeminal nerve (cranial nerve V_3).

In opening the mouth the lateral pterygoid muscle is assisted, at the beginning of the action, by the mylohyoid, digastric, and geniohyoid muscles. When the mandible is opened against resistance, the infrahyoid muscles are employed to stabilize the hyoid bone, establishing a stationary attachment for the suprahyoid muscles, which are actively involved in the opening process.

The suprahyoid muscles include the digastric, stylohyoid, mylohyoid, and geniohyoid muscles. All have attachments to the hyoid bone and act to move it. The digastric muscle is attached to the mandible and functions in the opening of the mouth. The digastric consists of two portions (bellies). The longer of the two, the posterior, arises from the mastoid notch of the temporal bone and passes anteriorly and inferiorly. The anterior belly arises from a depression on the inner surface of the inferior border of the mandible, close to the symphysis. It passes posteriorly and inferiorly. The two bellies, anterior and posterior, end in an intermediate tendon, which perforates the stylohoid muscle and has a fibrous connection to the hyoid bone. The action of the digastric is to raise the hyoid bone and assist in opening the mouth. The two bellies are innervated by different nerves and have different functions. The anterior belly draws the hyoid forward, whereas the posterior belly draws the hyoid backward. The anterior digastric is innervated by the inferior alveolar branch of the mandibular division of the trigeminal nerve (V_3). The posterior digastric is innervated by a branch of the facial nerve (cranial nerve VII). There are numerous anatomic variations in the digastric muscle, which will not be described here. It is recommended that an anatomy text be consulted for a comprehensive review of this complex anatomic region.

Hannam and co-workers are investigating the presence of distinct muscle groups within the mandibular muscles, which they feel are responsible for the precise functional movements of the mandible. Through the use of magnetic resonance imaging techniques, they are isolating these muscle subgroups.[16] The temporalis muscle attaches to the coronoid process of the mandible, which is the anterior terminal protuberance of the ascending ramus of the mandible. Hannam believes that it is the inner fibers of the anterior temporalis that contribute to the tenderness elicited by palpation of the area in the mouth described as the lateral pterygoid muscle. The area probably includes pterygoid and deep anterior temporalis muscle fibers.

History and Clinical Presentation

HISTORY

As with most illnesses, the history holds the key to a majority of diagnoses. Although clinical examination and bioelectronic testing play a large role in the confirmation of many of the diagnostic entities discussed here, the history provides definite clues to the etiology and natural history of the disease process.[17]

The history should include the patient's chief complaint and details from the past medical history that are relevant to that complaint. The examining physician should be cautioned, however, that a chief complaint may falsely localize the lesion to a particular organ when the pathologic lesion may be elsewhere. For example, a patient presenting with otalgia of 3 months duration may not have any otologic pathology but may instead have a pathologic lesion in the throat referred to the ear.

The interviewer should elicit the most definite historical information possible regarding the onset, duration, intensity, and changes in each presenting symptom. It is also important to note significant current or past medical conditions that may be relevant to the clinical picture.[18-20]

Patients presenting with complaints of chronic or atypical pain should be evaluated psychologically as well. A patient's current emotional or psychological state can influence the perception of pain and the reaction to pain. Likewise, chronic pain can have a profound effect on a patient's mood, affect, and perceptions.[21-28]

In eliciting a history of a craniomandibular disorder, it is particularly important to include any factors that may precipitate the pain or dysfunction. Patients should be questioned about events at the time of the onset of symptoms such as hyperextension of the mandible, medical or dental procedures involving the head and neck, or a specific traumatic episode. The interviewer should also inquire about possible noxious habits such as clenching and grinding of the teeth and postural habits that might be perpetuating factors in craniomandibular dysfunction.

Finally, the patient should be questioned about previous therapies and their effectiveness. This account should include a careful recounting of diagnostic tests, treatments, and medications that have been employed since the illness began.

CLINICAL PRESENTATION

The symptoms of temporomandibular joint dysfunction are pain, limitation of mandibular movement, sounds within the joint on mandibular movement, swelling, tenderness to palpation, and changes in dental occlusal relationships.

Temporomandibular joint pains have been described as somatic, deep, and of a musculoskeletal type. Such a description means that the pains are not neurogenic or psychogenic and are not cutaneous, visceral, or vascular. Pain in the temporomandibular joint can originate only in tissues that are innervated. These include the attachments of the disk (not the disk itself), the retrodiskal fibrous connective tissue, and the joint capsule. The articular surfaces of the condyle and the articular eminence are not innervated normally and therefore cannot be a source of pain unless the continuity of the surface has been destroyed, uncovering innervated bone below. Temporomandibular joint pains have, therefore, been classified as disk attachment pain, retrodiskal pain, capsular pain, and arthritic pain.

The clinical presentation of musculoskeletal disorders is far more varied than that of intrinsic joint disorders. Patients may present with isolated spontaneous pains seemingly unrelated to mandibular function or with muscular pain directly related to chewing, speaking, and yawning. Common symptoms include headaches, otalgia, muffled ears, pain in the area of the joints, facial and cervical pain, limited mandibular movement or opening, bruxism, and jaw clenching.[29-43] These disorders are discussed in more detail later in this chapter.

Clinical Examination

Clinical examination for craniomandibular disorders takes only a few minutes and can be performed by a physician or a dentist.[44-46] For the physician who is already performing an examination of the head and neck, the additional information that can be obtained from this enhanced examination will take a little extra time and provide valuable data. For the dentist who is performing an intraoral examination, the extraoral examination will likewise provide valuable diagnostic information.

OBSERVATION OF THE HEAD

Observe the position of the patient's head when viewed frontally and sagittally. Note the general body posture including curvature of the back, neck, and level of the shoulders and hips. Is the head level, or is it tilted laterally or tipped forward? Are the shoulders level, or is one higher (Fig. 8–5)? Does the neck have a normal curvature, and is the back straight? Look for symmetry or asymmetry in the facial contours, including the level and shape of the eyes and the lips. Ask the patient to rotate the head, observing indications of limitation, lack of fluidity, or discomfort associated with rotation and roll of the head.

OPENING AND CLOSING MOVEMENTS

Instruct the patient to open the mouth to the widest comfortable extent. Measure the distance between the incisal edges of the maxillary and

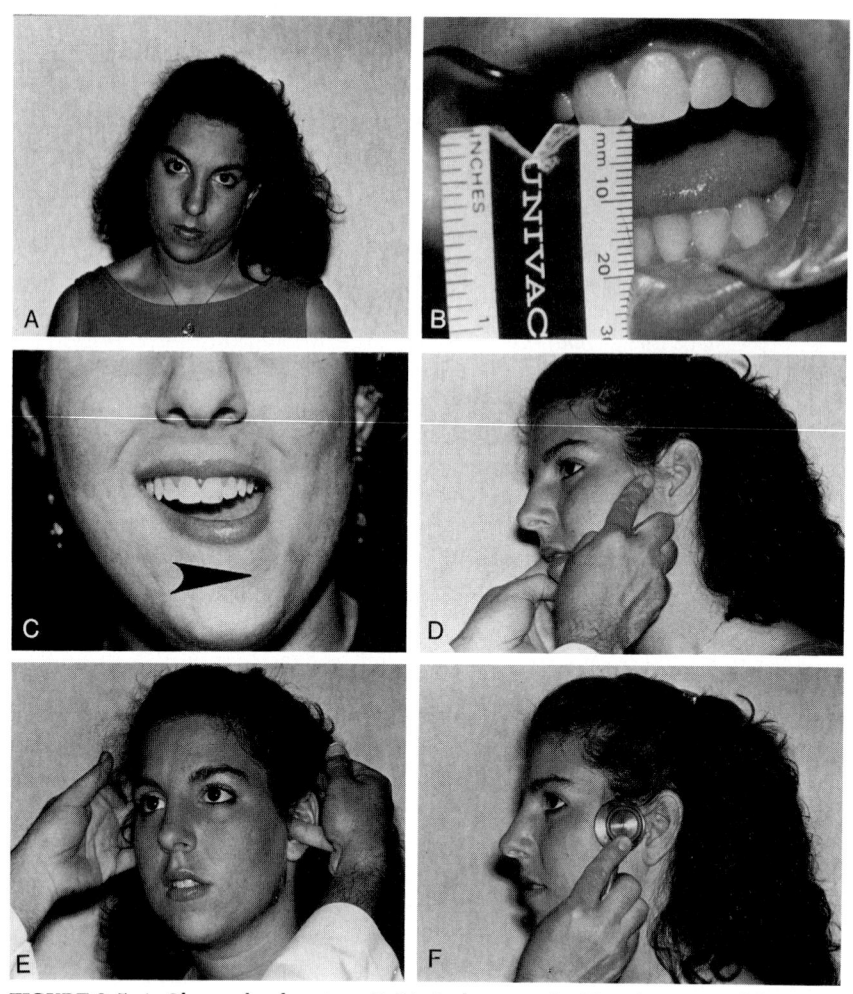

FIGURE 8–5. *A*, Observe head posture. *B*, Limited opening (< 35 mm). *C*, Lateral deviation on opening (arrow). *D*, Temporomandibular joint examination. *E*, External auditory canal. *F*, Listening for temporomandibular joint sounds with stethoscope.

mandibular central incisors. Healthy patients can typically open the mouth 35 to 50 mm, measured incisally (Fig. 8–5B).

While the patient opens wide and closes several times, observe any lateral deviations (Fig. 8–5C). These can be noted by comparing the opening with a vertical line, which you can provide with the edge of a 6-inch ruler used to measure the opening. Asymmetrical movement demonstrates bilateral imbalance in translational movement of the two condyles down the posterior slope of the articular eminences and is associated with either muscle dysfunction or internal derangement in the temporomandibular joint. The mandible often deviates to the side of greater dysfunction because opening is more limited on that side compared to the contralateral side. If equal dysfunction exists, this lateral deviation may not be seen. Muscle testing, which will be described later, can corroborate a muscle spasm associated with the deviate movement.

Fluidity and velocity of the opening and closing movements are also observed. Healthy muscle function together with normal joint function should permit smooth and rapid movements. Irregular, staggered (dyskinesic) movements or slow (bradykinesic) movements indicate muscle dysfunction (Fig. 8–6). The patient's facial expression as well as the verbal response often indicates painful movements. Patients' eyes also can show signs of discomfort.

MANDIBULAR EXCURSIVE MOVEMENTS
To analyze the various movements of the mandible associated with proper function, gently hold the lips apart with the index finger and thumbs of both hands while requesting the patient to bite down on the back teeth. From the posterior biting position, referred to as habitual centric occlusion (HCO) or intercuspal position (ICP), instruct the patient to slide the jaw forward while maintaining light tooth contact until the upper and lower teeth meet edge to edge, as if to bite a thread. Observe the relative position of the midlines of the upper and lower teeth in the initial posterior biting position and that in the protruded anterior position (Fig. 8–7). Note whether there is any pain associated with these movements either in the muscles or the joints.

Deviation to one side during protrusion of the mandible demonstrates more restriction of translation of the condyle on the side toward which the mandible deflects. Total symmetrical restriction of mandibular protrusion demonstrates bilateral equality of restriction. Once again, the restriction may have a muscular cause or may relate to internal derangements within the temporomandibular joint. If the examiner can cause pain by placing his hand against the patient's chin to resist protrusion, muscle spasm is likely to be the cause of the restricted or painful protrusion observed. Concerning the midlines of the anterior teeth, it should be noted that there need not

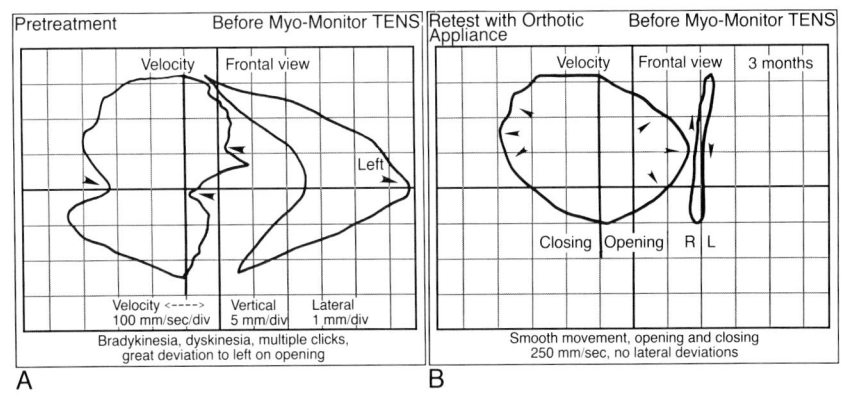

FIGURE 8–6. Mandibular kinesiograph (MKG) recordings of velocity of mandibular movement in opening and closing (left image) and frontal tracing during opening and closing (right image). *A*, Pretreatment velocity test demonstrates clicks on opening and closing (arrows). Frontal tracing shows marked deviation to left on opening. *B*, Following therapy, velocity is smooth with no clicks and no lateral deviation on opening. Patient was a 21-year-old female, whose mandibular dysfunction followed endodontic therapy (prolonged mandibular hyperextension) several months before. She also complained of jaw locking and temporomandibular joint pain.

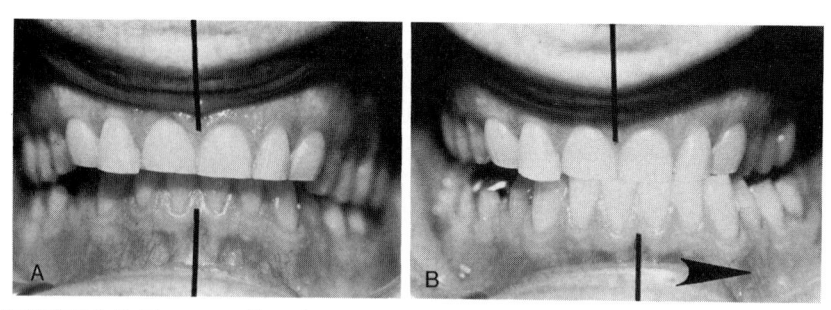

FIGURE 8–7. Observe midline change on protrusion of the mandible. *A*, Relative positions of midlines in habitual (natural) occlusion. *B*, Mandibular midline deflected to the left on protrusion of the mandible. Deflection is usually toward the side of more severe joint or muscle dysfunction.

be symmetry of the midlines of the upper and lower teeth. It is the change in the relative position of the two midlines in the habitual (posterior) and protruded (anterior) positions that is significant. This change is also observed in the wide opening movements. Question the patient about pain or tightness associated with this protrusive maneuver.

To complete the analysis of excursive mandibular movements, request the patient to move the jaw fully to the left and then to the right while keeping the teeth lightly in contact. Inability to perform lateral movement or temporomandibular joint pain associated with lateral excursion may indicate muscle dysfunction, usually in the lateral pterygoid muscles. These are the depressor or opening muscles, which by their position and angulation move the mandible anteriorly and down the slope of the articular eminence. Each lateral pterygoid moves the mandible to the contralateral side. The combined bilateral contraction of the lateral pterygoids results in a symmetrical anterior movement. If one of these muscles is in spasm the protrusive movement will deviate to the contralateral side with its joint acting only as a pivotal point. Once again, lateral deviations may be caused by either muscle dysfunction, joint dysfunction, or both.

TEMPOROMANDIBULAR JOINT EXAMINATION

Palpate the temporomandibular joints bilaterally with your index fingers, asking the patient to open the mouth wide and then close it (Fig. 8–5D). Observe any pain on palpation, swelling, and fluctuance. Question the patient about pain that occurs without palpation as well as pain associated with normal movement of the mandible, such as in eating, yawning, and speaking.

Pain in the ears is a common presenting complaint in patients with craniomandibular diseases. Otologic pathology must be ruled out if any ear-related complaint is made. Ear pain may be caused by pain in the temporomandibular joints or in the muscle system. Travell indicates that the area of the temporomandibular joint is a target area for trigger points in the lateral pterygoid muscles.[47, 48] The muscles in the ear and those associated with the function of the temporomandibular joint have a common innervation. The tensor tympani muscle is innervated by the fifth cranial nerve, as are the mandibular muscles. The tensor veli palatini, which is responsible for opening the pharyngeal end of the eustachian tube, is also innervated by the trigeminal nerve.[49-51]

Palpation of the external auditory canal has historically been part of the examination performed to determine temporomandibular joint dysfunction. The anterior wall of the ear canal is palpated with the ventral portion of the little finger of each hand (Fig. 8–5E). Press forward and observe whether that maneuver causes pain. Then instruct the patient to open wide and close on the back teeth. You may actually feel pressure against your fingers as the condyle presses posteriorly against the retrodiskal tissues. Pain may be elicited as well. You may also feel movement of the condyle-disk complex as a click. This click is sometimes palpable even if it is not audible with the stethoscope placed over the temporomandibular joint. The posterior wall of the temporomandibular fossa is so thin that a light, placed in the external auditory meatus can shine through it in a skull.

A patient may have temporomandibular joint dysfunction without palpable condylar pressure or pain. This is true of each of the clinical signs and presenting symptoms. Every one of the clinical signs and symptoms need not be present at the time of examination in order to make a clinical diagnosis.

TEMPOROMANDIBULAR JOINT SOUNDS
Sounds in the joint accompanying mandibular movement are a sign of dysfunction. Even with a stethoscope, the examining physician cannot always hear these sounds (Fig. 8–5F). Recently, more sophisticated instrumentation, including the Doppler and electric stethoscopes, have been used for observing sounds in the joint.

The most common joint sound observed is clicking, which can be caused by one of three phenomena. The first involves recapturing a disk. If the condylar position in the fossa is sufficiently displaced posteriorly, the disk that is supposed to be interposed between the condyle and the inferior surface of the fossa can become displaced anteriorly. As the mandible translates anteriorly with mouth opening, the disk may become recaptured, returning to its proper position on top of the condyle. As the condyle slips under the thickened posterior portion of the disk, a click may be heard. Conversely, as the mouth is closed and the teeth are returned to an occlusal position, the mandible is again displaced posteriorly, and the disk is returned to its anteriorly displaced position. This also may be accompanied by a click. Clicking on opening and closing is called *reciprocal clicking*. Many variations in observable clicks due to recapturing displaced disks occur. The timing of the clicks relative to the mandibular position is significant.[15, 52] Often clicks are observed on opening but not on closing. This may be due to the disk being gradually squeezed out on closing rather than to the abrupt snapping under the disk that occurs on opening. Reciprocal clicks are usually observed early in the opening cycle and late in the closing portion of the cycle.

A second cause of temporomandibular joint click is the passing of the condyle-disk unit beyond the prominence of the articular eminence or tubercle. This click does not represent recapture of a displaced disk but rather hyperextension of the mandible beyond the normal limits of the joint. It occurs near the widest opening and again at the beginning of the closing portion of the cycle.

The third cause of clicking, not frequently found, involves irregularity in the soft tissue lining of the posterior slope of the articular eminence, which articulates with the upper surface of the disk. As the mandible translates forward, it must ride down the eminence. If the lining of the eminence is thickened and irregular, a sound may be produced.

Crepitus or crackling indicates the presence of a destructive process within the joint and is caused by the rubbing together of bony structures. It signifies that either the integrity of the disk has been breached or that the disk, normally interposed between the condyle and the fossa, has been displaced, permitting direct contact between the bones. The bones in such a condition may undergo arthritic changes, becoming flattened or irregular, losing cortical substance, or sustaining osteophytic deposition. Crepitus is considered a sign of degenerative joint disease.

MUSCLE PALPATION

In a simple manner, all of the intraoral and extraoral muscles that move the mandible and skull can be palpated. Pain or tenderness on manual palpation demonstrates muscle hyperactivity or spasm. A 1 to 4 rating scale of intensity of pain on palpation may be utilized, No. 1 representing mild discomfort and No. 4 severe pain.

The intraoral examination begins with the lateral pterygoid muscle on the right side. Have the patient open the mouth wide. Press the soft tissue posterior and superior to the upper right last molar with your right index finger (Fig. 8–8A). You are pressing on fibers of the medial pterygoid superficially and the lateral pterygoid deep to that. The lateral pterygoid is a very significant muscle because it is most often tender to palpation in the patient with myofacial pain dysfunction.

The medial pterygoid muscle is palpated by pressing the tissue posterior and inferior to the last lower molar in the area of the inner aspect of the angle of the mandible (Fig. 8–8B). The attachment of the medial pterygoid is often tender in patients with myofacial pain disorder, although not as exquisitely tender as the lateral pterygoid.

Move anteriorly along the floor of the mouth and press downward on the mylohyoid muscle (Fig. 8–8C). Complete the intraoral muscle examination by pressing the masseter muscle between the forefinger on the inside and the thumb on the outside of the cheek, moving from its zygomatic attachment to its insertion on the outer aspect of the angle of the mandible (Fig. 8–8D). The masseter is usually quite large in patients who clench or grind (bruxism). It is not as frequently tender to palpation as the pterygoids because it is not a postural muscle, being utilized more for chewing and occluding the teeth in swallowing and in parafunctional actions such as clenching. More will be said about this muscle later in the discussion of electromyographic studies of muscles.

Craniomandibular Disorders

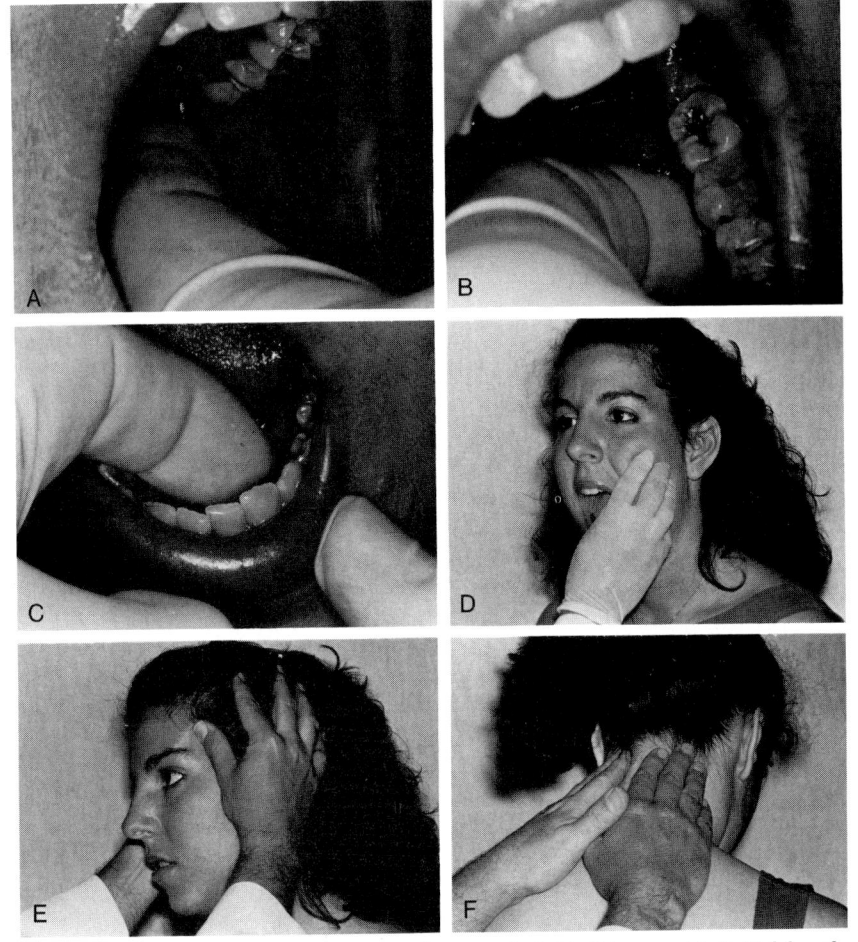

FIGURE 8–8. Muscle examination. *A*, Lateral pterygoid. *B*, Medial pterygoid. *C*, Mylohyoid. *D*, Masseter. *E*, Temporalis. *F*, Posterior cervical.

This intraoral four-muscle examination should be repeated on the left side of the patient's mouth, using the left hand.

The extraoral muscle examination can be performed bilaterally. Place both hands on the sides of the patient's head, fanning out your fingers, to palpate the full extent of the temporalis muscles (Fig. 8–8E). Beginning with your index fingers, press on the anterior fibers, located between the eyebrow and the beginning of the hairline. Ask the patient to clench the posterior teeth together to assist you in locating the fibers of the anterior temporalis. Proceed posteriorly, finger by finger, palpating all of this muscle through its posterior fibers, which are located above and just behind the ear. The temporalis muscle is the most important posturing muscle of the mandible, the most posterior fibers being more active when the occlusal position is most posteriorly displaced.

Palpate the posterior cervical muscles, beginning on the occiput and proceeding downward (Fig. 8–8F). Spasm in the posterior cervical muscles can cause stiffness in the neck and headaches in the occipital region that may radiate to the top of the skull. Spasm in the lateral cervical muscles may also limit cervical movement and, through pressure on the brachial plexus, may result in abnormal sensation in the arms and fingers.[53]

Palpate the sternocleidomastoid muscle between the forefinger and thumb from the mastoid process to the sternum (Fig. 8–9A). Limited ability to rotate and roll the head, which may have been observed at the beginning of this examination, may result from spasms in the sternocleidomastoid muscles.

The broad trapezius muscles can be palpated between the thumbs and other four fingers of each hand (Fig. 8–9B). Examine the suprahyoid and infrahyoid muscles. The mylohyoids attach to the mandible and are involved

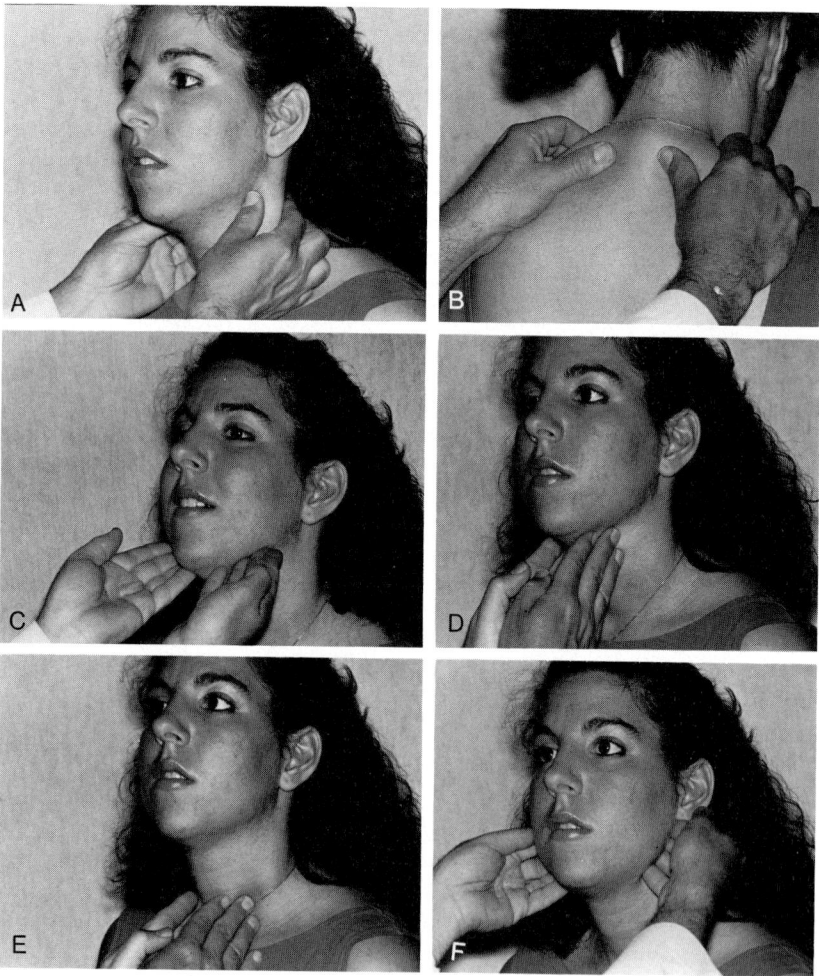

FIGURE 8–9. Muscle examination. *A*, Sternocleidomastoid. *B*, Trapezius. *C* and *D*, Suprahyoids. *E*, Infrahyoids. *F*, Angle of the mandible.

in opening the mouth. The stylohyoid is attached to the styloid bone, which projects from the undersurface of the skull, and the hyoglossus muscle attaches to the tongue. These muscles are therefore intimately associated with mandibular function, tongue activity, and cranial position. Abnormalities in any of these muscles affect tone in the suprahyoid muscles, which may in turn become dysfunctional and painful. Patients sometimes experience a cramp beneath the chin on wide opening of the mouth (Fig. 8–9C and D). Such a cramp is due to spasm in the suprahyoid muscles. These muscles should be palpated as well as the infrahyoids (Fig. 8–9E). Spasm in the infrahyoid and intercostal muscles may cause patients to complain of superficial chest pain or difficulty taking deep breaths. The infrahyoid muscles may become fatigued owing to prolonged stretching as the hyoid is elevated by foreshortened suprahyoids associated with mandibular overclosure.

Palpate the angle of the mandible with four fingers of each hand (Fig. 8–9F). Tenderness in this area indicates the presence of muscle spasm. The digastric, stylohyoid, and medial pterygoid muscles traverse this area, which is commonly tender to palpation in myofacial pain dysfunction patients. The parotid gland also is located in this area, and glandular pathology must be considered in a differential diagnosis. The angle of the mandible is commonly tender to palpation, although not as frequently as the pterygoid muscles.

INTRAORAL EXAMINATION

Many symptoms of extrinsic craniomandibular disorders involve the teeth and their supporting structures. Ask the patient to bite together on the back teeth in the normal bite that would accompany swallowing. A severely deep overbite in which the upper anterior teeth almost completely cover the lower anterior teeth may indicate an overclosed occlusive position (Fig. 8–10A and B). This position is also called a reduced vertical dimension of occlusion. Since the mandible hinges on the condyles in their temporomandibular joints, an overclosure of the mandible to reach the occlusal position may be accompanied by a posterior displacement of the condyle in the temporomandibular joint.

There are anatomic and developmental relationships between the contents of the temporomandibular joint and the ear. Unhealthy relationships

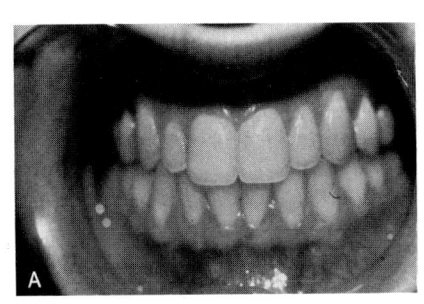

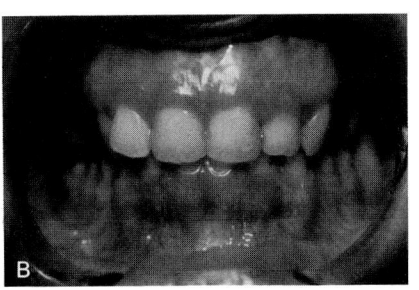

FIGURE 8–10. Intraoral examination. *A*, Normal anterior overbite. *B*, Deep overbite (overclosure of the mandible).

in the temporomandibular joint may be manifest as otologic symptoms because of the proximity of these structures and their common innervation. Palpation of the anterior wall of the external auditory canal, which was described in the extraoral examination procedure, is performed to determine whether the condyle is indeed palpable or to determine whether inflammation in the retrodiskal tissue exists.

It should be noted that all clinical signs and symptoms of myofacial pain dysfunction need not be present for the physician to make an initial clinical diagnosis of myofacial pain dysfunction. For example, a visible deep overbite with hidden lower anterior teeth need not exist, yet the position of dental occlusion might still result in a posteriorly displaced condyle, which can be observed on lateral transcranial radiographs.

The teeth in the position of occlusion, whether virgin natural teeth, artificially restored teeth, or orthodontically repositioned teeth, may appear to be in an ideal interdigitated position but may require unhealthy, strained, fatiguing muscle contraction to sustain it, resulting in myofacial pain dysfunction or at least a predisposition to it. Examine the lower arch of teeth, looking for a two-tiered occlusal plane (Fig. 8–11A). Is there an even curved plane to the entire arch of mandibular teeth or a sharp drop behind the six anterior teeth, with the bicuspids and molars on a lower plane? A two-tiered (bilevel) occlusal plane develops owing to downward pressure of the tongue on the lower teeth during the years of tooth eruption. It probably occurs during the time of deciduous (primary) tooth eruption.

In the healthy state the tongue lies in the center of the oral cavity gently touching the anterior palate. In the absence of a patent nasal airway, the mouth assumes the role of portal for respiration.[54, 55] The mouth is then usually open, the tongue assuming an unhealthy position covering the lower posterior teeth. This position permits air flow above the tongue but acts as a deterrent to normal eruption of the mandibular posterior teeth (Fig. 8–11B). It may also tilt the posterior teeth toward the tongue. Lingual tipping of the posterior lower teeth is often observed on clinical examination within the mouth (Fig. 8–11C). The unhealthy tongue position required for oral breathing may also result in a diminution in the normal lateral development of the palate and produce a characteristic scalloped lateral border of the tongue (Fig. 8–11D). In the healthy nasal breathing state, the tongue exerts a lateral force on the developing palate, resulting in the normal shallow roof of the mouth. In contrast, the mouth breather develops a narrow, constricted dental arch, a steeply vaulted palate, and a high nasal floor (Fig. 8–11E and F). The nasally obstructed obligate mouth breather also develops a decreased nasal air flow capacity. Here is an example of a functional disturbance, nasal obstruction, which can cause an oral cavity developmental abnormality, which in turn can result in a further functional disturbance, the overclosure of the mandible into occlusion. This abnormality may ultimately result in myofacial pain dysfunction or temporomandibular joint problems as well as cervical disorders. All of the systems interact.

The absence of posterior teeth in the maxilla or mandible, or both, either bilaterally or unilaterally, may result in both temporomandibular

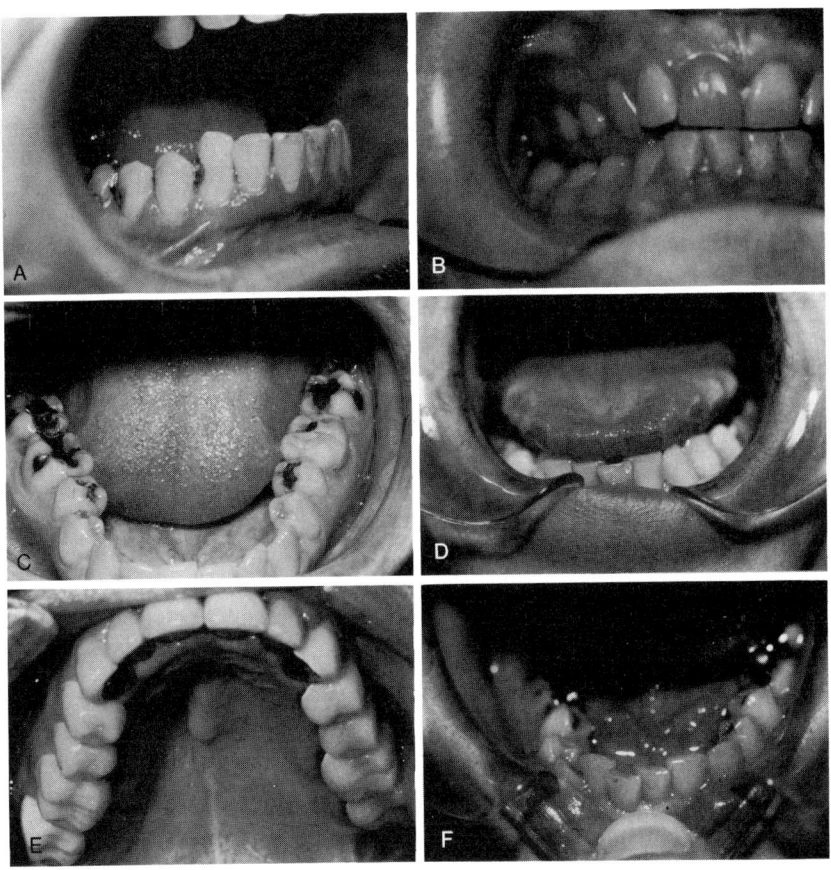

FIGURE 8-11. Oral breathing. Chronic placement of the tongue over the mandibular posterior teeth to provide an oral airway in patients with nasal obstruction can result in suppression of normal eruption of dentition. *A*, Two-tiered occlusal plane with posterior teeth depressed. *B*, Tongue placed between posterior teeth prevents normal eruption. *C*, Lingual (inward) tipping of the posterior teeth results from tongue pressure. *D*, Serrated lateral surface of tongue results from pressure against the surface of the posterior teeth. *E*, High vaulted palate with constricted dental arch is due to absence of normal tongue pressure, which acts as an outward counterbalance to muscle forces in the cheeks, which press inwardly. *F*, Narrow dental arch with lingually inclined posterior teeth.

joint disturbance and muscle dysfunction (Fig. 8–12).[56] It creates an unstable condition within the temporomandibular joint, which is built to function with the teeth in occlusion as an end-point in closing. Without teeth in the posterior region of the oral cavity, the muscles and soft tissues of the temporomandibular joint must support and stabilize the mandible. The absence of stability in the dental occlusal position is also a factor in the development of myofacial pain dysfunction in children. Youngsters go through a period in which teeth are being lost through exfoliation and new teeth are erupting into the oral cavity. This stage, called *mixed dentition*, is frequently associated with an unstable occlusal relationship composed of deciduous teeth, permanent teeth, and some missing ones as well (Fig. 8–13). Fortunately, most children are very adaptive and do not develop signs

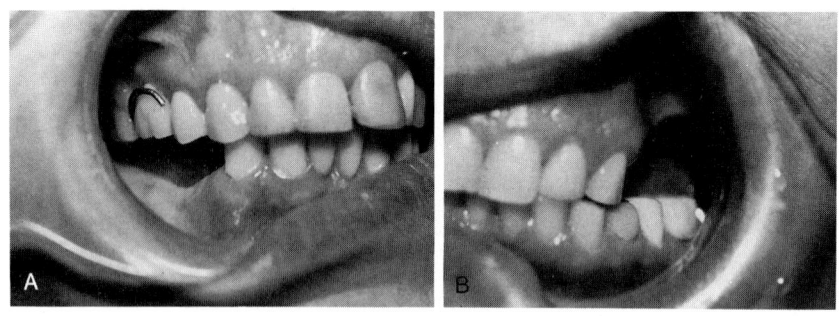

FIGURE 8–12. Missing posterior teeth (mandibular *A* or *B* maxillary) leave the mandible unsupported in occlusion, resulting in pressure within the temporomandibular joints.

and symptoms of myofacial pain dysfunction, which would be expected of an unstable occlusion. The possibility of myofacial pain dysfunction in a differential diagnosis in a child or adolescent should not be overlooked.[57, 58]

Instability in the dental occlusion may also result from flattened occlusal surfaces of the posterior teeth. This flattening may be caused by parafunctional grinding or clenching habits, the wear of artificial teeth restorations or denture teeth, or the fabrication of dental crowns, fillings, or denture teeth lacking in normal anatomic morphology (Fig. 8–14A and B). When flat teeth meet, the mandible must be muscularly braced to stabilize it to accompany the swallowing reflex. This is as fatiguing as bracing your legs on icy sidewalks when wearing smooth leather-soled shoes. Proper interdigitation of teeth requires far less muscle activity to stabilize the mandible

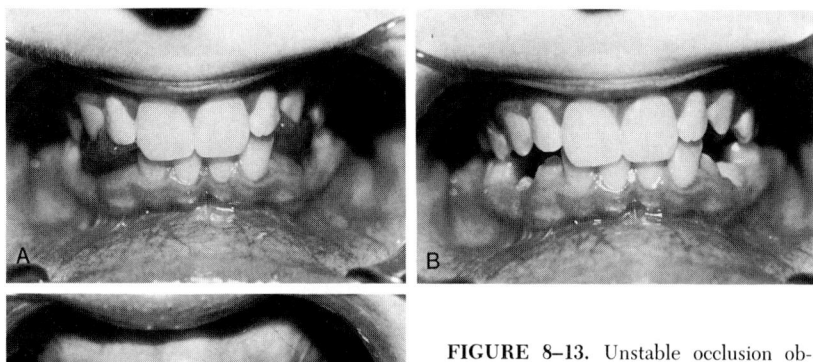

FIGURE 8–13. Unstable occlusion observed in child with mixed dentition (deciduous and permanent teeth). *A*, Tongue braces or stabilizes the mandible during swallowing, possibly resulting in *B*, Lateral tongue thrust habit. *C*, Locked occlusion in a child due to anterior crossbite can result in muscle fatigue because it restricts free entry into occlusion.

Craniomandibular Disorders

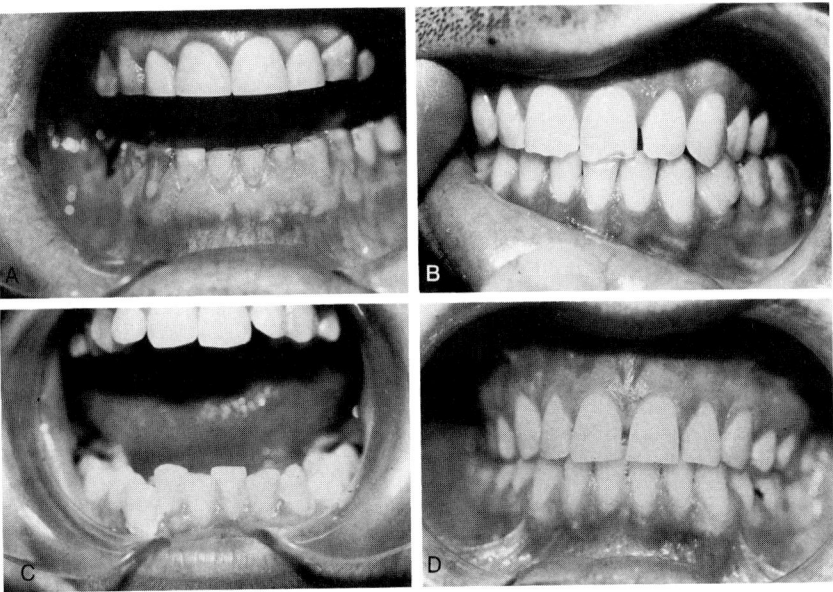

FIGURE 8–14. Muscle hyperactivity can cause pressure on teeth, resulting in the following conditions: *A*, Wear on anterior teeth (middle-aged adult). *B*, Worn anteriors in an 18-year-old. *C*, Crowding of mandibular (lower) anteriors as mandible is forced against the upper teeth due to muscle forces. *D*, Spreading maxillary (upper) anteriors in postorthodontic patient.

and is therefore less muscularly fatiguing. This concept will be discussed in detail in the therapy section.

The anterior teeth can reveal a great deal about the muscular health of the occlusion. The six mandibular teeth may show wear or crowding, which is indicative of a forward thrust of the mandible (Fig. 8–14C). If it occurs during bruxing, the same movement can force the maxillary anterior teeth apart (Fig. 8–14D). When these signs are observed, the patient should be questioned about:

1. Bruxing or clenching habits during the day or while asleep. A spouse often alerts the patient about the scratching noise, like chalk on a blackboard, which this habit produces. Patients often report a tired or stiff jaw in the morning on awakening. This can signify a night clenching or grinding habit.

2. Crowded, spread, or loose teeth. Ask whether these have been present for a considerable time or have been just recently observed, indicating changes. These signs too can be caused by pressure of the mandible against the maxilla, due to either muscle forces displacing the mandible from its tooth entrapment or merely nocturnal behavior patterns. Research on the interrelationships of bruxism, dream cycles, and REM activity is now being carried out. A great deal has been written about bruxism as a manifestation of emotional tension. This connection may be partially true, but such hyperactivity and muscular fatigue occur in the mandibular muscles because they are predisposed to spasm. The use to

which these muscles have been put in bringing about occlusion of the teeth produces this potentially explosive condition.

3. Finally, question the patient about recent breakage of fillings, teeth, crowns, or dentures. Such breakage indicate the presence of excessive maxillomandibular pressures, a sign of muscle hyperactivity, engendering potential fatigue and spasm.

Observe whether the patient has had modifications to the natural dentition, which could include single or multiple teeth reconstructed by fillings or crowns. Natural tooth structure may also have been modified by abrasion, either through bruxing or clenching or by dentists attempting to balance or equilibrate the bite, known as *coronoplasty*. Modifications to the dental occlusion may also be the result of orthodontic treatment.

If the patient reports painful teeth, find out whether a dentist recently performed an examination. Referred pain from other sites can be perceived as specific or vague dental pain in the absence of any dental problem. Seek dental consultation if doubt exists.

All these types of dentition, from natural virgin teeth to complete artificial dentures, or all of the other occlusal situations just enumerated, esthetic or unesthetic, may appear to mesh or interdigitate ideally or poorly. The key factor, which is not visible, is the effect of the existing occlusion on the delicate balance between neuromuscular function, the teeth themselves, and the temporomandibular joints. Clues to this effect are gained by palpating the muscles and the temporomandibular joint and observing mandibular movements.

SUMMARY OF CLINICAL EXAMINATION

The examination of the head and neck for signs of craniomandibular disorders involves observation of mandibular, head, and neck movements, palpation of the musculature and temporomandibular joints, auscultation of the joints for aberrant sounds, and observation of the dentition (Tables 8–1, 8–2). Deviations from normal jaw motions or pain on routine motions can be considered signs of craniomandibular disease, as can tenderness to palpation of the soft tissues. The mandibular muscles that provide the most important signs on palpation are the lateral and medial pterygoids and the temporalis.

The examination for craniomandibular disease must include an intraoral examination. Observe signs of wear on the teeth; look for missing posterior support in the absence of posterior teeth. Note whether the occlusion consists of crowns, natural teeth, or dentures, and if crowding of lower anterior or spreading of upper anterior teeth exists. Look for signs of wear or beveling on the incisal edges of the same anterior teeth and the plane of occlusion from anterior to posterior.

Failure to see any of these telltale signs does not mean that craniomandibular disease is absent. These disorders may be hidden, or the patient may harbor a predisposition to craniomandibular disease.

Craniomandibular Disorders

TABLE 8–1. Clinical Examination Summary

SUBJECTIVE PAIN AREAS

Top of skull	R [ ]	L [ ]	Orbit	R [ ]	L [ ]
Occipital	R [ ]	L [ ]	Suborbital	R [ ]	L [ ]
Cervical (rear)	R [ ]	L [ ]	Facial	R [ ]	L [ ]
Shoulder	R [ ]	L [ ]	Preauricular	R [ ]	L [ ]
Upper back	R [ ]	L [ ]	Auricular (ear)	R [ ]	L [ ]
Middle back	R [ ]	L [ ]	Cervical (side)	R [ ]	L [ ]
Lower back	R [ ]	L [ ]	Arm	R [ ]	L [ ]
Forehead	R [ ]	L [ ]	Finger	R [ ]	L [ ]
Supraorbital	R [ ]	L [ ]	Chest	R [ ]	L [ ]

EXTRAORAL EXAMINATION

Temporalis anterior	R [ ]	L [ ]	Sternocleidomastoid	R [ ]	L [ ]
Temporalis middle	R [ ]	L [ ]	Digastric	R [ ]	L [ ]
Temporalis posterior	R [ ]	L [ ]	Suprahyoid	R [ ]	L [ ]
Posterior cervical	R [ ]	L [ ]	Infrahyoid	R [ ]	L [ ]
Trapezius	R [ ]	L [ ]	Angle of mandible	R [ ]	L [ ]

TEMPOROMANDIBULAR JOINTS

Tender to palpation (closed mouth)	R [y] [n] L [y] [n]
Tender to palpation (on opening)	R [y] [n] L [y] [n]
No condylar movement on opening detected	R [y] [n] L [y] [n]
Stethoscope detected clicking (opening)	R [y] [n] L [y] [n]
Stethoscope detected clicking (closing)	R [y] [n] L [y] [n]
Stethoscope detected crackling (opening)	R [y] [n] L [y] [n]
Stethoscope detected crackling (closing)	R [y] [n] L [y] [n]

EAR EXAMINATION

Pain without palpation	R [y] [n] L [y] [n]
Pain on palpation (opening)	R [y] [n] L [y] [n]
Pain on palpation (closing)	R [y] [n] L [y] [n]
Palpable condylar head on closure	R [y] [n] L [y] [n]

HEAD MOVEMENT

Movement [normal, abnormal]   Cannot rotate [right, left, either]

INTRAORAL EXAMINATION

Lateral pterygoid	R [ ]	L [ ]	Masseter zygoma	R [ ]	L [ ]
Medial pterygoid	R [ ]	L [ ]	Masseter middle	R [ ]	L [ ]
Mylohyoid	R [ ]	L [ ]	Masseter mandible	R [ ]	L [ ]

Table continued on following page

TABLE 8-1. Clinical Examination Summary *Continued*

MANDIBULAR MOVEMENT

Interincisal opening [mm]	Limited opening (<35 mm) [y, n]
Lateral deviation on opening	[R] [L] [both]
Lateral deviation on closing	[R] [L] [both]
Staggered motion (dyskinesia)	[opening] [closing] [both]
Slow motion (bradykinesia)	[opening] [closing] [both]

EXCURSIVE MOVEMENTS

Protrusion—deviation to	[R] [L]
Right lateral motion normal	[y, n]
Left lateral motion normal	[y, n]

DENTAL EXAMINATION

[ ] Mobile teeth	[ ] Worn incisal edges [upper] [lower] [both]
[ ] Spaced upper anteriors	[ ] Complete dentures [upper] [lower] [both]
[ ] Crowded lower anteriors	[ ] Partial dentures [upper] [lower] [both]
[ ] Unstable occlusion	[ ] Clinically restorable teeth [upper] [lower] [both]
[ ] Hygiene poor	
[ ] Soft tissue problem	[ ] Missing posterior bite
[ ] Deep overbite [mm]	[ ] Unilateral occlusion
[ ] Severe overjet [mm]	[ ] Open bite
[ ] Crossbite	[ ] Bilevel bite
[ ] Midline discrepancy-related to upper, lower is [right] [left]	

y = yes; n = no; R = right; L = left.

Diagnostic Evaluation

Historically, clinical observation has been the basis for analysis of mandibular function. Subjective data derived from the patient combined with clinical information gathered by the examining dentist provided the basis for diagnosis and treatment planning. The same two sources of information, patient perception of symptoms and normalcy of function together with observation of function by the physician, have formed the basis on which treatment success or failure was judged.

The absence of objective data has led many practitioners to rely only on subjective criteria and empirical proof for treatment need, techniques, and the success or failure of therapy. Sometimes treatment produced comfort, and at other times it did not. Because the diagnosis was never quantified, neither was the treatment.

Since many craniomandibular disorders may involve muscle dysfunction that may be associated with mandibular movement, the instruments utilized to diagnose them must be capable of measuring mandibular movement and the muscle activity associated with mandibular function.

TABLE 8–2. Clinical Examination of 1647 Patients with Tenderness to Palpation

	PERCENT
EXTRAORAL MUSCLES	
Temporalis	51
Posterior cervical	36
Sternocleidomastoid	26
Angle of mandible	46
Trapezius	25
INTRAORAL MUSCLES	
Lateral pterygoid	81
Medial pterygoid	73
Any pterygoid	85
Masseter	17
OTHER CLINICAL OBSERVATIONS	
Pain in TMJ on palpation	64
Pain in ear on palpation	55
Palpable condylar heads (through ears)	47
TMJ sounds	32
Limited opening (<35 mm) interincisally	34
Lateral deviation on opening or closing	35
Dental findings (any of following): Worn incisal edges, deep overbite, depressed posterior teeth	49

From Cooper, B., and Cooper, D. Unpublished data on 1647 private and myofacial pain clinic patients, 1989.

MECHANICAL MEASUREMENTS OF MANDIBULAR FUNCTION

Since the late 1800s, concepts of perfect jaw function and dental occlusion have been based on mechanical models, derived from mechanical instruments used to record mandibular activity and maxillomandibular positions. Three-dimensional recordings were and still are made with writing instruments and graphic platforms attached to the mandible and head. These mechanical instruments can be used to transfer relationships recorded directly from the patient to the laboratory for analysis and fabrication of treatment appliances.[59]

Recordings made with these instruments are of the extremes in mandibular position, considered by some to be the borders of normal functional activity. Examples are the most forward position the patient could protrude the mandible while keeping the anterior teeth touching, and the most lateral excursive position possible. Measurements were also made of the most superior or posterior position of mandibular displacement, aided by pressure applied by the examining dentist to the patient's chin. Opening and closing movements were also included in the recordings. These positions are considered true functioning positions by some, as reference points by others, and irrelevant by the rest.

There are two problems with these mechanical models. First, the measurements are recorded with the patient reclining in a dental chair at exaggerated extremes of mandibular motion. Neither the setting nor the movements are natural. Simply the effect of gravity displaces the mandible posteriorly, bringing the posterior teeth into contact artificially.

The second problem involves the recording of mechanical measurements of mandibular motion through objects affixed to the teeth. These intraoral devices encumber the tongue and add weight to the mandible. In addition, recording outside the mouth compounds the degree of distortion in measurement.

BIOELECTRONIC MEASUREMENT TECHNIQUES

During the past two decades advances in computer science and medical instrumentation have led to the development of clinically useful instrumentation that can track mandibular motion three-dimensionally and simultaneously record electromyographic data on masticatory muscle activity.[60, 61] Technological advances have enabled clinicians to measure mandibular movement accurately without weighting down the jaw or adding artifact-creating distortion to the data.

Bioelectronic instrumentation permits accurate, reproducible, objective measurements that can be used in the clinical setting as well as for research. Dentists in universities, hospitals, and private offices in this country and abroad utilize these instruments to diagnose craniomandibular disorders and create precise occlusions.[62-64]

Mandibular Tracking

The first of these electronic mandibular tracking instruments to be developed was the Mandibular Kinesiograph (MKG) (Myotronics, Inc., Seattle, Washington).[65] A similar instrument is the Serognathograph (Siemans, West Germany). The MKG measures the position and movement of the mandible by tracking the movement of a small 0.1-ounce magnet temporarily affixed to the gingiva below the mandibular incisor teeth. As the mandible moves, the magnet's position is followed by magnetic sensors suspended on a sensor array worn on the patient's head (Fig. 8–15). Because nothing is attached to the mandible except the small magnet, no artifact to natural movement exists. Recordings are made with the patient in an upright seated position. Since there is nothing of any substance within the mouth during the recordings, the mandible, tongue, and muscles can act unimpeded in a natural manner, making the recordings valid.

The position of the magnet is determined by relating it to the various magnetic sensors suspended around the subject's head. The sensors are built into an object called the *sensor array.*

The precise tracking that is made can be explained by considering the magnet as the patient performs a simple task, such as opening and closing the mouth. As the mouth opens, the mandible moves downward and backward, possibly with a deviation to one side. As the mandible moves

Craniomandibular Disorders

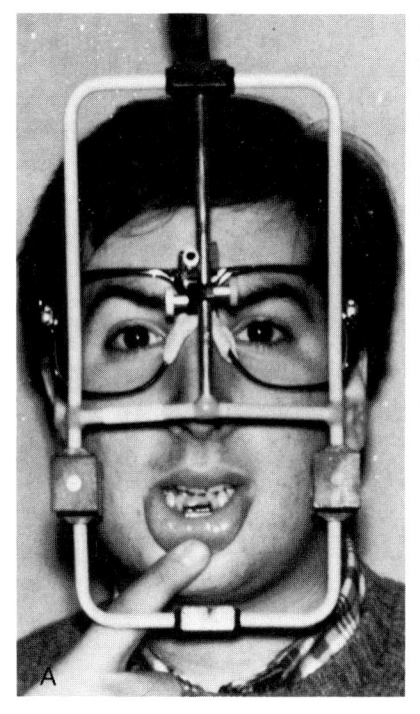

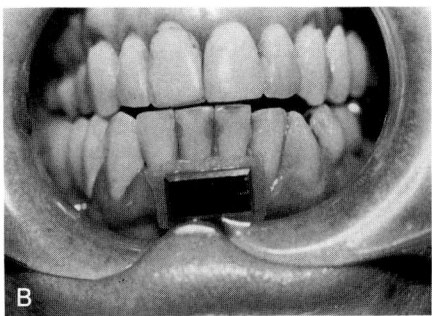

FIGURE 8–15. *A*, Mandibular kinesiograph sensor array. Observe the magnet affixed below the mandibular incisor teeth. Vertical, lateral, and AP sensors measure positional changes of magnet with mandibular movement as a function of changes in magnetic field strength. (Lip was retracted only to display the position of the magnet.) (From Cooper, B. and Rabuzzi, D. Myofacial pain dysfunction: A clinical study of asymptomatic subjects. Laryngoscope 94(1):68–75, 1984.) *B*, Close-up of magnet affixed with adhesive gel to gingiva below mandibular incisors.

along this trajectory, the magnet moves farther from the sensors in the front of the array and consequently closer to those below and lateral. In any mandibular position there are sensors or magnetic detectors lateral to, above, and below as well as anterior and posterior to the magnet. The magnet is located by measuring the differential magnetic field strength between the magnet and all of the sensors.

The accuracy of the MKG is 0.1 mm in the measurement of the mandible near the occlusal position.[66] The MKG is used to record the resting position of the mandible in the presenting patient as well as its movement from rest to occlusion. These positions can be recorded on a CRT screen, analyzed and stored on a computer disk, and printed on paper.

The data on the mandibular position in rest and occlusion can be displayed as a set of three individual vectors—vertical, horizontal (anterior and posterior), and lateral (Fig. 8–16).[67, 68] The actual movement of the mandible as it hinges and translates in the temporomandibular joint is curvilinear. Recorded data can be displayed in sagittal and frontal views simultaneously (Fig. 8–17). Finally, the movement of the mandible can be analyzed as a velocity measurement, demonstrating both speed and smoothness or irregularity of movement (Fig. 8–6).[69] Therefore, the MKG records mandibular movement in three dimensions and as movement in time. It is

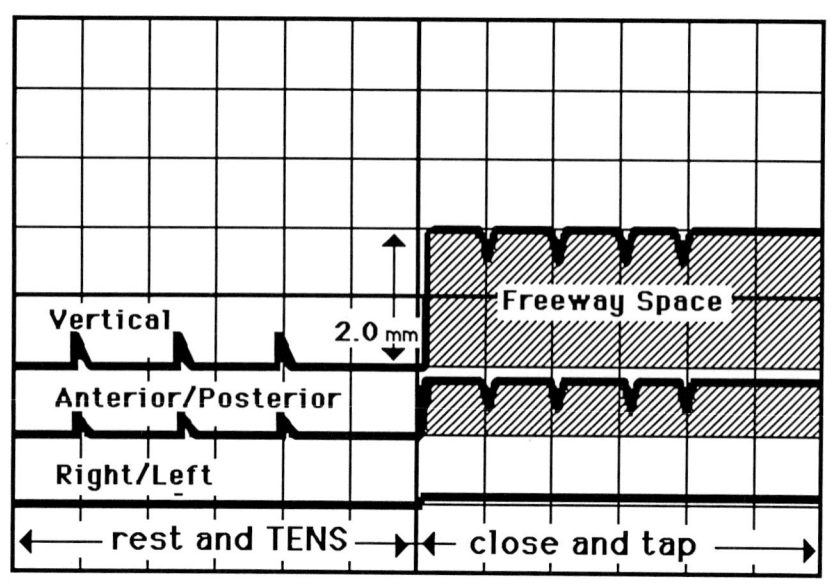

FIGURE 8–16. Schematic representation of mandibular kinesiograph (MKG) recording of movement of the mandible from rest to occlusion in the sweep mode. The left portion of the recording is the mandibular position at rest, the right portion represents the position of the mandible at closure (occlusion) with repeated tapping of the teeth together. The mandibular movement is displayed as three separate tracings, representing the three-dimensional vectors of movement. The upper tracing shows the vertical vector of movement (closure is upward). The center tracing shows the anterior-posterior vector of movement (anterior = upward deflection, posterior = downward deflection). The lower tracing represents the lateral vector (upward = right deflection, downward = left deflection). In all three tracings each box represents 1 mm vertically and 1 second on horizontal sweep.

a dynamic rather than a static recording device. The clinical significance of the MKG data in diagnosing particular disorders and abnormalities will be described later in the chapter.

Electromyography

Electromyographic recording of muscle activity related to mandibular function has been performed since the late 1940s.[70] During most of this time, electromyography (EMG) has been solely a research tool in dentistry. In later years researchers were involved in the study of muscle activity associated with mandibular function and dental occlusion. Recently there has been increased activity in dental research in the area of muscle function and the use of EMG in the study of craniomandibular disorders.[71–75]

A clinically utilizable EMG instrument was developed in the early 1980s, bringing EMG out of the research laboratory and into the office. Later improved and integrated with the MKG for simultaneous recording and analysis, the present EMG instruments can record the activity of up to eight muscle groups simultaneously.

The era of clinical bioelectronic measurement of muscle activity is now here. For the first time, muscle dysfunction associated with mandibular activity can be objectively quantified. EMG has greatly improved the efficacy of diagnosis and treatment of craniomandibular disorders.

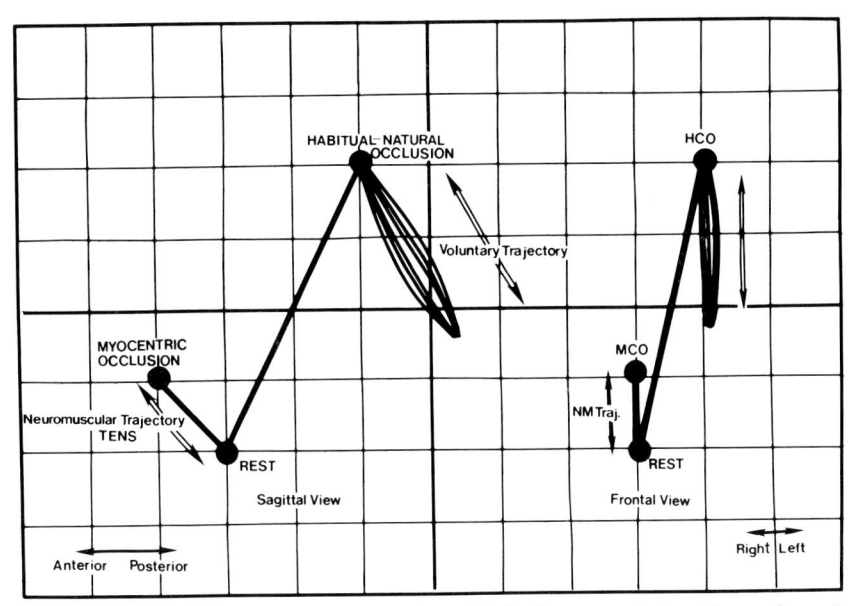

FIGURE 8-17. Schematic representation of mandibular kinesiograph (MKG) recording of mandibular movement trajectory from rest position to occlusion. This tracing compares the position of the voluntary closure trajectory into the natural occlusion (habitual centric occlusion—HCO) with an ideal neuromuscular trajectory from the true muscularly rested mandibular position to the ideal myocentric occlusion (MCO). The neuromuscular trajectory (NM Traj) reflects involuntary muscle contraction initiated by transcutaneous electrical neural stimulation (TENS) of the masticatory muscles. Simultaneous sagittal and frontal views are shown.

EMG recordings can be made utilizing either needle or surface electrodes. Needle electrodes are used to record nerve and muscle action potentials.[76] Muscle group activity can be better measured using surface electrodes, which sum the activity of many motor fiber units.[77, 78] For the diagnosis of musculoskeletal dysfunction, such information on the general resting state and contractile activity of this larger motor unit is more useful than single muscle fiber studies. Measurement is typically made of the anterior temporalis, posterior temporalis, middle masseter, and digastric muscle fibers (Fig. 8–18).[79] Depending on the diagnostician's needs, the instruments can also be used to record activity in other muscles, such as the posterior cervical, sternocleidomastoid, and trapezius.

Unfortunately, lateral pterygoid muscle activity cannot be measured with surface EMG. Needle electrode recordings of lateral pterygoid muscle activity have been made and have correlated with evidence of hyperactivity and muscle spasm in surface electrode measurements of the more superficial masticatory muscles.[80, 81]

EMG recordings are not absolute; they are relative to other measurements made on the same patient and to general standards for a particular instrument.[82] Measurements are also affected by such factors as skin conductivity and the quality of electrode contact with the skin. As relative measures they are of great value in assessing both bilateral symmetry of

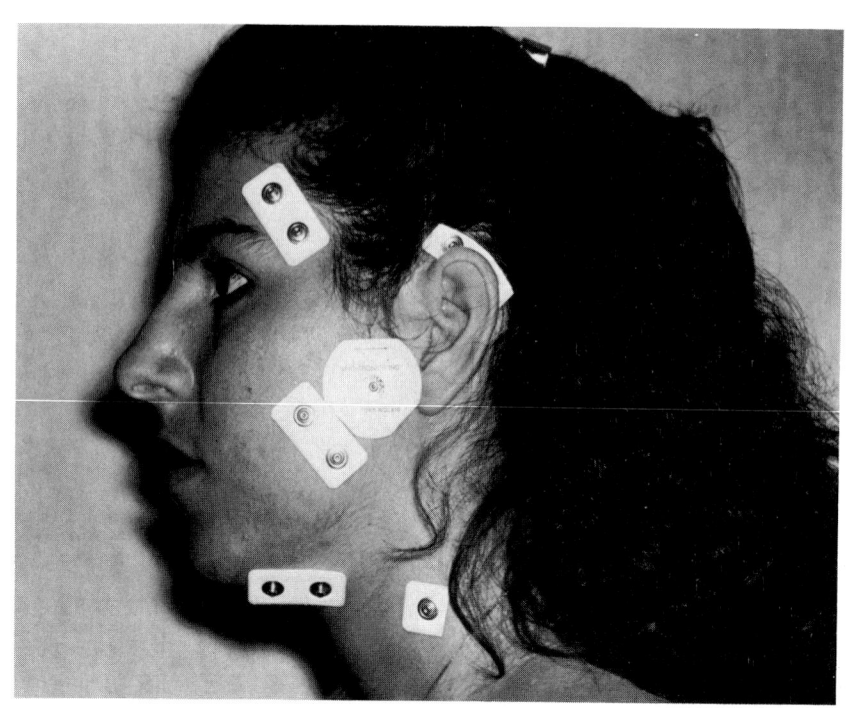

FIGURE 8–18. Placement of bipolar electromyography electrodes on anterior temporalis, posterior temporalis (above and behind the ear), masseter, and anterior digastric muscles (beneath the mandible). Also shown is the placement of a single ground electrode on the side of the neck.

activity and changes in electrical activity that occur in both muscle relaxation and therapeutic manipulations during the testing procedure.[83, 84]

EMG can be used to measure both muscle resting activity and activity associated with function. Resting levels help to assess whether the mandible is in a true resting position or an accommodative partially rested position (Table 8–3). This difference is significant because it is our hypothesis that the accommodative resting position is fatiguing to muscle. Incomplete resting in which the muscles are not allowed to relax to their full resting length predisposes a person to myofacial pain dysfunction.

Of equal importance is the ability of EMG to assess muscle function (Table 8–4) qualitatively and quantitatively.[85, 86] The temporalis and masseter muscles, which are mandibular elevators, can be measured as the patient clenches the teeth. The other mandibular elevators, the pterygoid muscles, cannot be assessed with surface electrodes. The symmetry of muscle activity can be assessed with EMG. Bilateral asymmetry in contraction of the muscles in occluding the teeth is frequently found in extrinsic (extracapsular) craniomandibular disorders. It accompanies lateral deviation or displacement of the mandible as it enters into occlusion. Instability of occlusion, often reported by patients as an "inability to find a comfortable bite," can also produce typical EMG recordings. Horizontal rotation of the mandible (torquing) may also be seen on EMG recordings of clenching. This will be illustrated later in this chapter.

TABLE 8–3. Typical Electromyographic Data of Presenting Patient[a] Resting Muscle Activity (in microvolts)[b]

MANDIBLE IN ACCOMMODATIVE REST POSITION				MANDIBLE IN TRUE REST POSITION AFTER TENS FOR 1 HOUR			
R		L		R		L	
Ta	Mm	Mm	Ta	Ta	Mm	Mm	Ta
6.2	5.0	4.2	5.9	2.1	1.0	0.9	1.7
Tp	Da	Da	Tp	Tp	Da	Da	Tp
4.7	2.8	3.1	4.5	2.3	1.8	1.7	2.2

[a]The patient was a 22-year-old female presenting with complaint of headaches, otalgia, dizziness, cervicalgia, clicking in the TMJ, backache, and numbness in the fingers.
[b]Averaged data of 1024 recordings made over 40 seconds. These EMG recordings of muscle electrical activity can also be displayed graphically on a computer screen.
Abbreviations: Ta, temporalis anterior; Tp, temporalis posterior; Mm, middle masseter; Da, anterior digastric; R = right; L = left.

TABLE 8–4. Typical Electromyographic Data of Presenting Patient[a] Muscle Clenching Activity (in microvolts)[b]

PATIENT CLENCHING IN NATURAL DENTITION (HABITUAL OCCLUSION)					PATIENT CLENCHING INTO ORTHOTIC APPLIANCE (NEUROMUSCULAR OCCLUSION)			
R		L			R		L	
Ta	Mm	Mm	Ta		Ta	Mm	Mm	Ta
4	0	1	7		1	0	0	1
4	0	7	28		13	52	22	6
22	0	15	31		93	214	166	82
84	4	47	55		145	247	203	131
13	0	21	72		145	255	223	183
7	0	11	85		196	255	249	215
75	4	34	71		178	255	240	201
117	17	61	75		192	241	251	191
83	12	27	47		181	251	214	206
98	7	12	26		152	223	213	171
55	4	26	54	averages	143	221	197	154

[a]The patient is the same 22-year-old female shown in Table 8–3. EMG data demonstrate weak muscle function with natural dentition that improves with creation of a neuromuscular occlusion by means of orthotic appliance.
[b]Each point is the average of 256 samples taken over 0.2 seconds.
Average printed below is the average of the 10 samples above. These EMG recordings of muscle electrical activity can also be displayed graphically on a computer screen.
Abbreviations: Ta; temporalis anterior; Tp, temporalis posterior; Mm, middle masseter; Da, anterior digastric; R = right; L = left.

Temporalis muscle fibers move the mandible upward and posteriorly, whereas the masseter fibers move the mandible upward and anteriorly.[87] EMG recordings that demonstrate temporalis dominance may represent posterior displacement of the mandible in occlusion, a condition often found in patients with craniomandibular disorders (Fig. 8–19).

EMG, therefore, provides essential diagnostic information about the resting activity of the muscles that control the posture of the mandible as well as their electrical activity during clenching. Compressive force studies have shown a positive correlation between the EMG-recorded activity level and compressive forces recorded between the teeth in occlusion.[88-93] These research studies are of great value because they validate the clinical EMG studies of electrical activity on clenching as representative of muscle strength.

Significance of Electronic Testing
Mandibular tracking and EMG measurements, together with transcutaneous electrical neural stimulation (TENS)-induced mandibular movement, make possible the diagnosis of muscle dysfunction associated with mandibular posture at rest, in movement, and in the dental occlusal position. The data obtained are used in diagnosis, to design therapy, and finally, to analyze the outcome of therapy.

Reliable, reproducible objective measurement is critical in the management of myofacial pain dysfunction (MPD) because most of the presenting symptoms of MPD involve subjective findings by the patient and subjective observations by the examiner. There are no objective tests for pain, whether in the form of headache, facial pain, temporomandibular joint pain, otalgia, pain on mandibular movement, or cervicalgia on movement of the head. The sensation described by patients as dizziness, lightheadedness, imbalance, or disequilibrium, in the absence of positive evidence of vertigo through an electronystagrogram (ENG), is not objectively measurable. Tinnitus also is not a symptom that is objectively recordable or quantifiable. This lack of verification has been a great problem in the diagnosis and treatment of complaints relating to musculoskeletal disorders in the past. No one could be certain what the nature of the problem was or what precisely should be done to cure it. Patient complaints, in the absence of documented pathology, were often considered emotional manifestations or psychosomatic pains and therefore untreatable. Sometimes treatments were performed empirically to see if symptoms were ameliorated. Proper treatment, however, should seek to eliminate a cause. Before that can be done, the cause must be capable of being isolated and objectively measured.

The ability to measure a dysfunctional state objectively, correct it, and record a healthy functional state following treatment is, therefore, essential to the practitioner attempting to treat craniomandibular disorders. Electronic testing performed during the course of therapy may demonstrate the necessity of modifying the therapy being used. For example, if occlusion is being altered to correct a muscle dysfunction, the occlusal-altering device may need to be modified or replaced if the test data dictate that need. Previously, a patient's report of comfort or a doctor's clinical observations

A. EMG Pretreatment before Myo-Monitor TENS Function-Clench Test

RIGHT			LEFT	
Ta	Mm		Mm	Ta
1	1		1	0
54	11		4	16
97	71		23	150
93	62		58	144
106	76		55	152
89	69		60	134
115	65		59	135
115	73		59	147
94	63		62	158
84	64		60	153
94	64	Average	47	132 ◄

Temporalis dominance shows posterior displacement, left temporalis dominance ◄ shows lateral displacement

Abbreviations: Ta, temporalis anterior; Mm, middle masseter. Averaged data.

B. EMG Pretreatment after Myo-Monitor TENS Function-Clench Test

RIGHT			LEFT	
Ta	Mm		Mm	Ta
0	2		2	0
7	12		17	10
89	68		53	38
101	108		85	124
129	120		78	141
125	98		80	146
121	120		86	163
121	115		82	100
101	123		89	162
116	104		82	157
101	96	Average	72	124

Muscles relaxed, occlusion released, mandible repositioned anteriorly, muscle function improved more evenly. Note improvement in masseters

Function as compared with before TENS function. Averaged data.

FIGURE 8–19. *A*, Electromyograph (EMG) of muscle activity on clenching in the presenting patient demonstrates dominance of the temporalis muscles (Ta) in comparison with masseters (Mm). *B*, Following transcutaneous electrical neural stimulation (TENS)–induced muscle relaxation, the mandible sometimes becomes repositioned, and the occlusal relationship is changed, showing improved masseter function in clenching (as illustrated here). The patient is an 11-year-old girl who complained of "violent earaches" with and without ear infection for the past 6 years accompanied by intermittent hearing loss. Complete remission of otalgia followed establishment of neuromuscular occlusion by means of an orthotic appliance.

were the only criteria available of treatment success or failure or the need to modify therapy. That type of information can be spurious.

The ability to subject treatment success or failure to objective scrutiny is essential. In treating a functional disturbance, the capability of recording healthy function following therapy is as important when the patient reports resolution of the clinical symptoms as when the therapy fails to eliminate symptoms.

If therapy fails to achieve symptom relief as reported by the patient, testing can determine whether the therapy did indeed successfully eliminate the physical dysfunction. If it did, the patient clearly requires further analysis and possible referral to other medical specialists to determine why symptoms have not been ameliorated. Objective analysis in the measurement of musculoskeletal diseases that involve subjective untestable symptoms is essential. Reliable, precise objective measurement in the management of craniomandibular disorders was lacking until bioelectronic testing procedures were introduced.

This capability of making objective measurements of mandibular function, dental occlusion, and associated muscle activity without mechanical artifacts, has revolutionized the management of craniomandibular disorders. Dentistry is the last of the health sciences to enter the electronic age. In all other areas of medical practice electronic measurement of body functions not only is utilized but is considered essential. The addition of bioelectronic testing to dentistry's armamentarium augments mechanical testing and provides objectivity in the management of musculoskeletal disorders of the head and neck. The neuromuscular status during the functional movements of the mandible can now be brought under scrutiny. The resting levels of muscles and their activity during compression with dental occlusion can be analyzed. Electronic tracking of the mandible throughout the various natural movements during mastication, deglutition, and speech as well as rest is possible. Bioelectronic instruments make the treatment of craniomandibular disorders more successful and more predictable.

IMAGING MODALITIES

Radiographic analysis is of great importance in making definitive diagnosis of temporomandibular joint pathology as opposed to muscle dysfunction. Radiographic imaging of the temporomandibular joint alone does not provide the comprehensive information necessary to diagnose and treat craniomandibular diseases. It is just one part of the diagnostic regimen.

A great many radiographic techniques are available for visualizing the temporomandibular joints. They have varying degrees of complexity in instrumentation and technique and show different structures within the joint. Some modalities such as transcranial radiographs are used in the dental office, whereas more expensive scanning equipment is used only in sophisticated radiology facilities.[94]

Transcranial Radiographs

Transcranial radiography is the radiographic modality most commonly employed for visualizing the temporomandibular joint.[95-97] Conventional

Craniomandibular Disorders

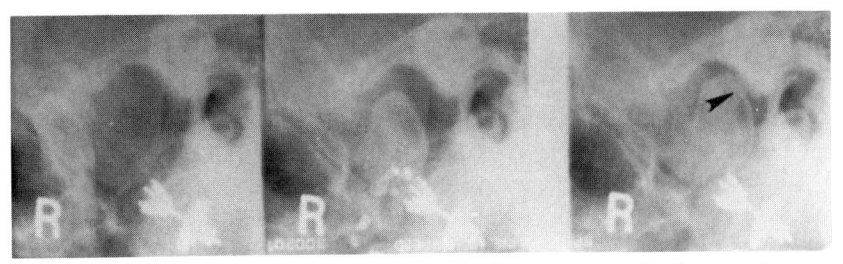

FIGURE 8-20. Lateral transcranial radiographs of right temporomandibular joint. Right is closed position (occlusion), center is 5-mm opened position, and left is the fully opened position. Osseous structures appear normal. Condyle is posteriorly displaced in occlusal position on the right (arrow). The condylar displacement is corrected in the 5-mm opened image (center) and translates normally anteriorly in the opened position (left image). (R is anterior in all images. Artifact is pierced earring.)

radiographs taken with modified dental x-ray equipment produce lateral transcranial radiographs. They are excellent first-imaging techniques and are used to confirm or diagnose osseous abnormalities in the joint (Figs. 8-20, 8-21, and 8-22). They are relatively inexpensive, utilize a low radiation exposure, and can often be taken in a dental office equipped to do so. Magnification techniques are available for improving visibility of the bony structures within the joint.

A variation of the lateral transcranial radiograph is obtained using a modified panoramic dental x-ray (Fig. 8-23A). The radiograph so produced is sometimes distorted and shows overlapping osseous structures but is again a good first-imaging technique. Cephalometric radiographs are a form of lateral transcranial radiograph; they are customarily used in orthodontic evaluation and are also used to visualize the joints.

Single plane radiographs of any type of the temporomandibular joint are of limited value because the osseous structures imaged are three dimensional and irregular in form. The mandibular condyle is an oblong object whose horizontal axis is not perpendicular to the surface of the face. To

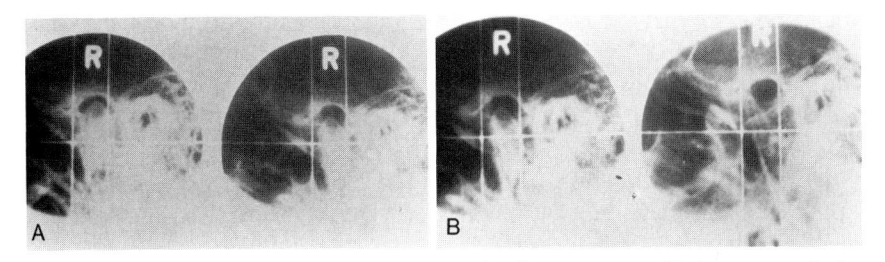

FIGURE 8-21. Lateral transcranial radiographs of right temporomandibular joint. In both pairs of radiographs, the left image shows the closed (occlusal) position, and the right image shows the opened position. A, The patient has severe muscle spasm. There is no anterior translation of the condyle, and opening is restricted. B, After TENS therapy the muscles became relaxed, and the condyle translates as the mouth opens normally. Patient was a 16-year-old girl with muscle dysfunction that followed a traumatic facial injury, not intrinsic joint dysfunction. (Radiographs courtesy B. Jankelson, D.M.D.)

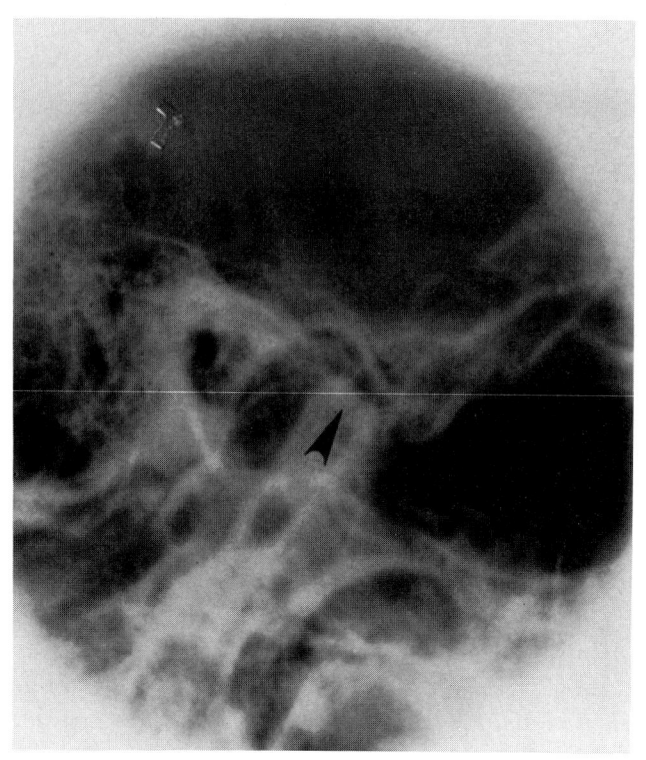

FIGURE 8–22. Lateral transcranial radiograph of the temporomandibular joint in the closed mouth position, showing irregularity along the cortex of the condyle (arrow). The joint space remains intact. Tomograms and CT scans of the same patient demonstrate data obtainable by each modality (see Figs. 8–24, 8–27, and 8–28). (Radiograph courtesy A. Liebeskind, M.D.)

align the x-ray properly, the angulation of the condyle must be determined using a submental vertex view (Fig. 8–23B). The temporomandibular fossa also has a complex architecture. The angulation of the x-ray cone used to take radiographs of the temporomandibular joint can affect the apparent relative position of the condyle in regard to the surface of the fossa and eminence. Varying the angulation of the cone varies the relationship of the bony structures being imaged. For that reason, diagnosis of mandibular displacement solely on the basis of conventional lateral transcranial radiographs is not absolutely accurate.

Diagnostic capabilities are improved if at least two different views of the joints are taken. They can be lateral transcranial, submental vertex, and frontal (Towne's) views.[98] The submental view can be used to establish the angulation of the condyle properly for more accurate lateral transcranial radiographs. Bony abnormalities may not appear on one view but may be evident on another.

Serial tomographs of the temporomandibular joint can be taken with specialized equipment to demonstrate the osseous architecture at various depths along the condyle and fossa (Fig. 8–24).[99–101] Conventional radiographs merely show one two-dimensional view of a three-dimensional joint.

Craniomandibular Disorders

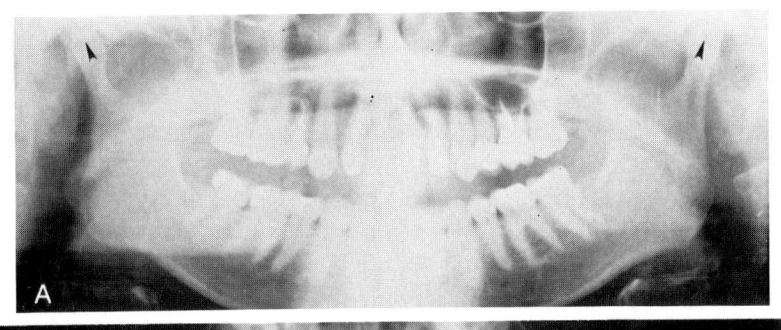

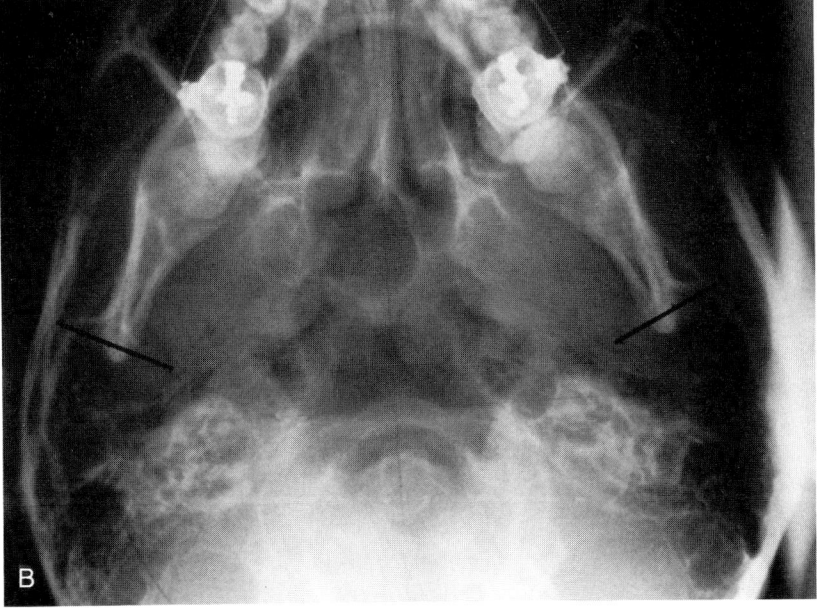

FIGURE 8-23. *A*, Panoramic radiograph of the skull and mandible demonstrates normal condyle (arrows) and fossa anatomy bilaterally. *B*, Submental vertex view is used to determine condylar angulation for proper lateral transcranial radiography. Black lines indicate condylar angulation.

Tomographs are focused narrowly on the temporomandibular joint and therefore avoid excess exposure of other adjacent tissues. Unfortunately, the images of osseous structures seen in tomographs lack clearly delineated borders.

Transcranial radiographs are used for screening the condition of osseous structures. If properly angulated, they provide a general indication of the condylar head position and the joint space around the condyle. It must be noted that the disk, which is located within the space between the condyle and fossa, is not visualized in these radiographs. Condylar position does not necessarily indicate disk position. A posteriorly displaced condyle is not always accompanied by an anteriorly displaced disk. The reverse is also true in that the disk may be anteriorly displaced even if the condyle is in a centered position in the fossa. The inability to demonstrate soft tissue,

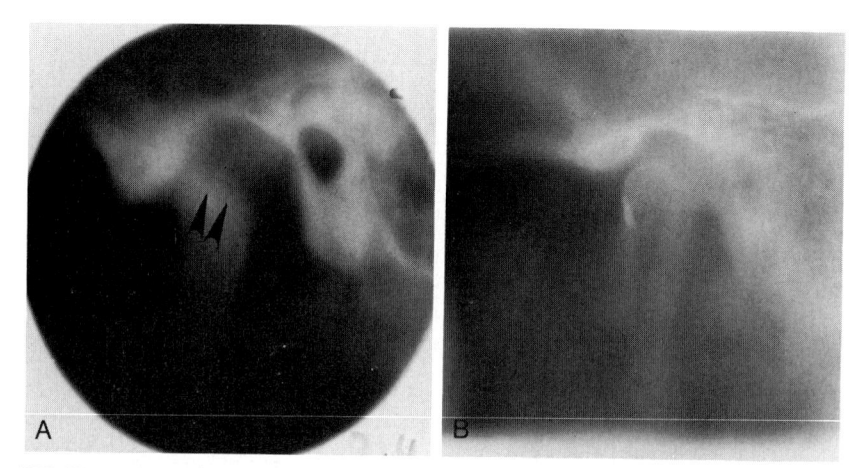

FIGURE 8–24. Evaluation of the temporomandibular joint in the closed mouth position, with multiple thin tomographic slices (2 mm thickness), shows the presence of two small subchondral cysts (arrows). Slight separation at the level of the joint space is noted. (This is the same patient as shown in Figures 8–22, 8–27, and 8–28.) *B*, Normal condyle seen on tomogram. (Radiograph courtesy A. Liebeskind, M.D.)

notably the disk, is the greatest shortcoming of conventional radiographs. Bony pathology is well shown. The cortex of the bones and their trabeculae is well represented. Arthritic changes, degeneration, and bone remodeling are visualized, as is the range of motion of the condyle in various positions. No representation of the dynamics of motion can be made by these fixed-position radiographs.

Radionuclide Scanning

To date, radionuclide scanning of the temporomandibular joint has been used solely as a research tool. It has been used to demonstrate alterations in blood flow to the joint capsule and surrounding tissues as well as to show abnormalities of metabolic activity within the temporomandibular joint system (Fig. 8–25). In the former, technetium-99 (^{99}Tc)-labeled red cells are utilized to "tag" the blood flowing to the area. In the latter, scans with gallium (Ga)- or technetium (^{99}Tc)-labeled metabolites are picked up differentially by more metabolically active tissues. The clinical application of these types of scanning has been traditionally limited to whole body radionuclide scans aimed at finding hidden or distant sources of infection and neoplasia. Scans of these types are nonspecific, showing only that a given area has increased blood flow, altered metabolism, or abnormalities of other parameters but not giving the clinician any insight into the pathogenesis of the alteration.

Arthrography

Arthrograms are radiographs taken after insertion of radiopaque material into the joint.[102-106] Several techniques are available for obtaining arthrograms of the temporomandibular joints. Since there are actually two joint spaces within the temporomandibular joint, one above and one below the disk, contrast material can be injected into the upper, the lower, or both

Craniomandibular Disorders 193

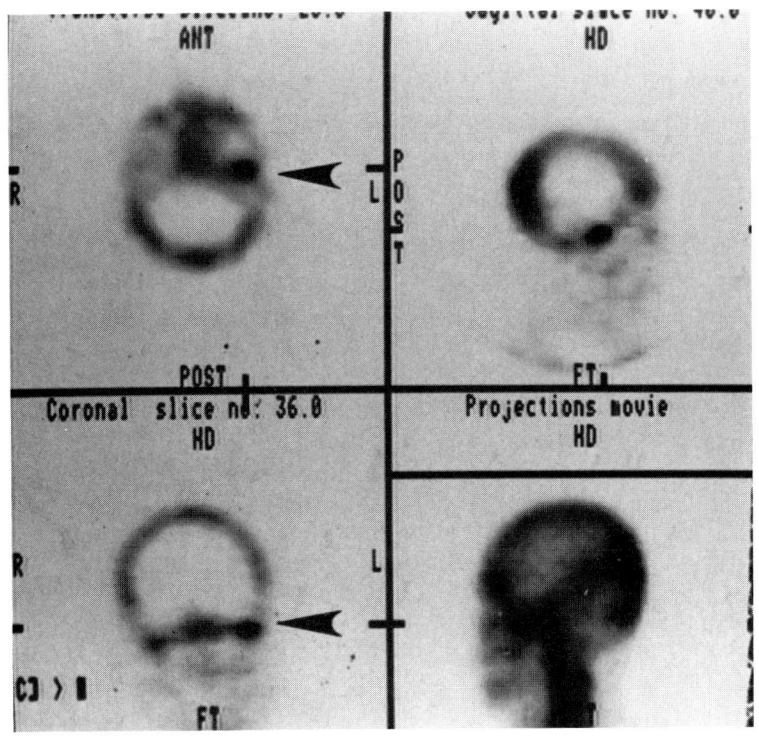

FIGURE 8–25. Radionuclide study. Technetium-99 (^{99m}Tc) bone scan study shows uptake at the level of the temporomandibular joint on the left, which is consistent with reactive bone changes on multiple images obtained. Arrows point to TMJ. (Radiograph courtesy A. Liebeskind, M.D.)

joint spaces. Some operators utilize a needle to insert the material, whereas others use a catheter. Some use single-contrast and others double-contrast materials. Finally, transcranial radiographs or tomographs as well as fluoroscopic recordings with videotapes can be taken of the joints for a permanent record of structure and function.

Arthrograms show detailed soft tissue anatomy (Fig. 8–26). Disk position, size, and shape as well as disk perforation and the posterior disk attachment can be visualized clearly with this modality. The only disadvantages of arthrography are that it requires the introduction of a foreign chemical agent into the joint, and technical expertise is necessary for its proper performance. The chemicals now being used do not seem to cause adverse effects. Improper injection into the soft tissues can result in pain. Properly done, with the newer radiopaque substances, the technique is not very uncomfortable to the patient. The discomfort that sometimes follows arthrographic studies may result from the intentional manipulation of the mandible by the operator during the procedure to demonstrate the disk and posterior attachments at the extremes of opening and closing. For the patient in whom limited mandibular movement secondary to muscle splinting is an accommodative response to avoid pain associated with movement, this forced movement under local anesthesia may precipitate pain.

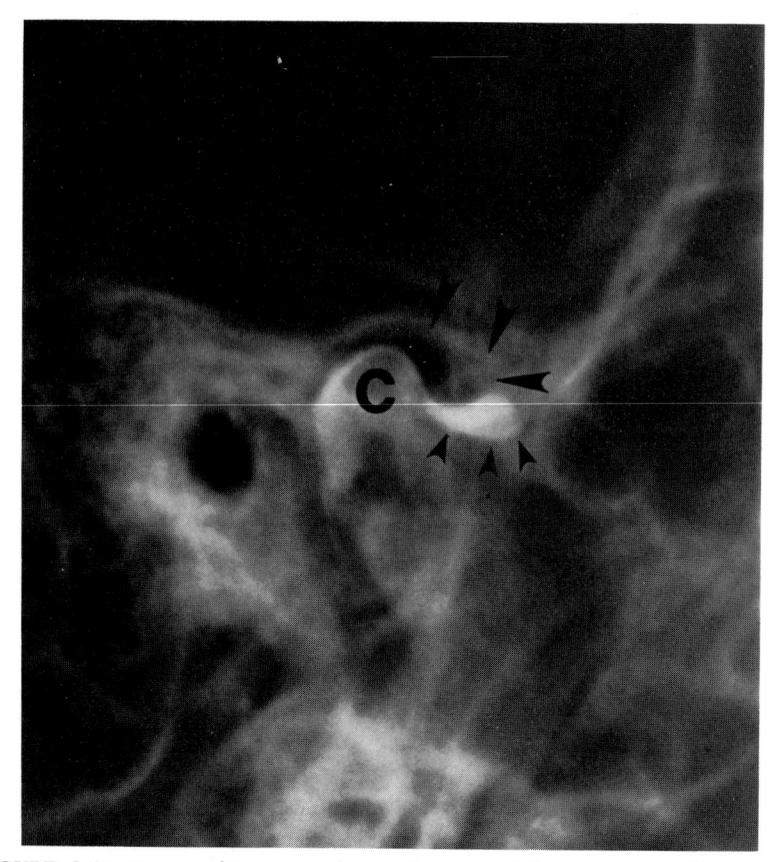

FIGURE 8–26. Tomographic image of an arthrogram of the temporomandibular joint. Radiopaque material is injected into the lower joint space and outlines the under surface of the disk, which is seen displaced anterior to the condyle (C). Smaller arrows point to opaque material in the inferior joint space. Larger arrows point to disk, which is the radioluscent area above. (Radiograph courtesy of M. Thomas, D.D.S.)

Although arthrography is an invasive technique, the arthrogram is an image that clearly demonstrates the position of the disk relative to the position of the condyle and eminence. It is also a reliable means of clearly showing the shape of the disk and the presence or absence of perforations in the disk or posterior attachment, and thus communications between the upper and lower joint spaces. It should be noted that arthrography does not actually demonstrate the disk because the disk does not become radiopaque; it is the joint spaces superior and inferior to the disk that become filled with the contrast material, thereby outlining the disk and retrodiskal fibers.

Arthrography provides verification of internal derangements that have been clinically observed. It aids in management decisions and in evaluating problem cases and treatment failures. In summary, the arthrogram is the only imaging modality that shows the configuration, location, and perforation of the disk with great detail. It is also the only radiographic test that shows the dynamics of joint function. With the new serial imaging techniques, which are not invasive, it is hoped that this important information about the disk status will be available to clinicians.

Computed Tomography

Computed tomography (CT) is particularly valuable in demonstrating osseous anatomy.[107] CT shows less soft tissue resolution compared with other scanning techniques. It is utilized when necessary as a followup to conventional radiography. It is a noninvasive procedure that requires sophisticated instrumentation that is available in most radiology facilities. Its clarity in visualizing osseous details is valuable in characterizing bony abnormalities such as fractures, arthritic changes, and osteophyte formations (Figs. 8–27 and 8–28). Through reconstruction of computerized data, it is possible to analyze structure on many planes. It can only suggest disk location on blink mode and provides no functional information because it images a static relationship only. Metal restorations in the teeth may create artifacts. CT scans are valuable in management decisions and in evaluating cases in which recapture of the disk has failed.

In the future, CT scanning will be improved by the availability of thinner sections with higher resolution. Three-dimensional CT scans and cine CT offer future possibilities.[108, 109]

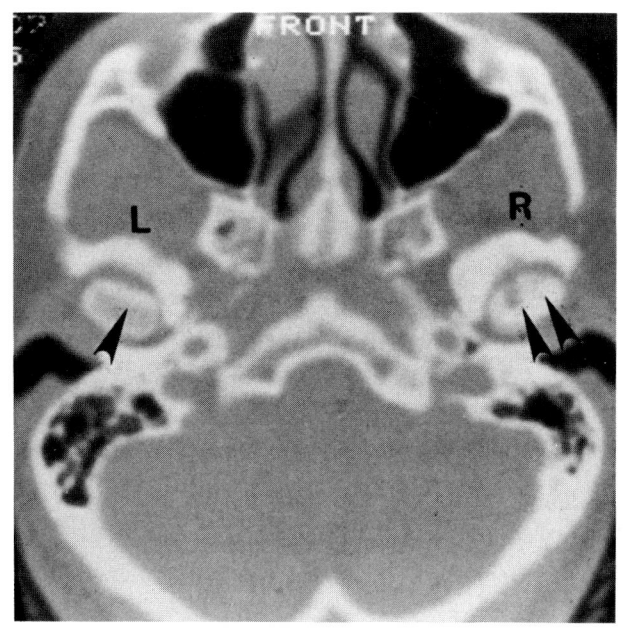

FIGURE 8–27. Computed axial tomographic (CT scan) evaluation of the right temporomandibular joint, with the left side for comparison, in the axial view (utilizing high resolution and high bone window) shows the presence of small, subchondral cysts, as well as irregularity along the cortex of the condyle (two arrows). The left condyle (one arrow) appears normal. (Radiograph courtesy of A. Liebeskind, M.D.)

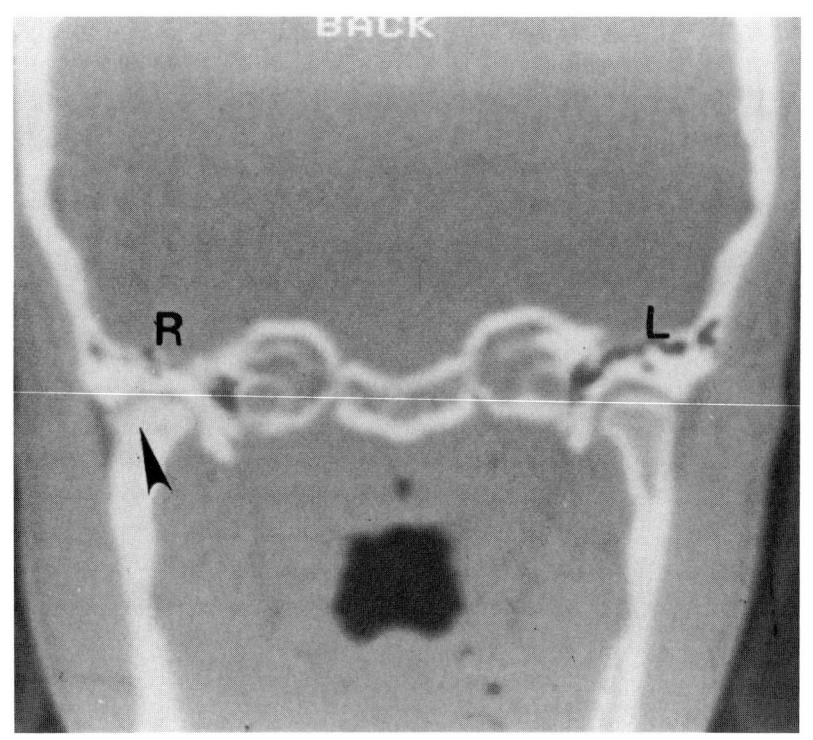

FIGURE 8–28. Computed axial tomographic (CT scan) evaluation of the right temporomandibular joint compared with the left joint (direct coronal views). This is the same patient as seen in Figures 8–22, 8–24, and 8–27. Again, small irregularities are seen along the cortex of the right condyle (arrow) compared with the left, which appears normal. (Radiograph courtesy A. Liebeskind, M.D.)

Magnetic Resonance Imaging

One of the newest forms of imaging the temporomandibular joint, magnetic resonance imaging (MRI, also called nuclear magnetic resonance), provides the high contrast in the soft tissues that is necessary for studying the temporomandibular joints.[110–112] MRI makes use of magnetic field effects on aligning the electrons spinning about the atoms that make up our bodies. Radiofrequency waves are directed at the spinning electrons, causing them to change their axis of rotation. As the electrons "relax," they give off a burst of radiofrequency energy equal to that of the wave absorbed. The content of certain key atoms in a tissue dictates how much energy is absorbed and released.

MRI affords multiplanar viewing directly, without reconstruction, and can demonsrate disk position but not disk shape or perforation (Figs. 8–29 and 8–30). Because of the high collagen content of the disk, the long echo or T2 relaxation time is short like that of bone, and both bone and disk appear black. This modality provides no dynamic information on joint function and does not show bone. Some patients, such as patients with permanent cardiac pacemakers, cannot undergo MRI studies.[113] MRI is beginning to be used on patients requiring additional diagnostic information.

Craniomandibular Disorders 197

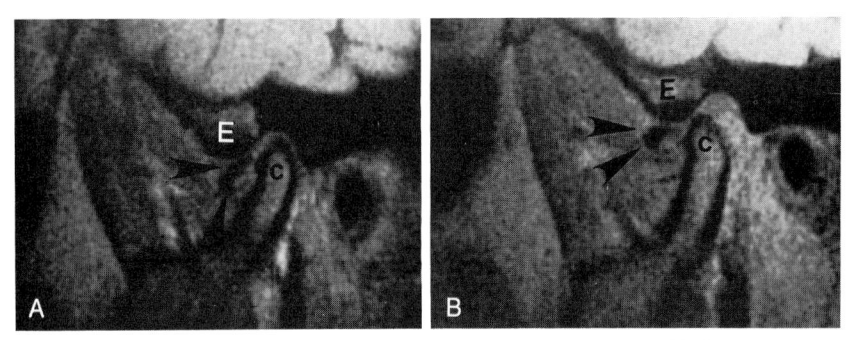

FIGURE 8–29. Magnetic resonance imaging (MRI) of the temporomandibular joint (using surface coil). A, In the closed mouth position, anterior displacement of the disk is seen. B, MRI image of the same temporomandibular joint in the open mouth position demonstrates the same anterior displacement of the disk observed in the closed mouth position (A). The disk is, therefore, not recaptured. E = articular eminence, C = condyle. Arrows point to disk. (Radiograph courtesy A. Liebeskind, M.D.)

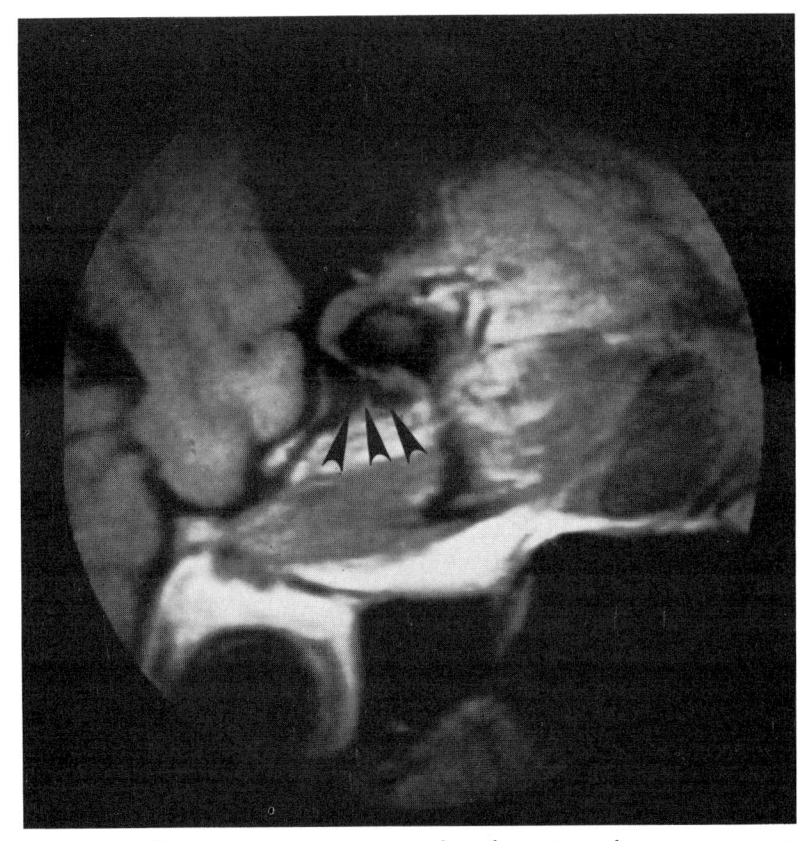

FIGURE 8–30. Magnetic resonance imaging of another patient shows anterior vertical displacement of the disk with thinning of the superior belly of the lateral pterygoid muscle. Arrows outline the disk. (Radiograph courtesy M. Thomas, D.D.S.)

It is an expensive modality and does not yield the quality of imaging of the disk that is provided by arthrograms. However, in the future, the detail of disk imaging in MRI may be improved.

MRI is now being used in research studies of muscle activity by Hannam and his coresearchers to demonstrate the size and location of various mandibular muscle groups. They are studying the form and function of the muscle fiber groups involved in mandibular function using MRI as well as other means.[16, 115]

OTHER DIAGNOSTIC MODALITIES

Arthroscopic examination of the temporomandibular joints is now being utilized to view the contents of the joint and perform simple surgical procedures, such as those used to eliminate fibroses. Electric microphones are being utilized to hear joint sounds. Doppler ultrasound is being applied to the study of temporomandibular function and dysfunction and provides additional information. Thermography is used in various parts of the body to monitor thermal changes in tissues as a function of vascular change. Surgical exploration of the joint is a diagnostic modality that usually accompanies surgical therapy of the joint.

Extracapsular Craniomandibular Disorders

MYOFACIAL PAIN DYSFUNCTION SYNDROME

Myofacial pain dysfunction results from an unhealthy working relationship between three groups of tissues in the head and neck. These are the dental apparatus, the temporomandibular joints, and the neuromuscular system, which acts as the motor unit for the mandible and head. Each of the three parts of this tripod depend on the others for stability and proper function. Dysfunction in one can affect the others.[115–119]

The term used here, *myofacial pain dysfunction* (MPD), is a descriptive term indicating a condition of pain or dysfunction in the facial musculature. It describes a form of musculoskeletal dysfunction involving the muscles of the head and neck, the skull, and the mandible that is related to an unhealthy dental occlusal position.

Craniomandibular disorders currently bear a multitude of names. These often describe the specific tissues involved, such as Schwartz's term *temporomandibular joint pain-dysfunction syndrome,*[120] Laskin's *myofascial pain-dysfunction,*[121] Arlen's *otomandibular syndrome,*[122] Lerman's *mandibular pain-dysfunction syndrome,*[123] Howe's *disorders of the masticatory apparatus,*[124] and lately, *craniomandibular syndrome.* Finally, the term used in the *Glossary of Prosthetic Terms* (1985 revision) is *Costen's syndrome,* a historical reference recognizing Costen's early observations (1930s) of symptoms within the ears, nose, and throat related to mandibular position and temporomandibular joint function in the dental occlusal position.[125]

Whatever the term used to describe the illness, the goal should be to isolate a clinical entity that can be objectively diagnosed, differentiated from other conditions, and ultimately managed successfully. If possible, successful treatment should include removal of etiologic factors, not merely relief of symptoms. The latter is important, of course, but is only transient if causal or aggravating factors are not eliminated or controlled. There are many ways to relieve pain and muscle tension, but they are short-lived if the cause of pain and muscle hyperactivity remains.

The head and neck is the most complex anatomic and functional region in the body. As such, it may be the site of a multitude of symptoms due to a wide variety of pathologic causes. Most of the symptoms of MPD may occur as manifestations of other diseases. It is essential, therefore, that the examining physician have an understanding of the clinical presentation of MPD as well as other conditions that can cause the same symptoms and physical signs.

Symptoms

The symptoms of MPD can be divided into three categories: those that produce pain, those associated with dysfunction, and those that destroy the dental apparatus (Tables 8–5 and 8–6). It should be noted that all patients do not report identical symptoms, and some report more symptoms than others. Many patients report that symptoms change over time in intensity, frequency, and even in type. The history is, therefore, quite important.

Painful Symptoms. The most common complaints of pain by MPD patients are otalgia, headache, pain in the temporomandibular joint area, and facial pain. Additionally, patients report cervical pain, oral soft tissue pain, dental pain, chest, back, and arm pain, pain on mandibular movement, and pain on cervical movement. Other symptoms, which are classified with pain symptoms, are barotrauma, or otalgia associated with changes in barometric pressure as in an airplane or during mountain climbing, and tinnitus. Tinnitus is not painful but does cause great discomfort in many patients.

Dysfunctional Symptoms. These symptoms relate to restricted or abnormal function. The movement of the mandible can be limited in the range

TABLE 8–5. Symptoms of Myofacial Pain Dysfunction

PAINFUL SYMPTOMS
- Headaches, tinnitus, barotrauma, dental pain, ear pain
- Facial, neck, back, shoulder, and chest pain
- Pain in the jaw joints or on jaw movement

DYSFUNCTIONAL SYMPTOMS
- Mandibular movement: limited, deviated, slow, irregular
- Head movement: limited rotation
- Ears: muffling, dizziness, hearing loss, clicking
- Throat: difficult swallowing, prolonged speech
- Jaw joint: dislocated jaw, facial asymmetry

SELF-DESTRUCTING DENTITION
- Wear on teeth, abrasion, chipping
- Looseness of teeth (bone loss)
- Movement of teeth, spreading, crowding

TABLE 8–6. Subjective Symptom Occurrence (Patient Perception Among 1647 Patients)

	PERCENT
HEADACHES	
Frontal	41
Temple	45
"Migraine"	24
Sinus	31
Occipital	41
Any headache	78
TEMPOROMANDIBULAR JOINT	
Limited opening	22
Clicking	37
Crackling	20
Pain in joint	48
Any joint symptom	66
EAR SYMPTOMS	
Tinnitus	38
Otalgia (without infection)	51
Dizziness	40
Muffled ears	37
Any ear symptom	81
THROAT SYMPTOMS	
Laryngitis	6
Dysphagia	17
Sore throat (noninfected)	25
Voice irregularity	12
Frequent cough	11
Sensation of object in throat	20
Prolonged speech difficulty	17
Any throat symptoms	46
OTHER SYMPTOMS	
Pain behind the eyes	36
Facial pain	42
Dental pain	22
Cervical pain	46
"Uncomfortable bite"	25

From Cooper, B., and Cooper, D. Unpublished data on 1647 private and myofacial pain clinic patients, 1989.

of opening and in the velocity, fluidity, and direction of opening and closing movements. Some patients report mandibular dislocation or locking. Restriction of mandibular movement associated with internal derangements within the temporomandibular joint must be considered here as contributing to or causing these symptoms, although muscle dysfunction may be the sole etiologic agent.

The movement of the head and neck may also be aberrant. Care must be exercised here in differentiating between muscle dysfunction related to craniomandibular disorders and muscle dysfunction related to cervical pathology or postural abnormality. In the ears, dysfunction has been described by patients as a sensation of blockage, clogging, fullness, or muffling. Patients frequently report a sensation of nonrotatory dizziness or disequilibrium, which is often associated with some hearing impairment and clicking sounds.[29–43, 126] In the throat, difficulty in swallowing, with the feeling of an object stuck in the throat, is noted by some patients, as is difficulty in prolonged speech.

Self-Destructing Dentition. The self-destructing symptoms of MPD rarely bring a patient to a physician, unlike the painful and dysfunctional symptom groups. These symptoms more often cause a patient to seek dental advice, although many times they go unnoticed because they do not cause pain or limit function. These symptoms include wear on the surfaces of the teeth (abrasion),[127] chipping of portions of teeth or restorations on the teeth, and loss of bony support around the teeth resulting in mobility, drifting, spreading, or crowding of some of the teeth.

Etiology

MPD as described here is a musculoskeletal dysfunction of the head and neck that is directly related to mandibular function and the unhealthy utilization of muscles associated with that function. The dysfunction results from a defective skeletal relationship between the mandible and the skull and between the skull and the cervical vertebrae. These unhealthy relationships are caused by the manner in which the maxillary and mandibular teeth interdigitate. Therefore, a neuromuscular malocclusion can cause muscle fatigue and ultimately dysfunction if the adaptive capacity of the tissues is exceeded.[128–132]

Dental Occlusal Position. The teeth are normally brought together in an intercuspal position (ICP) approximately 2000 times each 24-hour period to stabilize the mandible during the swallowing reflex.[133] That position of interdigitation of teeth, also called habitual centric occlusion (HCO), is the end-point of a cycle of mandibular movement, the beginning of which is the position of the mandible at rest. This is a very important point, because the two positions, occlusion and rest, are intimately related. Both can predispose an individual to MPD. Not only can the two end-points of the rest-occlusion cycle create a predisposition to MPD but also obstacles on the occlusal surfaces of the teeth, interposed between the teeth as the mandible moves from rest to the maximum intercuspal position, predispose to MPD.[134, 135]

Teeth are normally brought together in maximum intercuspation only in the empty mouth condition. When food is in the mouth, the teeth do not contact. The food bolus acts as an intermediary between the maxillary and mandibular teeth. The mandible is moved from the rest position to the biting position by muscle action. This function is accomplished by precisely coordinated contraction of the elevator muscles (temporalis, masseter, and medial pterygoids) and the relaxation of depressor muscles (lateral pterygoid, digastric, and suprahyoids). The pattern of muscle activity is determined by the ICP and by the dental structures, if any, that are interposed along the path to the maximal ICP. Dental occlusion, its position, stability, and entry path play an important role in muscle activity.

Rest Position of the Mandible. The position in which the mandible lies when not in the ICP is referred to as the *rest position* of the mandible. Studies have shown that the rest position is usually 0.75 to 2.0 mm from the ICP in a vertical dimension (Table 8–7). This vertical distance between the appositional surfaces of the upper and lower arches of teeth is measured at the midline of the dentition between the central incisor teeth. Changes in the occlusal position are followed by changes in the rest position of the mandible. This is significant because changes in occlusion that occur during life for a variety of reasons, including loss of teeth, wear of the tooth surfaces, and restoration and movement of teeth, can result in modification of the rest position of the mandible.

How does the mandible maintain a fairly stable rest position? It does so by coordinated postural activity by both elevator and depressor muscle groups. They receive information through a set of proprioceptive receptors in the muscles, peridontal ligaments surrounding the teeth, and the temporomandibular joints.[136-138]

Nasal Obstruction. The habitual resting position of the mandible is modified by physiologic needs and by habits. For example, in the presence of nasal obstruction, the oral cavity becomes the respiratory portal. The tongue, normally at rest against the upper surfaces of the mouth, is now positioned in the lower part of the mouth, overhanging the mandibular teeth. This is a natural accommodation to permit the flow of air over the tongue into the oropharynx. The mouth may rest at a position further from occlusion, with the lips apart so that air can enter and leave freely. The

TABLE 8–7. Mandibular Kinesiograph of Vertical Freeway Space Prior to Treatment (Measured Incisally)

BEFORE TENS	AFTER TENS
Healthy, 42%	Healthy, 24%
(average vertical 1.3 mm)	(average vertical 1.8 mm)
Unhealthy, 58%	Unhealthy, 76%
(average vertical 2.4 mm)	(average vertical 4.1 mm)

Healthy, 0.75–2.0 mm; unhealthy <0.75 mm or >2.0 mm (average ranges).
From Cooper, B. C., et al. Myofacial pain dysfunction: Analysis of 476 patients. Laryngoscope 96(10):1099–1106, 1986.

need for oral respiration may result in a set of adaptive developmental abnormalities including abnormal swallowing, undereruption and lingual inclination of mandibular posterior teeth (Fig. 8-11), abnormality of hyoid bone position, and development of an overly obtuse mandibular gonial angle. In addition, nasal obstruction can cause alterations in cervical and head posture, which can result in hard and soft tissue abnormalities in the cervical spine.

The interrelationship between function and development of the various structures in the head and neck cannot be overemphasized. In examining a patient, it may not be possible to establish an actual sequential order of development of abnormalities. For example, it may be impossible to determine with certainty whether the nasal obstruction observed in a patient caused undereruption of the posterior teeth, which then resulted in overclosure of the mandible in occlusion, putting pressure on the temporomandibular joints and excessive strain on the muscle system of the head and neck, resulting in stiffness and cervical pain and headache, and so on. The examining physician should know about these potential interrelationships. In therapy, multiple approaches may be necessary to solve the variety of unhealthy conditions that exist simultaneously. This will be discussed toward the end of this chapter.

Predisposition. From what has been said already, it would seem that everyone with some abnormality in occlusal alignment, improper vertical occlusal dimension, or unbalanced muscle function would exhibit the fullblown clinical picture of MPD. In fact, however, most people do not show such a clinical picture, and a larger percentage reveal only a few telltale signs of the illness.[139-141]

Perhaps because the masticatory system is used in so many ways, as in mastication, deglutition, vocalization, and respiration, it has been provided with tremendous functional adaptive capacity to remain effective under a variety of adverse conditions. It is only when this adaptive capacity is exceeded that the clinical entity of MPD becomes evident and requires treatment.

In the predisposed state, an individual has some malocclusion involving either interference with complete interdigitation or an excessive vertical, lateral, or anteroposterior distance from the rest position to complete closure. This neuromuscular "malocclusion" requires adaptive mandibular posturing and results in a lack of complete muscle relaxation.[142,143]

Although the patient may not be cognizant of this problem because of the adaptive capacity of the neuromuscular system, the strain on the neuromusculature may already be apparent. The experienced clinician may be able to detect subclinical signs of muscle fatigue and dysfunction and neuromuscular malocclusion. Clinical signs of stressed adaptive capacity include wear on the lower anterior teeth, a deep overbite, limited or deviated mandibular movements, bruxism or clenching habits, absent posterior teeth, or muscle tenderness to palpation.

Patients who are predisposed to MPD or who have a subclinical illness may indeed have had previous clinical manifestations that attest to the strain on the neuromuscular system. Information obtained through a comprehensive history may provide clues that the patient has symptoms of MPD such as otalgia, barotrauma, mouth locking open, and "migraine-line" or "chronic sinus" headaches.

Precipitating Factors. Given that many people in the general population are predisposed to craniomandibular dysfunction, it is important to realize that the active disease state may be precipitated by either physical or emotional stressors.[141] Physical stressors to the neuromuscular system may take the form of medical and dental procedures that require hyperextension with prolonged opening of the mouth. This can occur during difficult prolonged endotracheal intubations, essential surgical procedures in or through the oral cavity, oral surgery, extraction of impacted molar teeth, root canal therapy, or extensive dental reconstruction.

Psychological and emotional factors also play a role in precipitating MPD both by lowering the adaptive capacity of the neuromusculature and by increasing the muscle tone as a direct response to stress. Although some authors have postulated that myofacial pain occurs as a direct result of stress, stress is more likely a modulator of the adaptive capacity in the individual with a predisposing physiologic mechanism toward craniomandibular disease.[144, 145]

Perpetuating Factors. Once the adaptive capacity has been exceeded and a clinical picture of MPD is evident, certain factors tend to perpetuate the illness. Among these are overall posturing of the head in relation to the cervical spine, postural and other noxious habits, and stress.[146-149]

Any activity that involves constant muscle tension will fatigue muscles. This is especially evident in muscles that are already in a state of fatigue or spasm. For example, if a patient frequently clenches his teeth while awake or asleep, the muscle system is modified and becomes hyperactive and subject to fatigue (Fig. 8-31). A similar condition may occur in a patient who frequently chews gum or bites fingernails, pencils, or a pipe. Occupational habits may also modify normal muscle activity. Someone who spends hours on the telephone, who cradles the receiver between the neck and the side of the mandible, sets up an unhealthy postural muscle pattern, creating muscle fatigue and pressure on the joints, both the temporomandibular joint and the cervical vertebrae.

The physiologic response to movement-associated pain is muscle splinting—immobilization of the joint being moved by sustained muscle contraction of opposing muscle groups—to prevent further pain or joint destruction (Fig. 8-21). Chronic pain in the temporomandibular joint or cervical vertebrae can induce this protective muscle splinting. Pain from joint dysfunction thus stimulates muscle hyperactivity, resulting in chronic stress on the structures involved and eventual fatigue of the musculature. This becomes an endless cycle of dysfunction. The solution lies in interruption of the cycle by removal of predisposing or perpetuating factors.

Many patients have functional adaptations to habitual activities, such as mouth breathing in patients with nasal obstruction. Such a person must habitually posture the mandible so that the tongue lies over the mandibular posterior teeth, depressing these teeth or restraining their natural eruption. This posterior depression requires overclosure of the mandible to produce

Pretreatment EMG Test MANDIBLE IN REST POSITION

	RIGHT		LEFT	
BEFORE	Ta	Mm	Mm	Ta
TENS	2.7	3.3	2.9	6.2
	Tp	Da	Da	Tp
	2.5	1.6	1.7	3.0

High masseters activity level seen in bruxism; high left temporalis activity indicates elevated resting activity. Patient also demonstrated weak function in this muscle.

AFTER	Ta	Mm	Mm	Ta
TENS	1.5	1.6	1.9	1.9
	Tp	Da	Da	Tp
	1.7	1.3	1.4	2.2

Myo-Monitor TENS relaxed all muscles. Note lower activity levels after TENS
Abbreviations: Ta, temporalis anterior; Mm, middle masseter; Tp, temporalis posterior; Da, anterior digastric. Averaged data.

FIGURE 8–31. Electromyographic recording (EMG) of eight facial muscles while the mandible is at rest. Before TENS, the mandible is in an accommodative resting position. Hyperactivity in all muscles except the digastric muscle is observed. Excessive masseter activity is usually seen in patients who clench (bruxism). The masseters are not postural muscles, being active only in occlusion. TENS stimulation for a minimum of 60 minutes relaxed all masticatory muscles. The patient was a 47-year-old male with a grossly overclosed bite (7 mm) and posteriorly displaced natural occlusion. He had had severe headaches since childhood as well as cervical pain. Symptoms disappeared 1 week after insertion of a neuromuscular occlusion orthotic appliance. Long-term use of an orthotic device has maintained symptom relief for 5 years. Ta = anterior temporalis; Tp = posterior temporalis; Mm = masseters; Da = anterior digastric.

occlusion accompanying the swallowing reflex. To adapt to this overclosure, the tongue is used to stabilize the mandible during swallowing rather than the dental occlusion (Fig. 8–11B). Used in this manner, the tongue is restricted in its movements. Suprahyoid contraction is necessary, resulting in tension and displacement of the hyoid bone. This displacement in turn modifies the normal function of the superior constrictor muscles of the pharynx. The overall result is an aberrant swallowing pattern.

Some individuals clench or grind their teeth (bruxism) a great deal, either while awake or during sleep. This activity may have one or more causes. It may be a functional activity that occurs in an attempt to remove interceptive tooth-contacting occlusal prematurities, or it may be a manifestation of psychologic hyperactivity.[150] It may also be the result of prolonged muscle hyperactivity related to maintaining a mandibular rest position that is not at the resting length of the muscles.

The excessive pressures on the teeth can wear the enamel surface of the teeth or the surface of dental restorations, resulting in a loss of stabilizing occlusal dental anatomy. That is muscularly fatiguing because the mandible must be stabilized by the muscles in the occlusal position rather than by the interdigitation of teeth. The wear of the dental surface anatomy can eventually reduce the overall height of the teeth and lead to a reduced vertical dimension of occlusion, overclosure of the mandible, and compromised rest position of the mandible. These in turn can alter the position of the mandibular condyle in the temporomandibular joint fossa.

Intracapsular Temporomandibular Joint Disorders

DISORDERS OF THE ARTICULAR DISK
Etiology
The articular disk may undergo both temporary and permanent changes in morphology and integrity. Morphologic changes may be due to prolonged disk displacement associated with condylar displacement. The articular disk may become detached from its fibrous attachments by an external traumatic injury or by an internal chronic traumatic insult, such as excessive chewing habits, fingernail biting, gum chewing, or clenching and bruxing habits while awake or asleep. Other causes of chronic trauma to the joints affecting the disk attachments are interferences or instability in the dental occlusion.

Clinical Findings
When the disk is detached it may become displaced and may interfere with normal translatory mandibular movement by modifying the normal architectural compatibility of the disk, condyle, and articular eminence. It may also put pressure on other structures in the joint because of its presence and the presence of edema, which may accompany disk detachment, causing intermittent pain. Such pain occurs when the patient clenches the teeth with force and may be associated with dental occlusal interferences. It can be relieved by relieving the pressure between the condyle, disk, and eminence by biting on a tongue blade. This removes occlusal contact. As a normal accommodative reaction to pain on movement, muscle splinting may accompany this pain.

DISORDERS OF THE RETRODISKAL FIBERS
Etiology
The disk is attached to the posterior wall of the temporomandibular fossa by well-vascularized and well-innervated connective tissue fibers. If the mandible is displaced posteriorly in the fossa, the disk may be forced anteriorly, stretching or tearing the retrodiskal attachment fibers. Such an injury can occur abruptly in a traumatic injury to the mandible or skull (whiplash). In the latter case, the skull is first thrown backward as the car is forced forward and the victim's head remains in its original position due to inertia (a body at rest tends to remain at rest). The head is then secondarily thrown forward in a pendulum movement. The mandible, suspended from the skull by its muscles and ligaments, also is thrown. This "jawlash," as described by Kinnie, accompanies whiplash injuries and affects the retrodiskal fibers, resulting in their distortion or destruction.[151] Retrodiskal inflammation and pain result.

The mandible and its condyle may be chronically displaced posteriorly by the dental occlusal position. The occlusal plane is located inferior to the temporomandibular joints. If the vertical dimension of the occlusion is reduced, meaning that the mandible must close further to interdigitate the maxillary and mandibular teeth, the condyle is moved further posteriorly. Conversely, if the vertical dimension of occlusion is increased, the mandible does not close as far up to achieve occlusion, and the mandible moves forward. This fact is significant in therapy and will be discussed later in this section.

The vertical position of occlusion is not the only determinant of condylar position in the fossa. Actual inclined planes on the surfaces of the teeth may displace the mandible as the teeth are brought into occlusion. This abnormality can cause an unhealthy three-dimensional displacement. It is of great significance, since the teeth are occluded approximately 2000 times each day as an accompaniment to the swallowing reflex. Occlusal interferences may, therefore, cause chronic retrodiskal inflammation, edema, and pain.

Clinical Findings
Retrodiskal fiber pain is exacerbated by clenching the teeth with maximal tooth interdigitation. This pain, like disk attachment pain, is relieved by biting on a firm object such as a tongue blade. As described above, it serves to increase the vertical dimension of occlusion and also voids all occlusal interferences, thereby freeing the condyle to assume a new position that is less distorting to the retrodiskal fibers. Pain can be induced by forced mandibular movement on the side in which pain has been reported. Sometimes edema in the joint lowers the mandible, resulting in a lack of occlusion of the posterior teeth on the ipsilateral side.

If the examiner's hand is placed against the chin, restricting voluntary forward translation of the mandible, pain in the temporomandibular joint will not be elicited as the patient attempts to move the mandible forward. This maneuver differentiates retrodiskal pain from lateral pterygoid pain, which responds in the opposite fashion to resisted protrusion.

DISORDERS OF THE JOINT CAPSULE
Etiology
The capsule that incorporates the temporomandibular joint is composed of two layers. The outer layer is fibrous, providing support to the joint; the inner layer is synovial, providing lubrication. The pain that emanates from the capsule may arise in either or both of these tissues (capsulitis or synovitis). Both have the same clinical presentation. As with the other forms of temporomandibular joint pain already described, capsulitis may be caused by either external or internal chronic trauma of an occlusal or parafunctional nature. In addition, hypermobility of the joint may predispose to capsulitis. According to Roccobado, loose packed joints are more susceptible to traumatic injury than close packed joints.

Clinical Findings
A patient with temporomandibular joint capsulitis will experience pain on palpation of the joint, located anterior to the tragus of the ear. The examiner may feel fluctuance in the area as well. The capsular pain is exacerbated

by translational movements of the mandible on protrusion or opening. Clenching the teeth together and biting on a tongue blade do not alter the intensity of capsular pain. Stiffness in the joint and some sounds in the joint may be observed during the initial movements of the mandible due to alteration in the normal synovial fluid. Muscle splinting, as a protective reaction to pain induced by movement, may also account for the limitation of mandibular movement. If edema is present, the mandibular position may become altered, changing the relationships of the maxillary and mandibular teeth in occlusion.

INFLAMMATORY DISEASES OF THE JOINT
Etiology
Since the articular surfaces within the temporomandibular joints are not normally vascularized, inflammation cannot occur. If the integrity of the articular surfaces is compromised, inflammation is possible. Inflammation may result from either acute or chronic trauma to the joint, degenerative joint disease (osteoarthritis), immune-mediated arthritis, chronic infectious processes, or other causes.[152]

Traumatic arthritis presents typically as a unilateral arthritis following traumatic injury to one of the temporomandibular joints. The onset of pain can usually be traced back to some specific traumatic incident. Injury can be to the synovium, capsule, disk, retrodiskal tissue, or bony structures. Hemarthrosis may or may not be present. Traumatic arthritis is often associated with splinting, spasm, and inflammation.

Degenerative joint disease is a later stage of inflammatory arthritis.[153-156] It may follow chronic disk displacement that resulted in bone-to-bone contact. Stress and habits that cause increased pressure within the joint may also be involved in the pathogenesis of degenerative arthritis, as may occlusal interferences. Lack of posterior occlusal support can result in increased pressure on the joint that may eventually progress to degenerative joint disease.[157]

Infectious arthritis may be caused by contamination of the joint due to trauma involving perforation of the joint capsule or by direct extension from adjacent structures such as occurs with chronic otitis media. It may also occur in the spreading of sepsis.

The temporomandibular joints are frequently involved in the presentation of rheumatoid arthritis (RA). The etiology of pain in rheumatoid arthritic disease involves proliferation of inflamed synovial tissues and invasion of the disk space by this tissue. Pressure in the normally noninnervated joint is felt as pain owing to compression of this well-vascularized and well-innervated synovial tissue. RA can progress to condylar degeneration.

Other causes of inflammatory joint disease include systemic lupus erythematosus, polyarteritis nodosa, Reiter's syndrome, gout, and psoriasis.

Clinical Findings
Arthritis is accompanied by capsulitis and presents with palpable tenderness. Pain is increased by biting the teeth together and by rapid and resisted movements of the mandible. It is not reduced by biting on a

tongue blade. Restricted or difficult mandibular movement is observed as well as malocclusion because of effusion within the joint or osteolytic changes.

Clinical findings in traumatic arthritis may include localized pain and swelling of the joint, discomfort and limitation of joint function, and radiographic evidence of damage to one or more of the structures of the joint.

Degenerative joint disease is diagnosed on radiographic examination of the joints.

Rheumatoid arthritis of the temporomandibular joints is typically bilateral and usually occurs in patients with a previous history of rheumatic disease. In extreme cases in which condylar degeneration occurs, patients may present with anterior opening owing to vertical height reduction of the condyle.

NEOPLASMS INVOLVING THE TEMPOROMANDIBULAR JOINT

The temporomandibular joints are rarely involved as sites of primary neoplasia. All joint components may undergo neoplastic transformation, the most commonly seen forms of which are chondroma, osteoma and osteochrondroma, giant cell granuloma, and hemangioma. Secondary neoplastic involvement of the joints is more frequent, predominantly involving direct extension of the tumor from adjacent areas.

TRAUMATIC INJURIES TO THE JOINT

The delicate structures that comprise the temporomandibular joints are liable to injury, resulting in inflammation and pain. That injury may result from an acute traumatic episode or a chronic sutble noxious stimulus. A joint may be predisposed to injury either because its capsule is loose, which may be a systemic condition, or because it has already been the subject of chronic mild to moderate trauma and may become acutely painful and dysfunctional with additional trauma.

Trauma to the temporomandibular joint may result from prolonged hyperextension of the mandible in dental and medical procedures. Dental procedures that may precipitate temporomandibular joint dysfunction include extraction of teeth (impacted mandibular third molars in particular), root canal therapy, and any procedures that involve prolonged wide opening of the mouth. Similarly, medical procedures that require extreme and prolonged opening of the mouth either to perform diagnosis or surgery in or through the oral cavity or to maintain an airway and administer general anesthesia may precipitate temporomandibular joint and muscular dysfunction with their associated pain.

Injury may also occur following an innocent activity such as biting a large resistant object such as an apple or hero sandwich or merely yawning widely. In a patient predisposed to dysfunction, such a traumatic incident can precipitate temporomandibular joint dysfunction as well as muscle dysfunction. In a patient with no predisposition, such trauma will merely initiate a transient discomfort.

Chronic trauma to the temporomandibular joints may be caused by noxious stimuli such as frequent clenching and bruxing (grinding) habits while either awake or asleep. Postural abnormalities involving the head, neck, shoulders, and back as well as mandibular postural abnormalities associated with nasal obstruction may predispose to both temporomandibular joint and muscular dysfunction. Noxious habits such as fingernail biting, gum chewing, biting a pen, pencil, or pipe, cradling a telephone with the shoulder and side of the head without holding it, or carrying a heavy shoulder bag on one shoulder also traumatize the temporomandibular joint as well as the musculoskeletal system of the head and neck.

Therapeutic Approach to Craniomandibular Disorders

Sequential Approach to Therapy

The first priority in treatment is the amelioration or correction of emergent conditions. These include severe pain and mandibular immobility, infectious processes, fractures, and hemorrhage. Although amelioration of severe pain is considered a priority for treatment, the etiology of the illness must be determined by full diagnostic examination at the earliest opportunity.

Since neuromuscular and pure joint dysfunction often coexist and are intimately related, treatment of the patient should begin with treatment of the neuromuscular system. This treatment consists of muscle relaxation through transcutaneous electrical neural stimulation (TENS) and mandibular repositioning to a neuromuscularly based occlusal position. Because joint dysfunction can be caused by malocclusions of various types, correction of the occlusion will often result in stabilization of the joint, obviating the need for treatment of the joint itself.

If joint dysfunction still exists, or if radiologic examination reveals a joint lesion that must be treated (i.e., a neoplasm), further treatment of the joint itself can be instituted.

Musculoskeletal Dysfunction

THE PRIMARY DIAGNOSTICIAN
Craniomandibular disorders present with a predominant picture of medical symptoms and complaints and are thus most often seen first by a primary physician or medical specialist. The primary physician, most often not a specialist in treatment of craniomandibular disorders, must still have an appreciation for the etiologies of these disorders and be able to make the differential diagnosis of craniomandibular dysfunction. Following this diagnosis, the primary physician can provide ameliorative therapy for the patient's symptoms while organizing referrals to appropriate specialists for definitive diagnosis and therapeutic management.

Temporary ameliorative measures may include medications to relax muscles, nonsteroidal anti-inflammatory medications, sedatives, and tranquilizers. Patients may be counseled to use a soft diet and avoid gum chewing and extreme opening of the mouth. Hot wet compresses applied to the face and neck may be prescribed when pain and stiffness are felt.

These ameliorative measures are often beneficial and may mask the patient's presenting symptoms. They do not, however, effect a lasting cure for musculoskeletal dysfunction. In contrast, if the cause of the pain or dysfunction was indeed transitory, these therapies may suffice. When temporary efforts to treat muscle spasm produce some decrease in pain, this result can lend support to the diagnosis of musculoskeletal dysfunction.

When MPD is diagnosed clinically by the physician or dentist, definitive measures should be undertaken to afford the patient a lasting cure. When no pathologic cause is found, physicians unfamiliar with the spectrum of presentation of MPD frequently try to placate a patient complaining of pain, telling him or her that there is nothing seriously wrong and nothing to be concerned about. Physicians familiar with the presentations and etiology of MPD understand the importance of further diagnostic testing by bioelectronic instrumentation to diagnose MPD, since MPD may produce only symptomatic complaints and no apparent physical findings.

The physician or dentist who recognizes the clinical presentation, symptoms, and history of MPD and refers the patient for proper care performs a valuable service to the patient and engenders great respect. Patients who have been given ameliorative treatment do not always return when the prescription runs out and their symptoms return. All too often, they go to another practitioner in the quest for a durable cure.

THERAPEUTIC APPROACHES
Regardless of the specialty or philosophy of the treating clinician, the general approach to therapy for craniomandibular disorders should be one that emphasizes reversible, noninvasive techniques before those that are irreversible or result in permanent alterations to morphology or function.

A variety of therapeutic procedures are utilized today to treat the muscle spasm of MPD.[158] These include pharmacologic agents, physical means including application of heat or cold, stretching of muscles, ultrasound, electrical stimulation of several types, and injection with or without chemicals to release either muscles in spasm or myofascial trigger points.[159-162]

If it has been determined that mandibular function is compromised due to dental occlusal defects, most long-term therapies involve the use of mandibular orthopedic repositioning appliances. Their function is to change the maxillomandibular relationship at the position of closure. The variety of appliance designs reflects the variety of opinions that exist concerning the ideal position of the mandible from the viewpoint of temporomandibular joint and muscle function.[163-172]

The variety of appliances also reflects variations in the concept of the role of repositioning appliances. To be more specific, some practitioners feel that the mandible should be released from the constraints of dental occlusion and freed to reorient itself to a more physiologic position. These dentists create either maxillary or mandibular acrylic removable appliances with flat surfaces and only an anterior or posterior stop to end closure of the mandible.

So-called "pivotal appliances" provide a single tooth contact on each side of the mouth. Other appliances completely cover the posterior teeth or contain anterior inclines or ramps to guide the mandible as it closes. These appliances are worn for a time and modified, often on an empirical basis, as symptoms disappear, become worse, or remain unchanged. The end of therapy is either elimination of the appliance with a return to the original occlusal relationship or a modification, subtle or overt, of the occlusal relationships. Some clinicians who treat muscle dysfunction of this nature merely utilize semisoft acrylic coverings to reduce the pressure on the teeth as the patient clenches the teeth together. These appliances are similar to those worn by participants in contact sports to protect the teeth from trauma.

Some practitioners who believe that the exact three-dimensional occlusal position is intimately involved with the health of the neuromusculature create appliances to establish temporarily a specific neuromuscular occlusal position. Since these appliances provide an occlusal position near to the true muscle resting position, they eliminate the need for adaptive muscle function, thereby removing the cause of MPD. These orthotic appliances cover the lower teeth and provide a detailed occlusal surface that can interdigitate with the upper teeth for better mandibular stability and balanced muscle function. These appliances may effect the recapture of a displaced articular disk, obviating the need for temporomandibular joint therapy.[173, 174]

Therapy for temporomandibular joint disease can be both pharmacologic and surgical. Injection of anti-inflammatory agents into the joint space is sometimes employed to reverse inflammatory joint disease.

If surgery to the joint is indicated, it should be done only after conservative means have been employed first. If mandibular displacement caused an irreversible internal derangement and intraoral appliance therapy failed to alleviate pain, surgery will be more effective if the mandible is properly oriented in occlusion. This often requires continuation of intraoral therapy. Failure to correct the mandibular displacement will allow the original cause of the internal derangement to continue, which can result in relapse following surgery.

If intraoral orthotic appliance therapy does alleviate pain but the disk is not recaptured, a decision must be made as to whether to perform surgery. Studies by Isberg[175] and Isacsson[176] have demonstrated that in cases of anterior disk displacement without recapture, the elongated retrodiskal fibers sometimes become hyalinized, creating a pseudodisk.[177-179] If joint pain has been eliminated and good function restored, surgery may be electively omitted. If pain is not eliminated or if function cannot be restored, with compromised capacity to eat or speak, surgery or at least an arthroscopic procedure should be considered. Before surgical intervention is contemplated, comprehensive diagnostic evaluation is necessary. As described in the section on radiographic imaging, arthrograms are of tremendous value in evaluating treatment failure and should be considered before surgery.

Surgery of the temporomandibular joint involves several procedures of varying severity.[180-182] Plication of retrodiskal fibers, osteoplasty to remove bone irregularities, and removal and replacement of the disk may be performed. Allograft disk replacements were used previously, but homograft materials are now being utilized in the temporomandibular joint. It must be understood that a repaired joint is not an original joint. Surgical techniques include eminenectomy, condylectomy, and complete joint replacement. All conservative means should be employed before surgery is contemplated or performed.

Neuromuscular Approach to Therapy

TRANSCUTANEOUS ELECTRICAL NEURAL STIMULATION

Transcutaneous electrical neural stimulation (TENS) is an ancient therapeutic modality.[183] It is reported in the classic literature that electric eels were applied to the skin to treat patients in pain. In recent medical history, the concept of TENS has comprised two distinct meanings.

The first involved TENS as a pain suppressor. From the original work of Melzack and Wall[184] the gate theory of a barrage of afferent stimuli flooding the input pathways was developed.[185-187] This tremendous quantity of stimuli exhausted the input mechanism for the reception of noxious stimuli, resulting in an inability of the central nervous system to receive and perceive painful stimuli. This flooding of the afferent pathways with low-voltage, high-frequency stimuli is the basis for the present use of TENS as a pain suppressor. Such instruments are presently used on some patients with intractable pain to effect a reduction in the perception of pain.

TENS as utilized in the therapy described in this chapter is a low-frequency stimulator.[188-190] It is a neuromuscular stimulator that is designed to relax muscles that are in a state of hyperactivity, with decreased circulation, decreased energy supply (adenosine triphosphate and metabolites), and accumulation of the waste products of muscle contraction (adenosine diphosphate, lactic acid).[191-193] Muscles in this ischemic state may be mildly to severely fatigued and may even be in a state of spasm or contracture.[194-202] Fatigued muscles exhibit decreased contractile force.[203-205]

For the lymphatic system to debride a muscle of the end-products of metabolism, the muscle must be capable of alternating contraction and relaxation. The lymphatic system does not have muscle within its walls to pump itself. When a muscle is in a state of spasm, it does not alternately contract and relax, and the lymphatic system becomes inoperable. This results in accumulation of waste products, which chemically irritate the sensory nerve receptors and are perceived as pain in the muscle. Muscles in spasm exhibit two clinical features, pain and limited flexibility. These account for most of the symptoms associated with MPD. Low-frequency TENS has been shown to induce release of natural opiates (endorphins, enkephalins, etc.) from the pituitary gland.[206-214]

The TENS instruments described in this chapter are the Myo-monitor and BNS-40 (manufactured by Myotronics, Inc.). These instruments successfully reduce muscle hyperactivity and effect the relaxation of muscles by applying a brief microstimulus of 25 mA for 500 msec at a fixed rate of 40 per minute during a period of time ranging from 1 to several hours (Table 8–3). This relaxation capability has been proved by electromyographic recording of resting electrical activity before and following TENS stimulation (Table 8–8) as well as by spectral analysis of the peak frequency of muscle electrical activity (Fig. 8–32).[215-217]

The site of TENS stimulation is critical to the induction of relaxation of the muscles associated with mandibular function. These muscles are innervated by the mandibular division of the trigeminal (fifth cranial) nerve, which exits the skull from the foramen rotundum, as well as by the facial (seventh cranial) nerve, which is located superficially in the parotid gland.[218] The trigeminal nerve is accessible to stimulation applied to the skin through soft tissue conduction only in the area of the face between the condyle and the coronoid process of the mandible (Figs. 8–33 and 8–34). Soft tissue conduction of an electrical stimulus is 85 percent effective. Placement of the TENS stimulator on any other location on the side of the mandible to reach the mandibular division of the fifth cranial nerve would require bony conduction, which is only 5 percent effective. The electrodes are placed bilaterally on the face in the area described, and a third electrode is placed in the center of the neck as a common stimulator, so that simultaneous stimulation of left and right muscle groups can be performed. The neck electrode also brings the electrical stimulus to the cervical muscles.

The value of neural conduction of the electrical stimulus is its efficiency, in contrast to the direct muscle stimulation employed frequently in physical medicine. By stimulating muscles by means of their neural supply, many distant muscles can be stimulated almost simultaneously with a relatively small amount of electricity. Direct muscle stimulation would require larger

TABLE 8–8. Electromyographic Measurement of Resting Activity Prior to Treatment (Left and Right Anterior Temporalis and Masseters)

	PERCENT
BEFORE TENS	
Three of four muscles rested	17.1
Four of four	11.2
At least three of four	28.3
AFTER TENS	
Three of four muscles rested	11.8
Four of four	69.4
At least three of four	81.1

Rest = <2.5 μV on EM2 and <10 μV on EM1. Two different EMG instruments used throughout the study designated EM1, EM2.
From Cooper, B. C., et al. Myofacial pain dysfunction: Analysis of 476 patients. Laryngoscope 96(10):1099–1106, 1986.

Craniomandibular Disorders

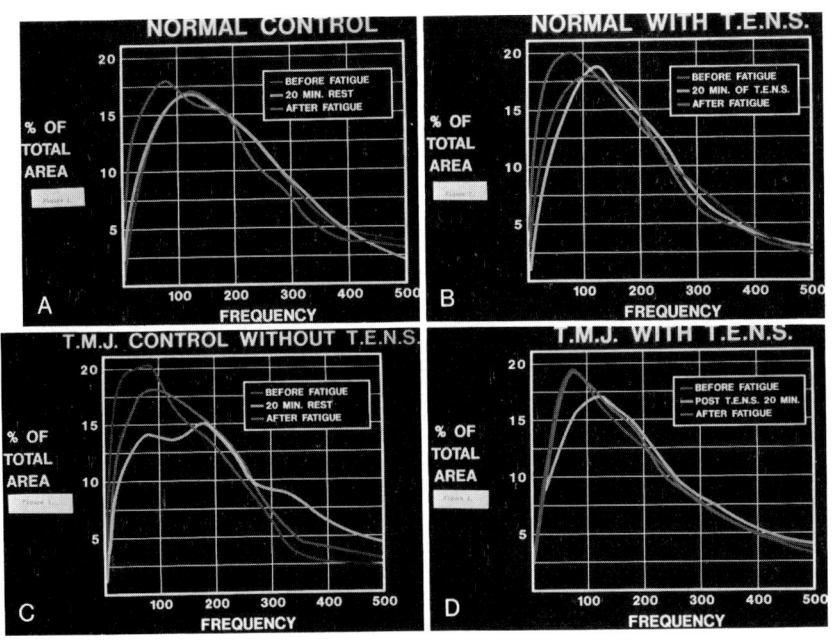

FIGURE 8–32. Spectral analysis of muscle. Comparisons were made between the power density frequency spectra of masticatory muscle electromyograms in 25 subjects with craniomandibular dysfunction and 25 control subjects. *A* and *B*, Resting peak frequency for controls appeared at 125 Hz. With sustained contraction, peak frequency shifted to 75 Hz. This shift was reversible with 20 minutes of rest with teeth disoccluded in control subjects. *C*, In patients with craniomandibular dysfunction, rest alone did not result in a return to normal peak frequency. *D*, However, after 20 minutes of TENS stimulation in these patients, peak frequency returned to normal. (Courtesy of Normal R. Thomas, B.D.S., B.Sc., Ph.D., University of Alberta, Edmonton, Canada.)

stimuli and contact with each and every muscle requiring stimulation. The lateral and medial pterygoid muscles, accessible either through the mouth or, in the case of the lateral pterygoid, by means of an entry through the coronoid notch, would be clinically difficult and impractical as a routine procedure. The neural pathway of muscle stimulation by the Myo-monitor has been documented.[219, 220] EMG data displayed on the MKG screen, as a recording of electrical activity in time, now also demonstrate the simultaneous electrical activity in the eight muscles being monitored with each stimulus of the TENS instrument (viewed four muscles at a time).

As stated, TENS stimulation causes muscles that are hyperactive to relax. As shown on the EMG and MKG instruments, the relaxation of the muscles is accompanied by a repositioning of the mandible from the accommodative postural rest position (Fig. 8–35).[221–225] The position of the mandible when the antagonistic elevator and depressor muscles are in a state of minimal electrical activity is considered the true *mandibular rest position*. TENS stimulation of the muscles whose function is to move the mandible does indeed move it upward and forward from the true resting position along an arc, known as the *neuromuscular trajectory of movement*. A position along this arc is selected to be the maxillomandibular position

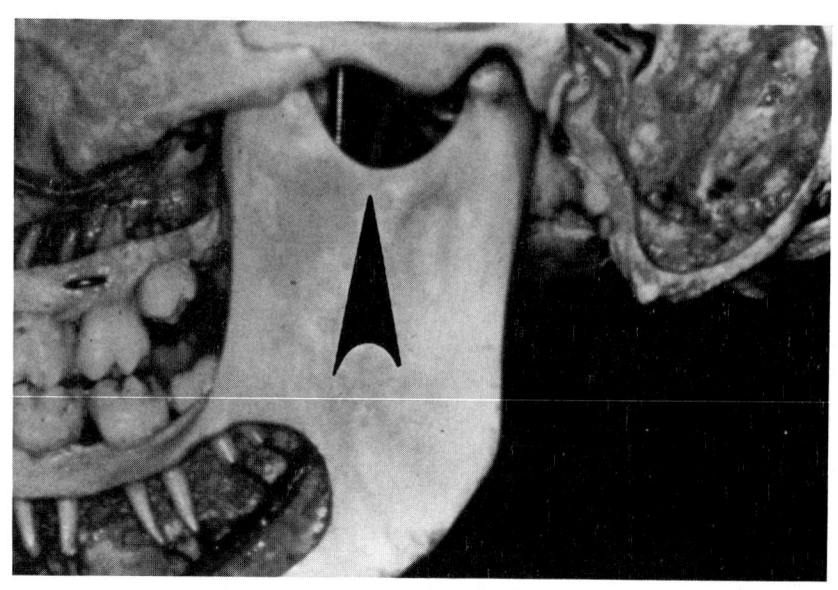

FIGURE 8–33. Lateral view of the skull. Electrode for TENS is placed over the mandibular notch between the condyle and the coronoid process (above arrow). This permits soft tissue conduction of the stimulus to the mandibular division of the trigeminal nerve (cranial nerve V) deep to the mandible directly behind the notch as well as stimulation to the facial nerve (cranial nerve VII) superficial to the mandible.

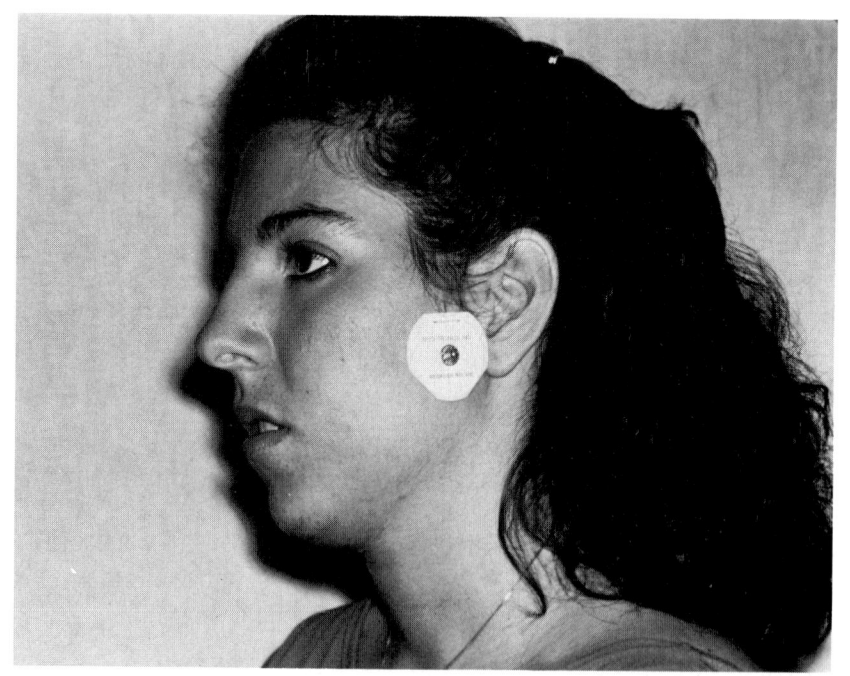

FIGURE 8–34. Placement of the TENS electrode on the face superficial to the mandibular notch as described in Figure 8–33. This is done bilaterally, and a third common electrode is placed on the rear of the neck.

Craniomandibular Disorders

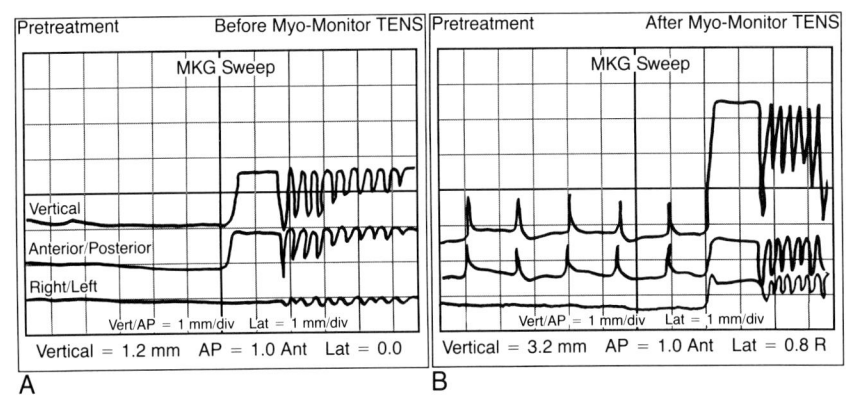

FIGURE 8–35. Mandibular kinesiograph (MKG) recording of mandibular movement from rest to occlusion. *A*, Accommodative rest before TENS. *B*, True rest position after TENS-induced muscle relaxation. EMG testing of muscle activity confirmed that muscles were rested following TENS. Note increased vertical freeway space as mandible rested further from upper teeth after muscles were relaxed by TENS. Patient also closes to the right (lower tracing) after TENS, which requires left lateral pterygoid contraction. Patient was 30-year-old female who complained of left facial and cervical pain, tinnitus, decreased hearing acuity, temporomandibular joint sounds, otalgia in airplanes, and limited mouth opening.

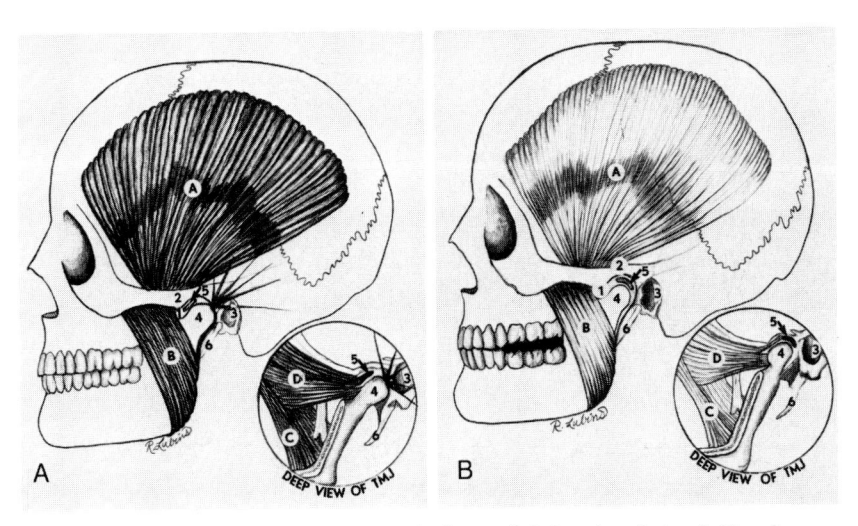

FIGURE 8–36. Diagrammatic representation of natural, habitual occlusion (left) and neuromuscular occlusion (right). Natural occlusion, though possibly esthetic, can be pathologic, requiring excessive muscle activity to produce it and causing pressures within the temporomandibular joint that result in myofacial pain dysfunction. Neuromuscular occlusal position (right), determined on the MKG/EMG, requires no accommodative fatiguing muscle activity and causes no pressure within the temporomandibular joint. There is no interdigitation of posterior teeth with mandibular stability, and occlusion is, therefore, initially maintained by a precise neuromuscular orthotic appliance. (1) Articular eminence, (2) glenoid fossa, (3) external auditory meatus, (4) head of condyle, (5) disk, (6) styloid process. Muscles: A = temporalis, B = masseter, C = medial pterygoid, D = lateral pterygoid. Radiating lines from TMJ in left diagram represent (symbolically) condylar pressure exerted posteriorly. (From Cooper, B. C., et al. Myofacial pain dysfunction: Analysis of 476 patients, Laryngoscope 96(10):1099–1106, 1986.)

for the occlusion that is to be therapeutically established. Therefore, TENS is utilized to relax hyperactive mandibular muscles and initiate involuntary mandibular movement along an arc or a pathway that is physiologically natural (Fig. 8–17). This function will be discussed further below.

NEUROMUSCULAR OCCLUSION

The starting point for determining the neuromuscular occlusal (NMO) position is the resting point of the mandible, a position achieved by TENS-induced relaxation of the musculature (Figs. 8–36 and 8–37). From this resting position, which is associated with minimal electrical activity measured on the EMG, the mandible should ideally move in a muscularly dictated arc to closure. This muscularly directed arc of movement can be stimulated only by involuntary muscle contraction achieved by TENS stimulation (Fig. 8–38A). This neuromuscular arc cannot be reproduced by willful effort of the patient, with his proprioceptive memories, or by the doctor.

With TENS stimulation, the mandible moves along a neuromuscular arc in a upward and anterior direction to closure. This arc can be traced on the MKG (Fig. 8–38B). Ideally, the perfect occlusal position would be about 1 mm from the muscular rest position along this physiologic closure trajectory.[226, 227]

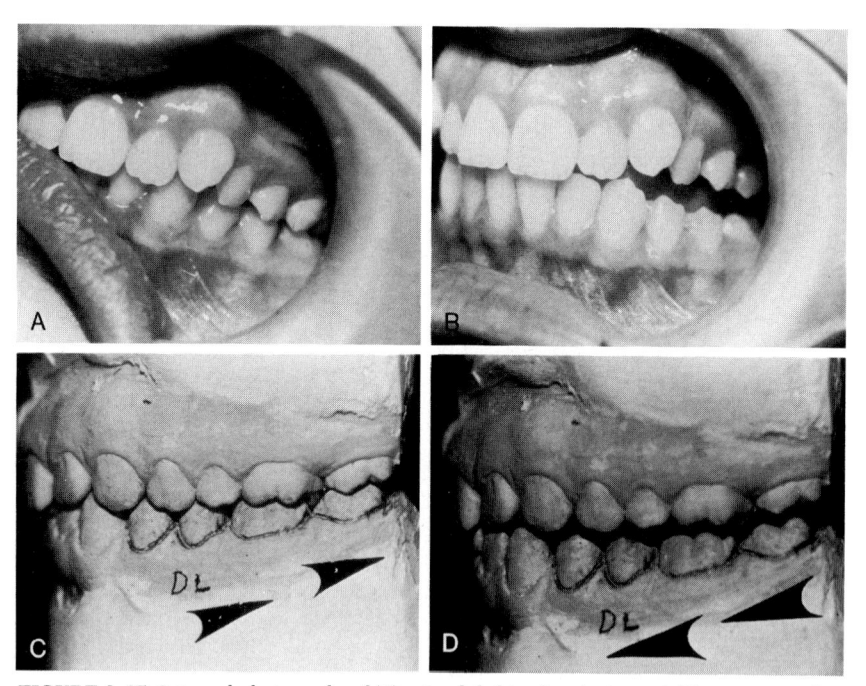

FIGURE 8–37. Intraoral photographs of (A) natural, habitual occlusion and (B) neuromuscular occlusal position. Models of dentition demonstrate (C) habitual occlusion and (D) neuromuscular occlusal position. Arrows signify the direction of mandibular movement to achieve each position. Habitual occlusion is more posterior, and the neuromuscular occlusal position is more anterior.

Craniomandibular Disorders

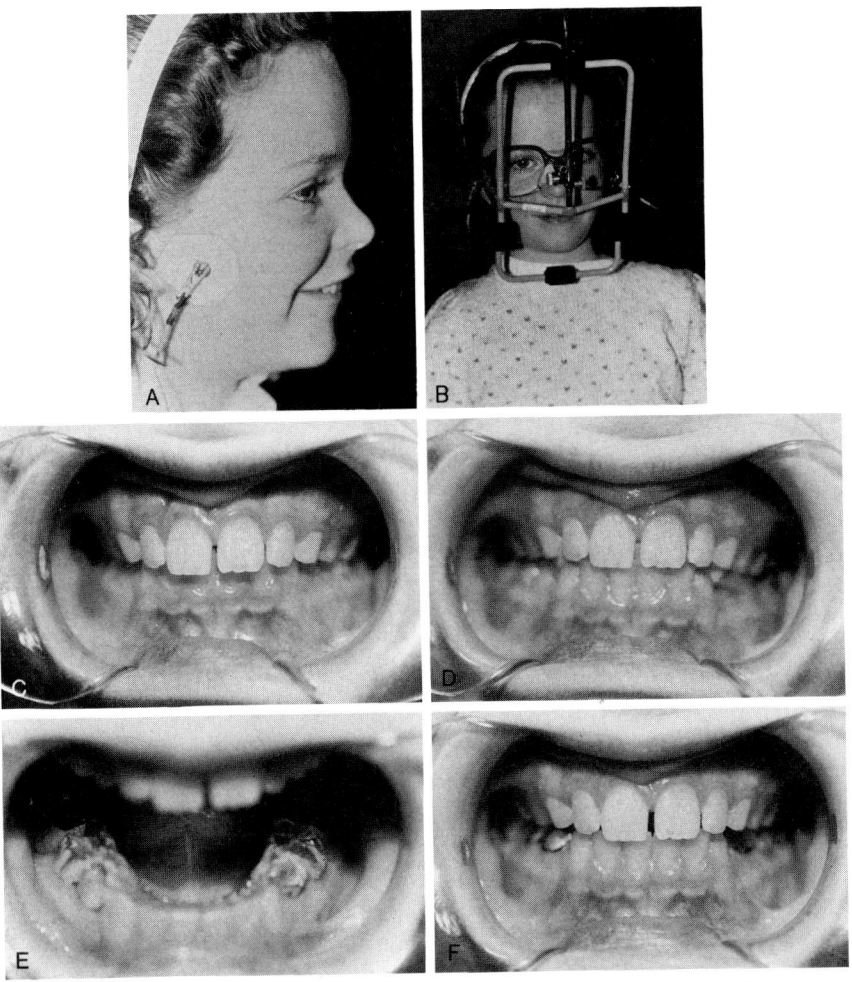

FIGURE 8-38. Illustration showing testing, recording of bite registration, and orthotic appliance insertion. *A*, TENS electrode during muscle relaxation portion of test. *B*, MKG sensor array in place during test to determine neuromuscular occlusal position. *C*, Natural, habitual occlusal position (pretreatment). *D*, Bite registration material in the mouth retested for accuracy. *E*, Acrylic orthotic appliance in place on mandibular teeth. *F*, Patient occluding with orthotic device. Patient was a 9-year-old child with chronic otalgia of many years' duration.

The position of occlusion as determined by MKG/EMG testing to be the optimum position is compared with the existing dental occlusal position by asking the patient to close the teeth voluntarily after the operator turns off the TENS stimulus (Fig. 8-38C). The two occlusal positions are then contrasted on the MKG—the natural (habitual, HCO) position and the ideal neuromuscular (myocentric, MCO) position.

The neuromuscular occlusal position can be localized with ease on mandibular tracings of the involuntary TENS-induced motion. This position can be more permanently recorded on a low-resistance impression material placed between the upper and lower teeth (Fig. 8–38D). TENS-induced stimulation brings the mandible toward the maxilla momentarily on the closure trajectory, 1 mm above rest, in this plastic medium. The semihardened impression material is removed from the mouth and further set on stone casts (models) of the patients's teeth. The bite registration can be reinserted into the mouth to test its accuracy. The mandibular position at this newly determined occlusal position can be compared on the MKG tracing and will be found to be exactly the same position as that recorded in the empty mouth as described above.

The establishment of this new occlusal position (Fig. 8–38E and F) allows maximum rest for antagonistic muscle groups (mandibular elevators and depressors) as demonstrated by electromyography.[43] However, in addition, this position provides better muscle health, which increases muscle compressive strength; this also is demonstrable by EMG (Fig. 8–39).[228] Muscle function is optimal near the resting length of the muscle fibers (Fig. 8–40).[229, 230]

Clinically, it has been observed that some patients exhibit a very narrow range of the ideal position of the mandible with resting levels of antagonistic muscle activity. In these individuals elevation of the mandible (closing) even 1 mm activates the temporalis muscles, whereas depression of the mandible (opening) even 1 mm activates the digastrics.[231-236] In these individuals the position of ideal neuromuscular occlusion is narrowly restricted to a specific vertical position (Fig. 8–41). In others there is a range of 2 or more mm in which equal levels of electrical activity, considered rest, exist. In these patients the doctor has some latitude in establishing the ideal vertical dimension of the new occlusion. A better term would be a range of longitude. Lateral and anteroposterior discrepancies cause muscular fatigue far more quickly than vertical discrepancies.[237]

If bilateral muscular balance is achieved at this point, with simultaneous initiation of electrical activity in both masseters on clenching, therapy will most likely result in good muscle function and patient comfort. If bilateral symmetry is not achieved at this point, the bite registration procedure is repeated. In addition to masseter strength and bilateral balance, the relative strength of the masseter and temporalis muscles is monitored. Temporalis muscles, owing to their anatomic orientation, pull the mandible posteriorly while elevating it. The masseters, on the other hand, direct the mandible anteriorly and upward.

Overall, temporalis dominance over the masseters in the bite registration, as in the testing of the natural occlusion previously performed, usually indicates a posteriorly displaced occlusion (Fig. 8–42). This dominance is not optimal because it usually indicates that the patient is still posturing or holding the mandible posteriorly. Since the lateral pterygoid muscles, which are responsible for the anterior movement of the mandible, are not being monitored during this EMG test, the masseter to temporalis relationship is monitored as an indication of posterior holding. If this temporalis dominance occurs repeatedly after additional bite registrations, the need for additional TENS stimulated muscle relaxation should be considered.

Text continued on page 225

Craniomandibular Disorders

A. EMG Pretreatment after Myo-Monitor TENS Function-Clench Test
NATURAL OCCLUSION

	RIGHT		LEFT	
	Ta	Mm	Mm	Ta
	0	2	2	1
	14	2	6	16
	41	5	17	92
	87	29	66	118
	102	38	46	153
	106	19	53	84
	100	26	58	74
	123	31	69	69
	104	22	49	85
	62	17	35	78
▶	82	21	Average 44	93 ◀

Temporalis dominance = posteriorly displaced occlusion in natural dentition.
Abbreviations: Ta, temporalis anterior; Mm, middle masseter. Averaged data.

B. EMG Bite Registration after Myo-Monitor TENS Function-Clench Test
NEUROMUSCULAR OCCLUSION

RIGHT		LEFT	
Ta	Mm	Mm	Ta
1	1	2	4
14	9	6	13
105	120	68	82
148	211	131	172
129	175	154	160
142	217	114	160
106	154	112	143
148	200	133	169
154	170	116	182
146	216	135	194
121	163	Average 107	141

Improved muscle function clenching in neuromuscular occlusion.
EMG confirms improved function in treatment occlusion
Abbreviations: Ta, temporalis anterior; Mm, middle masseter
Averaged data.

FIGURE 8–39. Electromyograph (EMG) of anterior temporalis (Ta) and masseter (Mm) muscle function in clenching. *A,* In natural dentition temporalis muscles dominate (arrows) and masseters are weak, indicating posterior occlusion. *B,* Following TENS, maxillomandibular bite registration taken in the neuromuscular occlusal position (also called myocentric occlusion [MCO]) demonstrates improved muscle function with new occlusion. The patient was a 14-year-old girl who had otalgia (intensified on airplanes), pain behind her eyes, and facial, head, and throat pain. She had missed 25 school days in one year due to head pain. (Each point is the average of 256 samples taken over 0.2 second. Average of 10 samples is printed below.) Ta = temporalis anterior; Mm = masseters.

A. Pretreatment EMG Test before Myo-Monitor TENS
MANDIBLE IN REST POSITION

RIGHT			LEFT		
Ta	Da	Mm	Mm	Da	Ta
2.1	1.3	▶ 4.0	0.8	2.6	▶ 7.2

Many muscles have high resting activity levels. Averaged data.
Bilateral asymmetry left temporalis anterior pain is left sided
Abbreviations: Ta, temporalis anterior; Mm, middle masseter; Da, anterior digastric

B. EMG Pretreatment Before Myo-Monitor TENS Function-Clench
TEST OF MUSCLES IN OCCLUSION

RIGHT			LEFT	
Ta	Mm		Mm	Ta
0	0		0	4
9	8		6	5
21	9		19	6
48	17		25	10
72	20		42	5
70	22		42	4
85	33		50	5
82	40		81	5
67	31		63	5
48	24		40	5
55	23	◀ Average	40	5 ◀

Bilateral asymmetry; note weakness of left temporalis anterior, which had highest resting activity level. Averaged data.
Abbreviations: Ta, temporalis anterior; Mm, middle masseter
Arrows indicate text emphasis

FIGURE 8–40. Electromyographic (EMG) recording of muscles with mandible at rest. *A*, Pretreatment bilateral asymmetry with high resting activity levels in left temporalis and right masseter (arrows). *B*, Function test demonstrates weakness in those muscles that had the highest resting activity (arrows). Ta = temporalis anterior; Mm = masseters; Da = anterior digastric.

Craniomandibular Disorders

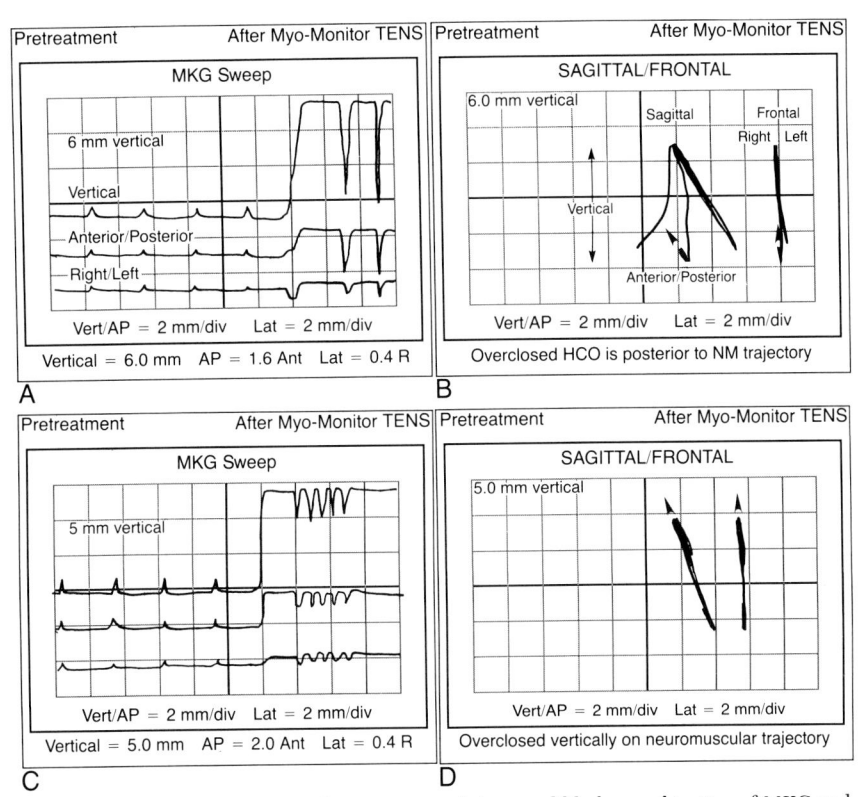

FIGURE 8-41. Determination of rest position of the mandible by combination of MKG and EMG testing. Patient exhibited two distinct resting positions of the mandible following TENS-induced muscle relaxation. *A* and *B*, In one position there was 6 mm of vertical freeway space between the upper and lower teeth. *C* and *D*, In the other position there was 5 mm of space between the dental arches.

Illustration continued on following page

E. Pretreatment EMG Test After Myo-Monitor TENS
MANDIBLE IN REST POSITION

	RIGHT		LEFT	
	<u>Ta</u>	<u>Mm</u>	<u>Mm</u>	<u>Ta</u>
6 MM	3.5	2.2	2.3	2.7
VERTICAL		<u>Da</u>	Da	
		▶ 7.7	6.8 ◀	

Mandible is overopened; note high resting activity levels for digastric muscles
All muscles are in high-activity state

		<u>Ta</u>	<u>Mm</u>	<u>Mm</u>	<u>Ta</u>
5 MM		1.4	0.4	0.2	0.9
VERTICAL			<u>Da</u>	Da	
			▶ 1.2	0.9 ◀	

Mandible at more rested position EMG normal for all antagonistic muscles. EMG is utilized to determine freeway space at true rest position. Data is integrated with MKG data. Note low activity in digastrics at this vertical.

Abbreviations: Ta, temporalis anterior; Mm, middle masseter; Da, anterior digastric. Averaged data.

FIGURE 8–41 *Continued E,* The determination of the optimum rest position was made utilizing EMG data. All muscles rested at lower levels of activity at 5 mm. The 6-mm vertical space was, however, an active open position, in which protrusion of the mandible was accompanied by higher EMG activity in both temporalis and digastric muscles. Patient was a 25-year-old male presenting with bilateral eye and ear pain and a history of frequent breakage of many dental crowns (evidence of self-destructing dentition). HCO = habitual natural occlusion; NM = neuromuscular; Ta = temporalis anterior; Mm = masseter; Da = anterior digastric.

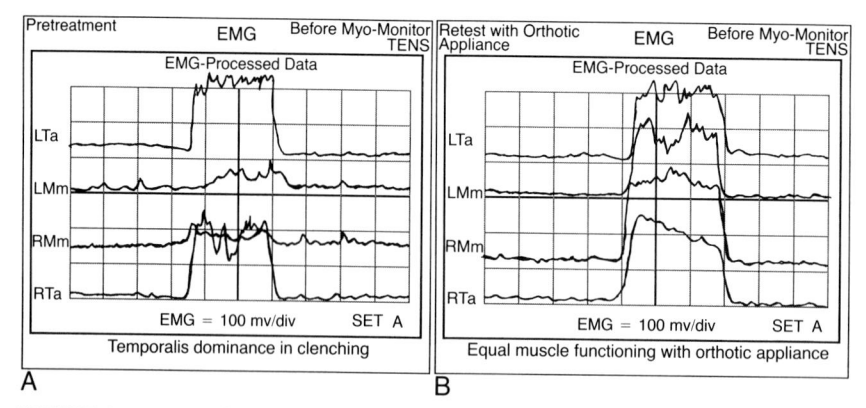

FIGURE 8–42. EMG data can be displayed either as numerical values, as seen in previous figures, or graphically on the computer screen. Here EMG processed data of the temporalis and masseter muscles show the electrical activity involved in a single clench. *A,* Natural dentition (before treatment) shows temporalis dominance and masseter weakness. *B,* Under active treatment, the patient, utilizing an orthotic appliance to establish neuromuscular occlusion, demonstrates equal bilateral four-muscle function in clench. (Data are displayed on an MKG computer screen.) LTa = left temporalis anterior; LMm = left masseter; RMm = right masseter; RTa = right temporalis anterior; SET A = EMG instrument's designation of anterior temporalis and masseter muscles.

As an additional test of the accuracy of the bite registration, the patient is given dental cotton rolls on which to clench. EMG function testing is performed to measure the capacity of the muscles to function without the constraints of the natural dentition or the bite registration (Fig. 8-43). Good muscle function and bilateral symmetry with masseter strength equal to or dominant over the temporalis is an indication of excellent muscle capacity. This capacity should be obtainable with the bite registration already made. If it is not observed, the bite registration should be repeated until good function is achieved. After therapy, better function may become evident, since a muscularly healthy occlusion has existed for several months.

ESTABLISHMENT OF NEUROMUSCULAR OCCLUSION

Coronoplasty

It is important to note that not all MPD patients require orthotic therapy. Some individuals require only minor correction of specific interfering surfaces on one or more teeth to eliminate the etiologic agent that has caused muscle fatigue due to patterns of avoidance conditioning (Figs. 8-44 and 8-45). Once these premature occlusion contacts have been identified, often on the sloping inclines of the teeth, and eliminated by prudent reshaping of the teeth, the muscular dysfunction disappears permanently. The operative word here is *identified*.[238-242]

Coronoplasty and *equilibration* are the terms used in dentistry to describe the process of reshaping the natural contours of teeth. Unfortunately, much tooth grinding has been performed with the ostensible purpose of solving muscular dysfunction but in the absence of objective measurement of muscle function. Tooth grinding is an irreversible procedure that should be performed only when conclusive objective evidence supports the need.

Such evidence can be obtained with the electronic data discussed here. When the muscles are fully relaxed, as determined on EMG, and the vertical space between the upper and lower teeth (vertical freeway space) is within acceptable parameters (0.75 to 2.0 mm), consideration should be given to correcting the natural occlusion by means of coronoplasty rather than an orthotic appliance.

Prudence is advised. Once removed, tooth structure cannot be replaced naturally. If there is any possibility of further relaxation, which would lead to increased vertical freeway space and the possibility of an orthotic appliance to correct the vertical space, coronoplasty should not be performed. It is preferable to utilize an orthotic appliance temporarily, even if it is very thin, to aid in achieving maximum muscle relaxation and physiologic mandibular repositioning before irreversible changes in tooth morphology are implemented. It is a critical decision and has been the subject of litigation recently.

The coronoplasty procedure is extremely precise and effective. It utilizes the TENS instrument first to relax the mandibular muscles. Following relaxation, with MKG/EMG determination that the mandible is in its true resting position, TENS initiates involuntary mandibular movement along

A. EMG Pretreatment before Myo-Monitor TENS Function-Clench Test
NATURAL DENTITION

RIGHT			LEFT	
Ta	Mm		Mm	Ta
4	0		0	2
11	0		1	12
17	3		5	90
33	18		10	117
32	16		4	55
39	16		7	46
41	14		6	62
35	20		6	53
28	15		6	64
37	20		4	64
30	13	◄ ►	5	62

Temporalis dominance indicates posterior displacement. Masseter weakness (arrows)
Note bilateral discrepancy. Averaged data.

B. EMG Pretreatment before Myo-Monitor TENS Function-Clench Test
BITE ON COTTON ROLLS

RIGHT			LEFT	
Ta	Mm		Mm	Ta
58	138		91	120
57	152		68	91
73	163		68	122
62	125		69	98
57	134		65	118
61	97		65	114
47	97		51	102
64	111		81	94
55	97		55	91
45	67		61	82
57	118	◄ ►	66	102

Cotton roll test bypasses occlusion. Improved masseter function (arrows)
Abbreviations: Ta, temporalis anterior; Mm, middle masseter. Averaged data.

FIGURE 8–43. EMG recording of muscle action in clenching. *A*, In natural dentition all muscles are weak, but temporalis muscles dominate, the left temporalis (Ta) being the strongest. *B*, Patient is instructed to clench on dental cotton rolls to test the capacity of four muscles to function when dental occlusion is eliminated as a factor. Great improvement in all muscles is observed, suggesting a good prognosis for therapy that improves occlusion. Patient was a 49-year-old woman who had facial and cervical pain and otalgia (which became acute on airplane flights). Establishment of long-term neuromuscular occlusion resulted in relief of all symptoms (6-year follow-up). Ta = temporalis anterior; Mm = masseter.

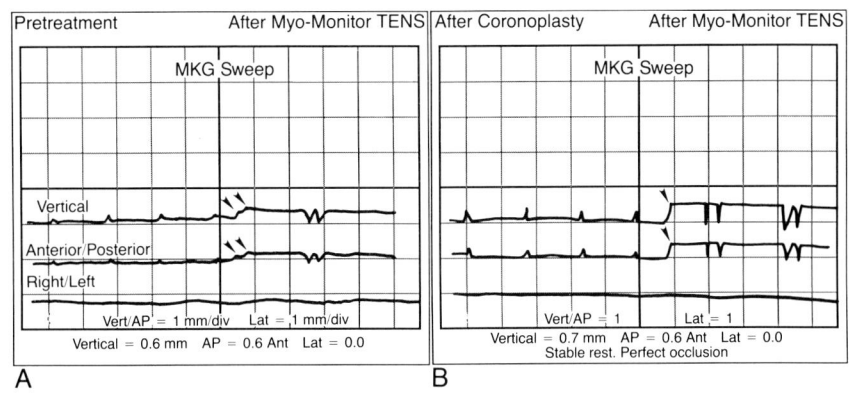

FIGURE 8–44. MKG recording of movement of mandible from rest to occlusion. *A*, Closure into natural occlusion position reveals a premature contacting point, which deflects the mandible during closure into full occlusion of the teeth (indicated by arrows) into full occlusion, seen on vertical (upper) and anteroposterior tracings (center). *B*, Following coronoplasty procedure using TENS, premature tooth contacts have been eliminated, and patient closes perfectly into total occlusion without impediment. Patient was a 31-year-old male who complained of "blinding headaches," cervical and sinus pain, dizziness, and temporomandibular joint clicks. All symptoms disappeared following coronoplasty procedure. No orthotic appliance therapy was required.

EMG Pretreatment Before Myo-Monitor TENS Function-Clench Test
NATURAL AND RESTORED DENTITION

	RIGHT		LEFT	
	Ta	Mm	Mm	Ta
	1	0	0	0
	11	3	0	3
	22	20*	1	17
	66	42	36 ◄	69 ◄
	64	37	46	66
	96	58	48	69
	68	59	49	106
	76	67	50	78
	80	49	55	101
	61	49	56	80
	60	42	Average 36	67

Abbreviations: Ta, temporalis anterior; Mm, middle masseter. Averaged data.

FIGURE 8–45. Electromyographic recording of muscle activity during clench. Patient occluded first on right side (observe right masseter activity), and then left temporalis activity occurs (arrow) as mandible is elevated on left to bring about secondary occlusion on left. The occlusal contact is indicated by activity in left masseter muscle (arrow). Patient was a 61-year-old male who had left temporal headaches, muffled and painful ears. He was aware that his left rear teeth, which consisted of severely worn partial denture teeth, did not easily come together as he tried to bite together. The left temporalis muscle was the most tender to palpation, was identified as the painful area by the patient, and showed the highest activity levels at rest on EMG. Ta = temporalis anterior; Mm = masseter muscles.

the neuromuscular trajectory (arc) from rest to the first premature point of occlusion. That point or points can be demonstrated by first applying a thin wax coating on the teeth on one arch, either upper or lower. This wax is first warmed in hot water before being applied to the teeth. The TENS stimulus gently projects the mandible by isotonic contraction of its muscles into the softened wax. Tiny perforations or indentations in the wax mark the premature occlusal contacts. These are marked through the wax with a wax marking pencil, the wax is removed, and the tooth surface where marked with the wax pencil is carefully polished. The test is repeated until no premature contacts are observed on TENS-induced mandibular movements. In this part of the coronoplasty procedure, the patient is not asked to close voluntarily into occlusion because learned avoidance conditioning through proprioception prohibits voluntary contact in an uncomfortable position. To illustrate this, consider a splinter in the sole of your foot. Once you have experienced pain accompanying stepping on that splinter, you will not voluntarily place your foot squarely on the floor. You will, rather, establish a pattern of walking that avoids the painful contact. The TENS instrument bypasses the proprioceptive learning and sends the mandible gently and freely into the first tooth contact. That unmasks the occlusal prematurity.

The second part of the coronoplasty procedure does involve voluntary chewing. The patient is instructed to perform a few rapid chewing strokes. Here laterally inclined interferences can be visualized in the wax. They are identified, marked with the wax pencil, and eliminated carefully with a fine carbide finishing bur in the dental high-speed handpiece. Judiciously performed, this procedure is not harmful to the teeth. This procedure is again repeated, great care being taken not to eliminate any important vertical holding points in the entire occlusion. These are the cusp tips of the outer (buccal) cusps of the lower teeth and their corresponding fossae or concavities in the centers of the upper posterior teeth. Similar essential vertical holding stops are the cusp tips on the inner (palatal) cusps of the upper teeth and their corresponding fossae located in the centers of the lower posterior teeth. Similarly, there are essential vertical holding stops on the inner palatal surface of the upper anterior teeth and the corresponding incisal edges of the lower anterior teeth. All tooth surfaces are carefully shaped to create the natural curved spheroidal form of the teeth.

The goal of this procedure is the establishment of a secure, stable interdigitation of the teeth that can be freely entered and freely exited. It is a dental occlusal position that is synchronized with healthy balanced muscle function near the rest position of the mandible and at which its antagonistic muscles can be at their full resting length.

The coronoplasty technique described here is utilized to modify the morphology of natural teeth to perfect the occlusion. It is also employed in adjusting orthotic appliances and in secondary long-term treatment forms as described below.

Orthotic Appliances
When MKG/EMG analysis demonstrates that the vertical freeway space between the maxillary and mandibular teeth is greater than 2.0 mm after

the muscles have been adequately relaxed, the new neuromuscular occlusal relationship cannot be established by modification of the surfaces of the natural teeth alone (Fig. 8–46). An appliance must be fabricated to alter the maxillomandibular relationship totally. The function of the orthotic appliance is to establish a healthy occlusal position that is synchronized with balanced muscle function near the point of muscle relaxation and healthy joint function.[243]

Fitted over the mandibular posterior teeth, the removable orthotic appliance is made of a transparent acrylic material (Fig. 8–47). The uppermost surface of the orthotic device is contoured to simulate the anatomy of the natural teeth, which can intercuspate or interdigitate with the opposing upper teeth. It provides a "home plate" on which the mandible can comfortably land as it moves to occlude the teeth. Use of the appliance all day and all night provides the stable occlusal position necessary for swallowing and chewing food while allowing the muscles to remain continually in a relaxed condition.

The orthotic appliance is worn for a period of at least 3 months. Initially, patients return for additional TENS therapy to aid in relaxing the musculature. Small changes are made if necessary in the orthotic appliance's occlusion to correct for ongoing modification in the rest position as the muscles continue to relax. These corrections are usually completed in a few weeks with several visits. The patient then continues to wear the neuromuscular orthotic appliance for the remainder of the 3-month period, returning only if symptoms persist and the patient requires additional TENS therapy or adjustment of the orthotic device.

MONITORING THERAPEUTIC RESULTS

At the end of the third month of orthotic therapy, the patient returns for a second MKG/EMG study to monitor the results of therapy. Ideally, this retest should demonstrate that the occlusal position provided by the orthotic device is synchronized with balanced muscle function and that muscle function is strong and also rested in the relaxed position of the mandible. It should also show that the occlusal position is accurately located on the neuromuscular trajectory at a proper vertical height above the true rest position of the mandible (Tables 8–9 and 8–10).

If the appliance does not provide a neuromuscularly balanced occlusal position 1 mm from the muscular rest position, it must be replaced. Inaccuracy of the appliance at the 3-month test may reflect excessive wear on the acrylic material, resulting in a change in the occlusal position. In this case, the occlusal position may be too far from the rest position, but it is most likely still on the same neuromuscularly determined closure trajectory.

When muscles relax further during the 3-month interval, the mandibular rest position may change. As a result, the occlusal position of the orthotic appliance may appear posteriorly or laterally displaced from the neuromuscular trajectory (Figs. 8–48 and 8–49). These patients sometimes report initial remission of symptoms, with a return to some symptoms in the later

Text continued on page 234

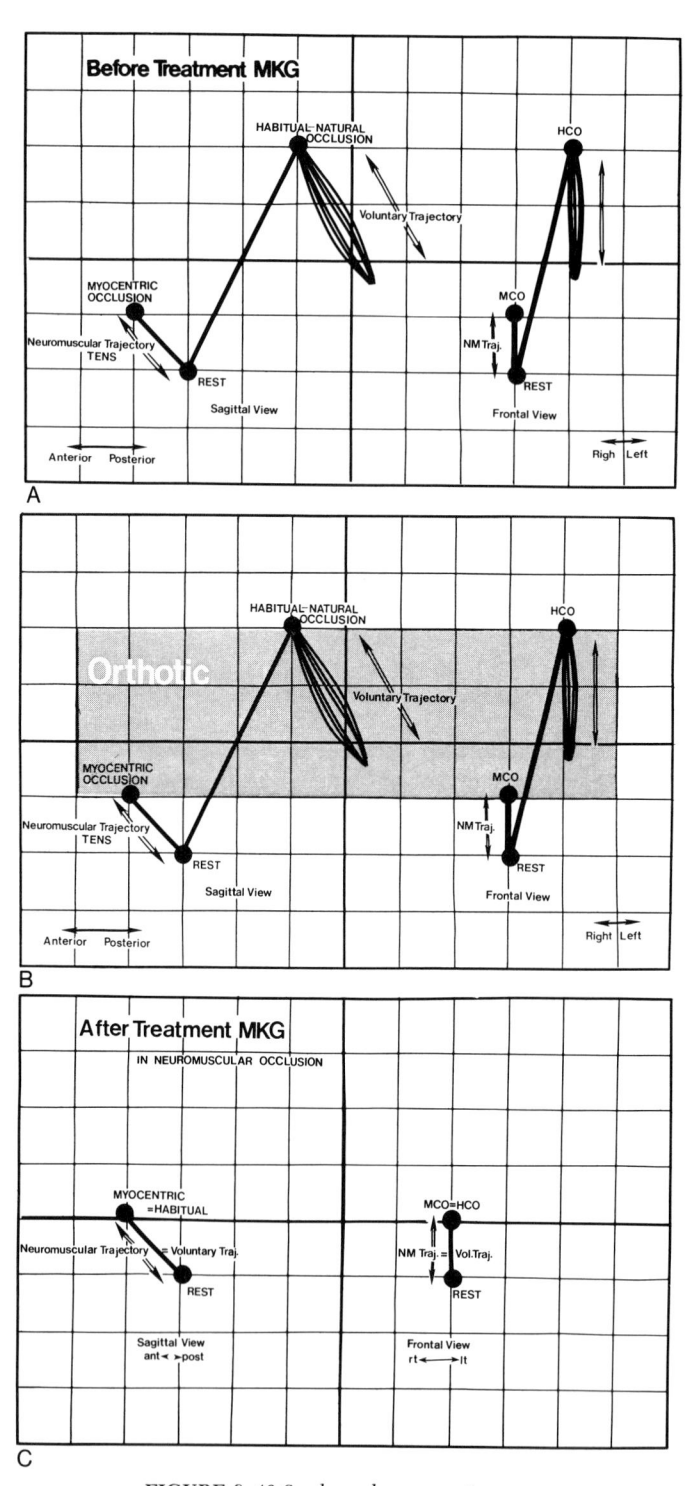

FIGURE 8–46 *See legend on opposite page*

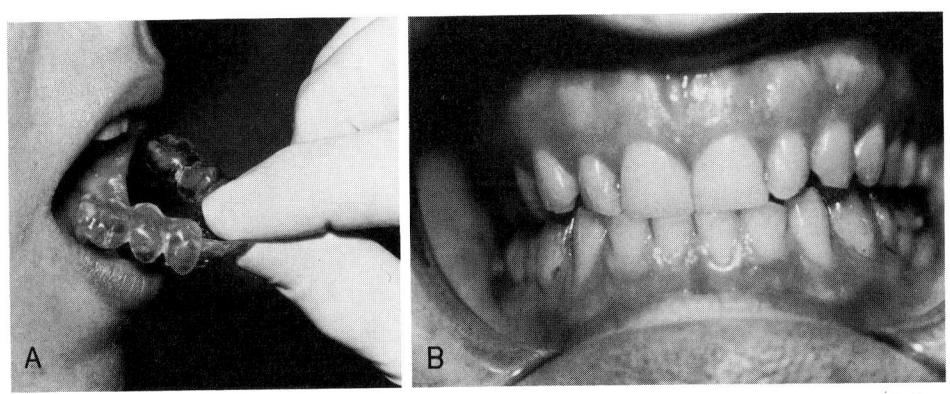

FIGURE 8–47. *A,* Insertion of precision neuromuscular occlusion orthotic appliance over the mandibular posterior teeth. *B,* Orthotic appliance in place with patient biting in therapeutic maxillomandibular relationship.

TABLE 8–9. Mandibular Kinesiograph of Vertical Freeway Space (Measured Incisally)

BEFORE TREATMENT (476 PATIENTS)	UNDER TREATMENT (300 PATIENTS)	LONG-TERM TREATED (125 PATIENTS)
Healthy 24% (avg vertical space 1.8 mm)	Healthy 87% (avg vertical space 1.2 mm)	Healthy 100% (avg vertical space 1.1 mm)
Unhealthy 76% (avg vertical space 4.1 mm)	Unhealthy 13% (avg vertical space 2.7 mm)	Unhealthy 0%

From Cooper, B. C., et al. Myofacial pain dysfunction: Analysis of 476 patients. Laryngoscope 96(10):1099–1106, 1986.

FIGURE 8–46. Schematic representations of mandibular kinesiograph tracings of the mandible at rest and in occlusion. *A,* After TENS-induced muscle relaxation, the mandible assumes a true resting position (confirmed by EMG recordings). There is excess vertical freeway space between upper and lower teeth. *B,* The excess freeway space will be occupied by the neuromuscular orthotic appliance, represented by the shaded area, leaving a healthy freeway space of 1.0 mm between the upper surface of the orthotic device covering the lower teeth and the occlusal surface of the opposing upper teeth. *C,* A retest of the patient after 3 months, with the orthotic appliance in place, demonstrates a healthy freeway space of 1.0 mm between the occlusal surface of the mandibular orthotic appliance and the surface of the maxillary teeth. HCO = habitual natural occlusion; MCO = myocentric occlusion.

TABLE 8–10. Comparison of Occlusal Position with Ideal Myocentric Occlusion

	PRETREATMENT NATURAL (476 PATIENTS)	UNDER TREATMENT ORTHOTIC (300 PATIENTS)	LONG-TERM MYOCENTRIC (125 PATIENTS)
On neuromuscular trajectory	25%	76%	100%
Overclosed	64%	11%	0%
Displaced posteriorly	65%	16%	0%
Displaced laterally or A/P	74%	25%	5%

From Cooper, B. C., et al. Myofacial pain dysfunction: Analysis of 476 patients. Laryngoscope 96(10):1099–1106, 1986.

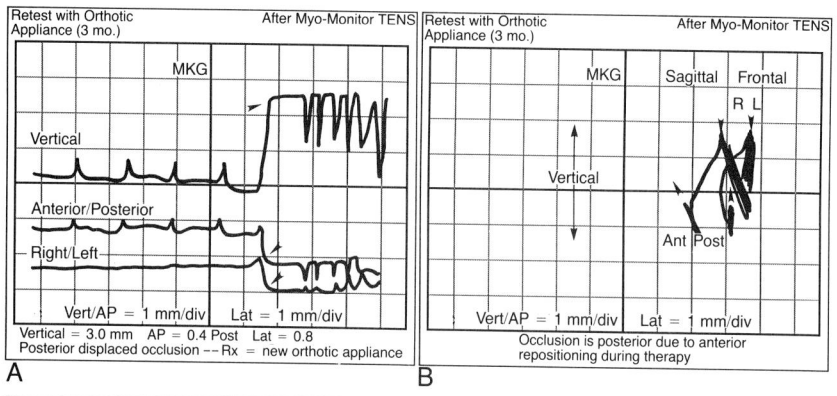

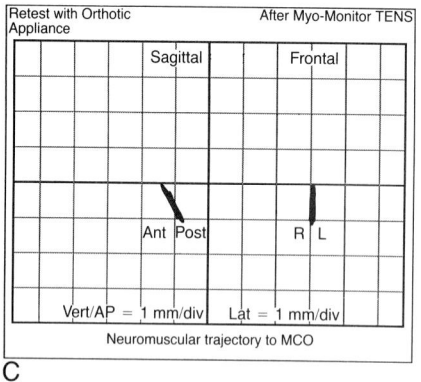

FIGURE 8–48. MKG monitoring of patient with orthotic appliance worn 3 months. Testing is performed with the orthotic device in the mouth to check for accuracy. *A*, Data reveal that the occlusion position provided by the orthotic device is excessively far from the rest position of the mandible (> 2.0 mm) in the upper tracing and displaces the mandible posteriorly (center) and left (lower tracing). *B*, The same MKG data, displayed on an X–Y graph, illustrate the overclosure, posterior, and lateral (left) displacement of occlusion from the neuromuscular ideal position. With use of the neuromuscular orthotic appliance, the muscles relaxed further, and the mandibular rest position changed. Therefore, closure into the orthotic device required displacement. At the time of this retest, this 16-year-old girl complained of temporal headaches on the left side. This complaint was corroborated on EMG, which showed hyperactivity in the left anterior temporalis muscle. *C*, A new accurate orthotic appliance was fabricated. Tested after insertion, occlusion was shown to be precisely on the neuromuscular trajectory.

Illustration continued on following page

D. EMG Retest with New Orthotic Appliance After Myo-Monitor TENS

	RIGHT			LEFT	
MANDIBLE AT REST	Ta	Mm		Mm	Ta
"REST TEST"	1.0	0.9		0.5	1.5
(AVERAGED DATA)	Tp	Da		Da	Tp
	1.2	1.5		1.3	1.3
MANDIBLE IN FUNCTION	Ta	Mm		Mm	Ta
"CLENCH TEST"	99	133	◄ ►	124	96
(AVERAGED DATA)					

Balanced function bilaterally; masseter slightly stronger (arrows) in function
EMG confirms healthy muscle function through therapy
Abbreviations: Ta, temporalis anterior; Mm, middle masseter; Da, anterior digastric; Tp, temporalis posterior

FIGURE 8–48 *Continued D*, EMG testing of the new orthotic device proved the presence of muscular rest and balanced activity in function. Patient became symptom free.

EMG Pretreatment After Myo-Monitor TENS Function-Clench Test
NATURAL DENTITION

	RIGHT			LEFT	
	Ta	Mm		Mm	Ta
	0	0		0	0
	26	1		3	8
	53	4		42	23
	56	15		47	25
	71	17		46	23
	65	19		50	24
	76	23		54	27
	66	25		63	24
	61	16		54	24
	45	18		46	16
►	57	15	Average ►	45	21

Dominant muscles in function are right Ta, left Mm (arrows).
Note torque on closure, right Ta pulls back, left Mm pulls forward
Abbreviations: Ta, temporalis anterior; Mm, middle masseter. Averaged data.

FIGURE 8–49. EMG testing demonstrating horizontal rotation (torque) of the mandible in occluding the upper and lower teeth. This torque is shown on the function test as dominant activity of the right temporalis (posterior pull) and left masseter (anterior pull). Patient was a 20-year-old male who had headaches (principally right temporal), limited opening of the mouth, uncomfortable bite, tinnitus, dizziness, clicking in the temporomandibular joint, and cervical, back, chest, and throat pain.

weeks of therapy. This event can be explained by understanding that the orthotic device initially aided in obtaining additional relaxation of muscles, which were in a state of hyperactivity or spasm and were producing pain. As these muscles relaxed and the mandible was repositioned to a new resting place, the occlusal position provided by the orthotic appliance required lateral or posterior movement of the mandible to enter occlusion. It has been demonstrated that even slight lateral or anteroposterior displacement of the mandible into occlusion is a greater cause of muscle fatigue than slight overclosure vertically.[237] If lateral or anteroposterior discrepancies are found on MKG testing, replacement of the orthotic appliance with a more accurate one is indicated. The corrected occlusion usually relieves muscle hyperactivity and results in relief of pain.

If testing reveals that the occlusion provided by the orthotic device is neuromuscularly healthy but the patient feels no relief of the original symptoms, either painful or dysfunctional, it is appropriate to consider other diagnoses and if necessary make appropriate referrals. Therapy up to that date was noninvasive and fully reversible. It should be understood that there can be multiple causes of the same symptoms. The correction of one physical dysfunction may not eliminate other possible causes of the patient's symptoms. Testing at this time is, therefore, valuable in assessing treatment success as well as treatment failure. Without this capacity to objectively monitor treatment results, endless useless treatments could be undertaken and proper essential diagnoses delayed.

When retesting of the initial appliance or a second one reveals that the neuromuscular occlusion is accurate and the patient reports significant or complete symptom relief, a treatment plan for long-term perpetuation of the new neuromuscular occlusal position should be made. Patients are given the option of discontinuing use of the orthotic appliance and returning to the pretreatment occlusal position. This is not encouraged, since it is felt that the original occlusal relationship predisposes the patient to MPD. Some patients do discontinue full-time use of the orthotic device, and some completely discontinue wearing it, electing to readapt to their pretreatment occlusion and experiment to see if their adaptive capacity can enable them to function comfortably with an occlusion that is not neuromuscularly perfect. Some are comfortable and others are not. Most patients want long-term perpetuation of the new occlusal relationship, which may take many forms.

LONG-TERM TREATMENT OPTIONS
Following successful treatment of MPD, the best way to prevent recurrence is to eliminate any predisposing factors and perpetuating factors. Noxious habits that fatigue the muscles should be avoided if possible. These include postural abnormalities, frequent biting on pencils, fingernails, or pipes, telephone cradling with the side of the head and shoulder, and carrying heavy shoulder bags. Clenching and bruxing (grinding the teeth) habits are difficult to eliminate especially when they occur during sleep. During sleep these habits are associated with hyperactivity in the central nervous system.

These particular habits are fatiguing to muscle and destructive to the teeth and surrounding bone structure. When such habits occur during the day, patients can often learn to avoid them. By becoming aware of the damage that clenching or grinding the teeth can do, patients learn to part their teeth when they are aware of holding them tightly. The mouth does not have to be opened; the jaw can merely be allowed to drop slightly so that the teeth do not touch. When bruxing habits are caused by the presence of occlusal interferences, removal of the interference may eliminate the bruxism.[244-247]

Most important, when occlusion is the cause of the muscle fatigue that results in MPD, the long-term success of treatment requires modification of the occlusion. This means perpetuating the temporarily created bite with a long-term appliance or modifying the teeth. Failure to perpetuate the neuromuscular occlusion merely returns the patient to the status that existed before the precipitation of the illness. That adaptive state may have existed for many years without causing problems of sufficient magnitude to lead the patient to seek care. There is no way of knowing what precipitating events lie ahead for that patient, nor how well his adaptive capacity will allow him to cope with a fatiguing muscle use.

Permanent elimination of the neuromuscular occlusal disequilibrium, which predisposes to MPD by changing the occlusion of the teeth, can take on many forms. Individual teeth can be changed morphologically, as previously described, utilizing the coronoplasty procedure. If total change in the maxillomandibular relationship is necessary, either orthodontic treatment is instituted to move many teeth[248] (Fig. 8–50), or passive eruption procedures are initiated to erupt single teeth gradually to the neuromuscular occlusal position while the orthotic appliance is worn. As posterior teeth erupt into new positions, adjacent ones are uncovered by removal of a portion of the orthotic appliance so that they too can erupt.

The unhealthy occlusion can be changed into a healthy neuromuscularly balanced occlusion by the fabrication of crowns on certain teeth or by bonding new porcelain occlusal surfaces on top of the natural teeth (Fig. 8–51). In patients who wear dentures, either partial or complete, new dentures can establish healthy muscle function (Fig. 8–52). All of these procedures, which seek to create healthy muscle function through proper neuromuscular occlusion, can be performed by implementing the same electronic measuring modalities that were originally used to treat the MPD. Therefore, long-term therapy, if performed with the aid of objective measurements, is an extension of the initial orthotic therapy with more durable materials. The key to long-term cure is precise, objective measurement. Trial and error treatments with empirical treatment modalities produce unpredictable short-term and long-term results. No treatment is totally effective in every patient. The anatomic region in which MPD exists is far too complex to be able to ascribe a single diagnosis and treatment for pain and dysfunction in it. MPD does, however, occur commonly; it has a typical clinical presentation, history, and symptoms and can be objectively identified and quantified with bioelectronic testing. The greatest chance of

Text continued on page 240

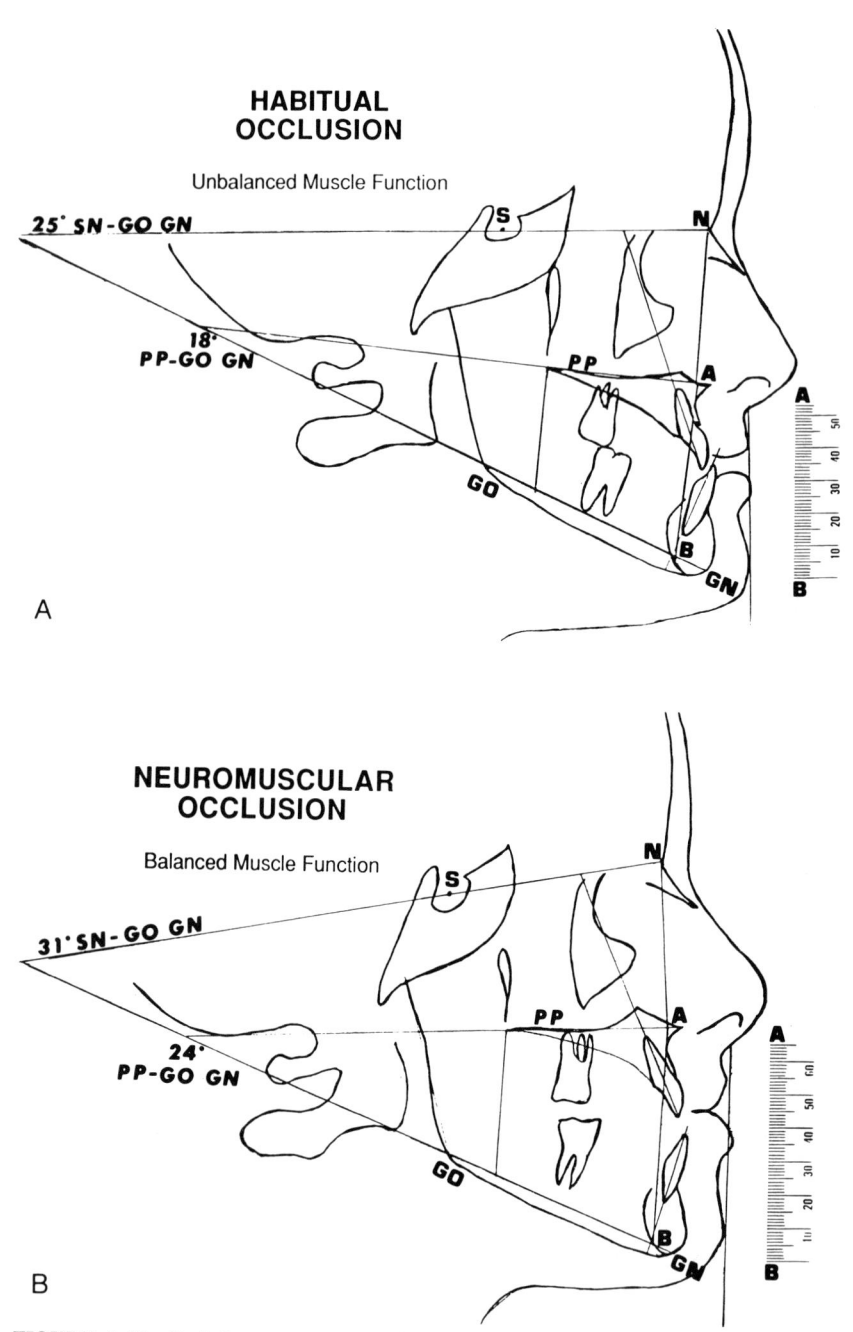

FIGURE 8–50. Cephalometric tracings of the lateral transcranial radiograph utilized in orthodontic evaluation and treatment planning. Observe the difference in vertical height of the lower third of the face (A to B) in the habitual (natural) occlusion with accommodative muscle function (A) and the neuromuscular occlusion with relaxed muscles (B). Alphabetical designations represent standard skeletal landmarks used in cephalometric analysis. (Courtesy of William Shipley, D.D.S.)

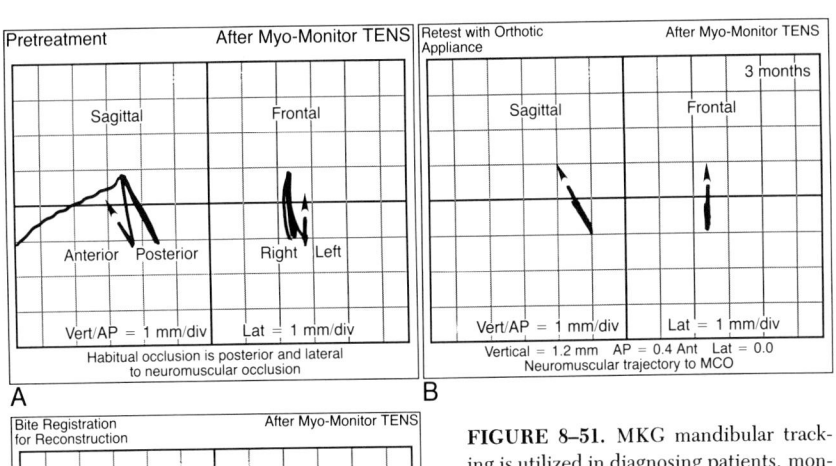

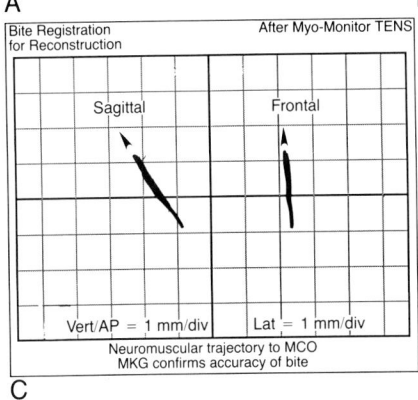

FIGURE 8–51. MKG mandibular tracking is utilized in diagnosing patients, monitoring therapy, and designing and testing long-term treatment modalities. *A*, X–Y recording of mandibular movement from rest to occlusion shows posterior and lateral discrepancy, seen on sagittal and frontal tracings. *B*, Testing with orthotic appliance in place for 3 months reveals that the occlusal position is on the neuromuscular trajectory with the proper vertical freeway space from rest to occlusion. *C*, MKG testing of bite registration for oral reconstruction (crowns) to establish long-term neuromuscular occlusion proves that this is in the position of neuromuscular occlusion.

A. EMG Clench—Pretreatment After Myo-Monitor TENS
Patient With Two Different Biting Positions in
Natural Dentition

| BITING POSTERIORLY |||| | BITING ANTERIORLY ||||
| Right || Left || | Right || Left ||
Ta	Mm	Mm	Ta		Ta	Mm	Mm	Ta
0	0	0	0		0	0	0	0
0	9	3	0		0	13	5	0
1	4	2	0		4	101	97	8
0	0	0	0		9	129	170	17
0	0	0	0		9	158	163	9
26	3	1	20		11	152	177	7
126	9	8	92		11	144	143	10
152	14	8	84		10	159	146	10
88	8	4	61		10	161	133	7
64	8	4	44		10	129	146	8
▶ 50	6	3	33 ◀ Average		8 ▶	122	131 ◀	8

In posterior biting, Ta dominate (arrows). In anterior biting, Mm dominate (arrows) in function shown on EMG.

Abbreviations: Ta, temporalis anterior; Mm, middle masseter. Averaged data.

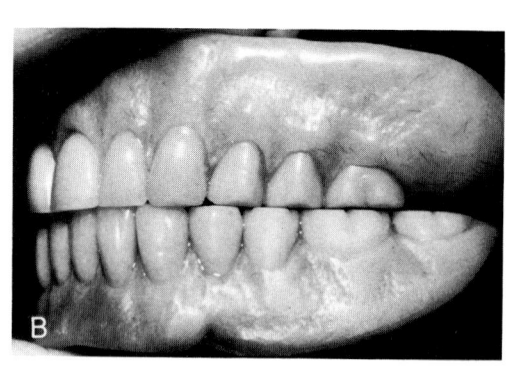

FIGURE 8–52. *A*, EMG function testing of patient with unstable occlusion, as demonstrated by multiple biting patterns. Anterior and posterior oriented occlusions are possible as is seen in patients who wear old, worn dentures (*B*).

Illustration continued on following page

C. Bite Registration After Myo-Monitor TENS EMG Clench Neuromuscular Occlusal Position

RIGHT			LEFT	
Ta	Mm		Mm	Ta
0	0		0	0
6	10		2	5
32	54		18	25
86	93		78	60
128	118		111	78
122	148		135	71
115	173		143	88
138	155		146	83
159	166		160	94
<u>107</u>	<u>139</u>		<u>142</u>	<u>74</u>
99	103	Average	103	64

Symmetrical muscle function.
Abbreviations: Ta, temporalis anterior; Mm, middle masseter. Averaged data.

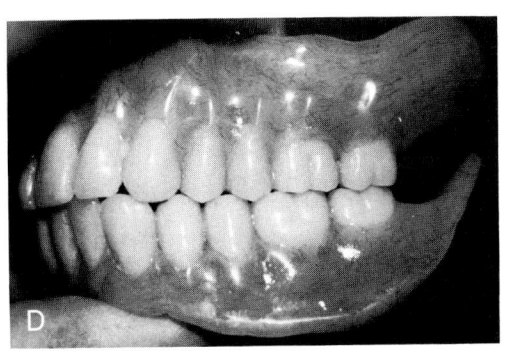

FIGURE 8–52 *Continued* C, After TENS and MKG/EMG testing, a neuromuscular occlusion position is established in an acrylic imprinting material intraorally. The bite registration is tested on EMG. Note balanced muscle function, with masseter dominance. *D*, New dentures provide a stable neuromuscular occlusion with proper interdigitation of teeth. The instability described can be observed in natural or restored teeth, which are worn flat.

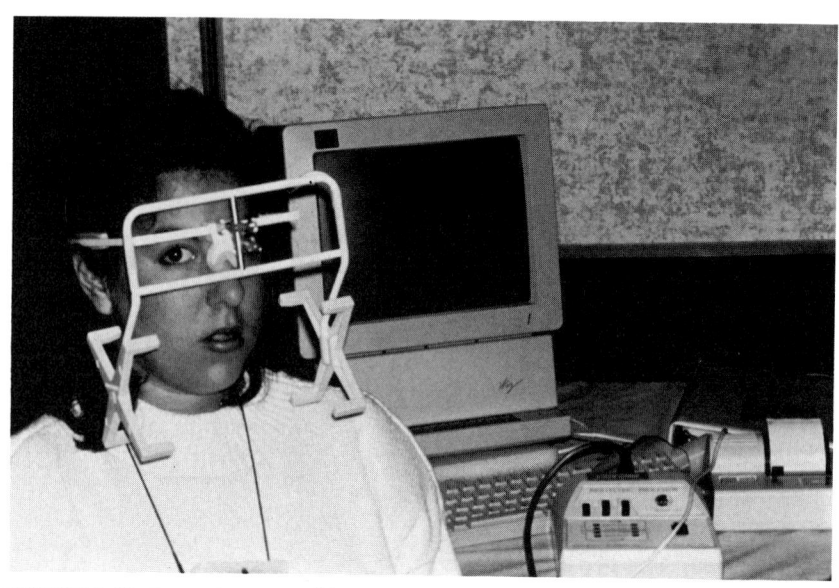

FIGURE 8–53. Patient being tested by mandibular kinesiograph (MKG) and electromyograph (EMG) instruments. EMG and TENS electrodes have been removed from the patient's face for this photograph to more clearly show the MKG magnetic sensor array.

success should accompany the most accurate diagnosis and precise therapy (Fig. 8–53).

EVALUATION OF TREATMENT RESULTS
In evaluating treatment results, one has to consider both the therapeutic effect of treatment and the patient's compliance with that treatment. Patients reporting little or no improvement in symptoms may have a remaining problem with their occlusion or another concurrent medical problem, or simply may not be wearing their orthotic appliance.

Prognosis

Musculoskeletal Dysfunction

The prognosis of therapy for MPD, properly diagnosed and treated and predisposing factors eliminated, is excellent. Sometimes complete diagnosis and treatment require the coordinated participation of various health care providers. Overall cure rates through establishment of a neuromuscular occlusion have been shown to range from 85 to 90 percent following 3 months of therapy (Table 8–11).[43]

Temporomandibular Joint Disorders

The prognosis for temporomandibular joint dysfunction is favorable if there has been no destruction of the hard and soft tissues within the joint and if

TABLE 8–11. Patient Evaluation of Symptom Status

1 month progress: significant improvement or cure	79%
3 month progress: significant improvement or cure	88%
Long-term treated subjects: significant improvement or cure	100%

From Cooper, B. C., et al. Myofacial pain dysfunction: Analysis of 476 patients. Laryngoscope 96(10):1099–1106, 1986.

the etiologic agent has been permanently removed. This frequently requires a permanent alteration in the maxillomandibular functional relationship in the dental occlusion if that was the cause of the joint dysfunction. If noxious or parafunctional habits were the cause, they must be eliminated. If systemic disease, either physical or emotional, is an etiologic or contributing agent, it must be controlled or cured. Failure to remove the cause predisposes to recurrence. The prognosis becomes increasingly guarded with increasing degrees of destruction of the joint components. Parts of the joint do have the capacity to regenerate normal bony anatomy through remodeling if the etiologic agents of the dysfunction are removed.[249, 250]

Interdisciplinary Approaches

Team Approaches to Diagnosis

Sometimes complete diagnosis and treatment of patients with complaints of pain and dysfunction in the head and neck require the coordinated efforts of various health care providers. Sometimes a single practitioner can begin the process of diagnosis and can even institute therapy and await a response before calling on others to become involved.

It is up to the first diagnostician who recognizes the nature of the craniomandibular disorder to institute treatment or refer the patient to another physician. It is the goal of this text to provide the primary examining physician and dentist with sufficient information to make a primary diagnosis or at least know in what area of medicine the patient's problem lies. Proper referral may be the finest service that can be provided by that first examiner.

It is always preferable to diagnose before treatment. Sometimes ameliorative measures must be implemented before diagnosis is complete. Care must be taken not to rely merely on amelioration, neglecting to obtain an adequate diagnosis.

Once a diagnosis of a craniomandibular disorder is made and other diseases have been eliminated, treatment is begun. Since the symptoms of craniomandibular disorders are so varied and potentially can mimic so many other pathologic conditions, caution must be exercised throughout therapy to be certain that other conditions are not overlooked. Patients rarely are fully screened with all available tests for neurologic, otorhinolaryngologic, psychiatric, orthopedic, and medical diseases. It is therefore important for the dentist who treats craniomandibular diseases to be aware of other possible complicating conditions that might coexist.

Often consultation with other medical practitioners is valuable during the early stages of diagnosis or therapy. Depending on the medical screening tests that have preceded the dentist's entry into the case, early referral may be necessary. The history of the illness, diagnostic tests already performed, and the quality of symptoms reported initially are significant in determining the need for referral.

Coordination of Treatment and Referral

After therapy is instituted, careful monitoring in the earliest stages is important. If symptoms are not relieved within a few weeks, a decision must be made about the need for consultation with other specialists. In this manner, while one form of therapy proceeds, other diagnostic possibilities can be investigated.

An example of such coordination may be seen in a patient with nasal obstruction in association with mouth breathing, postural abnormality, and muscular fatigue in the mandibular muscles. Successful comprehensive therapy requires the establishment of a patent nasal airway, which might require the surgical intervention of an otolaryngologist or treatment of an allergy that is contributing to the nasal obstruction.

The cervical problem, frequently found in musculoskeletal dysfunction of the head and neck along with MPD, may require the diagnostic skills of a neurologist and the intervention of an orthopedist or rehabilitative medical specialist. These treatments can be carried out while the problem of MPD is being treated.[251]

Obviously, any symptom of pain that does not respond to treatment of MPD should be evaluated quickly by an appropriate specialist. After reading this entire text, it is the hope of all the contributing authors that readers will have a better understanding of the tremendous variety of pathologic conditions that can be manifested as pain in the face, head, and neck. With good medical judgment and an effective diagnostic team, patients can be quickly and effectively diagnosed and treated.

Successful management of pain requires more than technical diagnostic and therapeutic skills. It requires compassion, understanding, and patience. Success is greatly enhanced if a positive facilitative interaction is developed between therapist and patient.[252, 253]

References

1. Dorland, Illustrated Medical Dictionary, 26th ed. Philadelphia, W. B. Saunders Co, 1985.
2. Cooper, B. C. Craniomandibular disorders. In Lucente, F. E., and Sobol, S. M., (eds.). Essentials of Otolaryngology, 2nd ed. New York, Raven Press, 1988.
3. Bell, W. E. Orofacial Pains: Classification, Diagnosis, Management, 3rd ed. Chicago, Year Book, 1985.
4. Farrar, W. B., and McCarty, W. L., Jr. Outline of Temporomandibular Joint

Diagnosis and Treatment, 6th ed. Montgomery, Ala., Normandie Study Group, 1980.
5. Lunn, R. H., Cooper, B. C., Coy R. E., et al. Principles, concepts and practices of the management of craniomandibular diseases. American Equilibration Society Compendium 20:180–227, 1987.
6. Hunter, J. The Natural History of the Human Teeth. London, J. Johnson, 1771, p 9.
7. Bell, W. E. Temporomandibular Disorders: Classification, Diagnosis, Management, 2nd ed. Chicago, Year Book, 1986.
8. Moss, M. L. A functional cranial analysis of centric relation. Dent Clin North Am 19:431, 1975.
9. Moss, M. L. The functional matrix concept and its relationship to temporomandibular joint dysfunction and treatment. Dent Clin North Am 27(3):445–455, 1983.
10. Pinto, O. F. A new structure related to the temporomandibular joint and middle ear. J Prosth Dent 12:95–103, 1962.
11. Ioannides, C., and Hoagland, G. A. The disco-malleolar ligament: A possible cause of subjective hearing loss in patients with temporomandibular joint dysfunction. J Maxillofac Surg 11:227–231, 1983.
12. Goss, C. M. (ed.). Gray's Anatomy. 29th American ed. Philadelphia, Lea & Febiger, 1973.
13. Hairston, L. E., and Blanton, P. L. An electromyographic study of mandibular position in response to changes in body position. J Prosth Dent 49:2, 1983.
14. Rocabado, M. Biomechanical relationship of the cranial, cervical and hyoid bones. J Craniomandibular Pract 1(3):62–66, 1983.
15. Mahan, P. E. The temporomandibular joint in function and pathological function. In Solberg, W., and Clark, G. (eds.). Temporomandibular Joint Problems: Biological Diagnosis and Treatment. Lombard, Ill., Quintessence Publishing Co, 1980, Chap 2.
16. Hannam, A. G. Magnetic resonance imaging of the jaw muscles. Presented at the 40th Annual Midwest Seminar of Dental Medicine, Bailey's Harbor, Wisconsin, 1987.
17. Mikhaib, M., and Rosen, H. History and etiology of MPD. J Prosth Dent 44:438, 1980.
18. Sonkin, L. S. Endocrine disorders, locomotor and temporomandibular joint dysfunction. In Gelb, H. (ed.). Clinical Management of Head, Neck and Temporomandibular Joint Pain and Dysfunction. Philadelphia, W. B. Saunders Co., 1977, pp. 140–180.
19. McNeill, C. Craniomandibular (TMJ) disorders—the state of the art. Part II: Accepted diagnostic and treatment modalities. J Prosth Dent 49(3):393–397, 1983.
20. Lazar, M. L., Greenlee, R. G., and Naarden, A. L. Facial pain of neurologic origin mimicking oral pathological conditions: Some current concepts and treatment. J Am Dent Assoc 100:884–888, 1980.
21. Remick, R. A., Blasberg, B., Campos, R. E., et al. Psychiatric disorders associated with atypical facial pain. Can J Psychiatry 28:178–181, 1983.
22. Gibilisco, J. A., Goldstein, N. P., and Rushton, J. G. The differential diagnosis of atypical facial pain. Lancet 85:450–454, 1965.
23. Rushton, J. G., Gibilisco, J. A., and Goldstein, N. P. Atypical facial pain. JAMA 171:545–548, 1959.
24. Engel, G. L. Primary atypical facial neuralgia: An hysterical conversion syndrome. Psychosom Med 13:375–396, 1951.

25. Alling, C. C. The diagnosis of chronic maxillofacial pain. J Prosth Dent 45(3):300–306, 1981.
26. Marcovich, S. E. Pain in the head: A neurological appraisal. In Gelb, H. (ed.). Clinical Management of Head, Neck and Temporomandibular Joint Pain and Dysfunction. Philadelphia, W. B. Saunders Co., 1977, Chap 5.
27. Smith, B. H. Anatomy of facial pain. Headache 9:7–13, 1969.
28. Kienast, H. W. Psychological aspects of facial pain. Headache 9:31–35, 1969.
29. Costen, J. B. A syndrome of ear and sinus symptoms dependent upon disturbed function of the temporomandibular joint. Ann Otol Rhinol Laryngol 43:1–5, 1934.
30. Alpher, E., Epstein, S., and Stack, B. C. Hearing loss treated by decompression of the temporomandibular joint. Ear Nose Throat 61:214–217, 1982.
31. Bernstein, J. M., Mohl, N. D., and Spiller, H. Temporomandibular joint dysfunction masquerading as disease of the ear, nose and throat. Trans Am Acad Ophthalmol Otolaryngol 73:1208–1217, 1969.
32. Wright, W. H. Deafness as influenced by malposition of the jaws. J Nat Dent Assoc 1:979, 1920.
33. Uhlemeyer, H. A. Combined dental and ENT approach to TMJ dysfunction. Basal Facts 2:2, 1977.
34. Hansson, T., and Milner, M. A study of the occurrence of symptoms of diseases of the temporomandibular musculature and related structures. J Oral Rehab 2:313–324, 1975.
35. Heyck, H. Headache and Facial Pain. Chicago, Year Book, 1981.
36. Kemper, J. T., and Okeson, J. P. Craniomandibular disorders and headaches. J Prosth Dent 49(5):702–705, 1983.
37. Magnusson, T., and Carlsson, G. E. Recurrent headaches in relation to temporomandibular joint pain dysfunction. Acta Odontol Scand 36:333, 1975.
38. Reik, L., Jr., and Hale, M. The temporomandibular joint pain dysfunction syndrome: A frequent cause of headache. Headache 21(4):151–156, 1981.
39. Saper, J. H. Headache Disorders. Boston, John Wright-PSC, 1983, p. ix.
40. Ziegler, D. K., Hassancia, R. S., and Couch, J. R. Characteristics of life headache histories in a nonclinic population. Neurology (Minneapolis) 27(3):265–269, 1977.
41. Brookes, G. B., et al. Costen's syndrome—correlation or coincidence: A review of 45 patients with temporomandibular joint dysfunction, otalgia and other aural symptoms. Clin Otolaryngol 5:23–36, 1980.
42. Myrhaug, H. The incidence of ear symptoms in case of malocclusion and temporomandibular joint disturbances. Br J Oral Surg 2:28–32, 1964.
43. Cooper, B. C., Alleva, M., Cooper, D. L., et al. Myofacial pain dysfunction: Analysis of 476 patients. Laryngoscope 96(10):1099–1106, 1986.
44. Cooper, B. C., and Mattucci, K. Myofacial pain dysfunction: A clinical examination procedure. Int Surg 72:165–169, 1985.
45. Snow, D. F. Initial examination. In Morgan, E. (ed.). Diseases of the Temporomandibular Apparatus: A Multidisciplinary Approach. St. Louis, C. V. Mosby, 1982, Chap. 6.
46. Hoppenfeld, S. Physical examination of the cervical spine and temporomandibular joint. In Hoppenfeld, S. (ed.). Physical Examination of the Spine and Extremities. Norwalk, Conn., Appleton-Century-Crofts, 1976, Chap 4.
47. Travell, J., and Rinzler, S. H. The myofascial genesis of pain. Postgrad Med 11:425–434, 1952.
48. Travell, J. Temporomandibular joint pain referred from the muscles of the head and neck. J Prosth Dent 10:745–763, 1960.

49. Misurya, V. K. Functional anatomy of tensor palatini and levator palatini muscles. Arch Otolarngol 102:265, 1976.
50. Weaver, E. G., and Lawrence, M. L. Functions of round window. Ann Otolaryngol 57:553–556, 1978.
51. Proctor, B. Anatomy of the eustachian tube. Arch Otolaryngol 97:2–8, 1973.
52. Bell, W. E. Understanding temporomandibular biomechanics. J Craniomandibular Pract 1(2):28–33, 1983.
53. Dugal, G. L., and Anseman, V. E. The entrapped greater occipital nerve and internal derangement of the temporomandibular joint. J Craniomandibular Pract 2(1):51, 1984.
54. McNamara, J. A., Jr. Neuromuscular and skeletal adaptation to altered orofacial function. Monograph No. 1, Craniofacial growth series. Ann Arbor, University of Michigan, Ann Arbor Center for Human Growth and Development, 1972.
55. McNamara, J. A., Jr. Naso-respiratory function and craniofacial growth. Monograph No. 9, Craniofacial growth series. Ann Arbor, University of Michigan, Ann Arbor Center for Human Growth and Development, 1979.
56. MacDonald, J. W. C., and Hannam, A. G. Relationship between occlusal contact and jaw-closing muscle activity during tooth clenching. Part I. J Prosth Dent 52(5):718–728, 1984.
57. Blake, P., Thorburn, D. N., and Stewart, I. A. Temporomandibular joint dysfunction in children presenting as otalgia. Clin Otolarngol 7:237–244, 1982.
58. Williamson, E. H. Temporomandibular dysfunction in pretreatment adolescent patients. Am J Orthodont 72:429–433, 1977.
59. Guichet, N. R. Applied gnathology: How and why. Dent Clin North Am 13(3):687, 1969.
60. Glickman, I., Pameijer, J. H. Roeber, F. N., et al. Functional occlusion as revealed by miniaturized radio transmitters. Dent Clin North Am 13(3):667–679, 1969.
61. Messerman, T., Reswich, J. B., and Gibbs, C. Investigation of functional mandibular movements. Dent Clin North Am 13(3):629–642, 1969.
62. Yamashita, A., and Inoue, H. Mandibular kinesiograph (MKG)—The principles, directions and clincal application. J Dent Engineering 4:1, 1977.
63. Hannam, A. G., Scott, J. D., and DeCou, R. E. A computer-based system for the simultaneous measurement of muscle activity and jaw movements during mastication in man. Arch Oral Biol Great Britain 22(1):17–23, 1977.
64. Neill, D. J., and Howell, D.D. Kinesiograph studies of jaw movement using the Commodore Pet microcomputer for data storage and analysis. J Dent 12(1):53–61, 1981.
65. Jankelson, B., Swain, C. W., and Crain, P. F., and Radke, J. C. Kinesiometric instrumentation: A new technology. J Am Dent Assoc 90:834–840, 1975.
66. Jankelson, B. Measurement accuracy of the mandibular kinesiograph—a computerized study. J Prosth Dent 44(6):656–666, 1980.
67. George, J. P., and Boone, M. E. A clinical study of rest position using the kinesiograph and myomonitor. J Prosth Dent 41:456, 1979.
68. Wessberg, G., et al: Comparison of mandibular rest positions induced by phonetics, transcutaneous electrical stimulation, and masticatory electromyography. J Prosth Dent 49(1):100–112, 1983.
69. Hannam, A. G., Inster, W. C., DeCou, R. E., et al. Speed of jaw movement during mastication and clenching tests in man. J Dent Res 56(4):442, 1977.
70. Moyers, R. E. Temporomandibular muscle contraction patterns in Angle Class II, division I malocclusions: An electromyographic analysis. Am J Orthodont 35:837, 1949.

71. Moyers, R. E. Electromyographic analysis of muscles in temporomandibular movement. Am J Orthodont 36:481–500, 1950.
72. Shpuntoff, H., and Shpuntoff, W. A study of physiological rest position and centric position by electromyography. J Prosth Dent 6(5):621–628, 1956.
73. Perry, H. T., Jr. Muscular changes associated with temporomandibular joint dysfunction. J Am Dent Assoc 54:644–653, 1957.
74. Moller, E. The chewing apparatus: An electromyographic study of the action of the muscles of mastication and its correlation to facial morphology. Acta Physiol Scand (Suppl. 280), 69:229, 1966.
75. Basmajian, J. V. Muscles Alive: Their Function Revealed by Electromyography, 4th ed. Baltimore, Williams & Wilkins, 1978.
76. Basmajian, J. V., and Stecko, G. A new bipolar electrode for electromyography. J Appl Physiol 17:849, 1962.
77. Kotani, H., Kawazoe, Y., Hamada, T., and Yamada, S. Quantitative electromyographic diagnosis of myofascial pain dysfunction syndrome. J Prosth Dent 43(4):450–456, 1980.
78. Dahan, J., and Boitte, C. Comparison of the reproducibility of EMG signals recorded from human masseter and lateral ptyergoid muscles. J Dent Res 65(3):441–447, 1986.
79. Vitti, M., and Basmajian, J. Integrated actions of masticatory muscles: Simultaneous EMG from eight intramuscular electrodes. Anat Rec 187:173–190, 1976.
80. Lehr, R. P., and Owens, S. E. An electromyographic study of the human lateral pterygoid muscle. Anat Rec 196:441–448, 1980.
81. Mahan, P. E., and Wilkinson, T. M. Superior and inferior bellies of the lateral pterygoid muscle: EMG activity at basic jaw positions. J Prosth Dent 50:710–718, 1983.
82. McCarroll, R. S., Honee, G. L., and Naeije, J. M. Relationship of electromyographic parameters in jaw dysfunction patients classified according to Heikimo's index. J Oral Rehabil 110:521–527, 1984.
83. Camacho, L. An investigation of the relationship between electromyographic findings and unilateral chewing in children. J Pedodont 8(3):293–299, 1984.
84. Mushimoto, E., and Mitani, H. Bilateral coordination pattern of masticatory muscle activities during chewing in normal subjects. J Prosth Dent 48:2–7, 1982.
85. Jarabak, J. R. An electromyographic analysis of muscular and temporomandibular disturbances due to imbalances in occlusion. Angle Orthodont 46:170–190, 1956.
86. Tallgren, A., Holden, S., Lang, B. R., et al. Correlations between EMG jaw muscle activity and facial morphology in complete denture wearers. J Oral Rehab 10(2):105–120, 1983.
87. Williamson, E. H., and Lundquist, D. O. Anterior guidance: Its effect on electromyographic activity of the temporal and masseter muscles. J Prosth Dent 49:813–823, 1983.
88. Lippold, O. C. J. The relation between integrated action potentials in human muscle and its isometric tension. J Physiol 117:492–499, 1952.
89. Bigland, B., Lippold, O. C. S. The relation between force, velocity and electrical activity in human muscles. J Physiol 123:214–224, 1954.
90. Ahlgren, J., and Owall, B. Muscle activity and chewing force: A polygraphic study of human mandibular movements. Arch Oral Biol 15:271–280, 1970.

91. Yemm, R. The orderly recruitment of motor units of the masseter and temporalis muscles during voluntary contraction in man. J Physiol (London) 265:163–174, 1977.
92. Kawazoe, Y., Kotani, H., and Hamada, T. Relation between integrated electromyographic activity and biting force during voluntary isometric contraction in human masticatory muscles. J Dent Res 58:1440, 1979.
93. Palla, S., and Ash, M. Effects of bite force in the power spectrum of the surface electromyogram of human muscles. Arch Oral Biol 26:287–295, 547–553, 1981.
94. Schelhas, K. P., Wilkes, C. H., Omlie, M. R., et al. Temporomandibular joint imaging: Practical application of available technology. Arch Otolaryngol Head Neck Surg 113:744–748, 1987.
95. Dixon, D. C., Graham, C. S., Mayhew, R. B., et al. The validity of transcranial radiography in diagnosing TMJ anterior disk displacement. J Am Dent Assoc 108:615–618, 1984.
96. Updegrave, W. M. Temporomandibular articulations: X-ray examination. Dent Radiog Photog 26:41–46, 1953.
97. Farrar, W. B., and McCarty, W. L. A Clinical Outline of Temporomandibular Joint Diagnosis and Treatment, 7th ed. Montgomery, Ala., Montgomery Walker Printing Co., 1983, p. 111.
98. Williamson, E. W., and Wilson, C. W. Use of submental vertex analysis in producing quality temporomandibular radiographs. Am J Orthodont 20:200–207, 1976.
99. Pullinger, A. G., Hollender, L., Solberg, W. K., et al. A tomographic study of mandibular condyle position in an asymptomatic population. J Prosth Dent 53(3):706, 1985.
100. Yale, S. H., Rosenberg, H. M., Ceballis, M., et al. Laminate cephalometry in the analysis of mandibular condyle morphology. Oral Surg 14:793–805, 1961.
101. Omnell, K. A., and Peterson, A. Radiography of the temporomandibular joint: A comparison between oblique lateral and the tomographic image. Odont Rev 27:77–92, 1976.
102. Katzberg, R. W., Dolwick, M. F., Helms, C. S., et al. Arthrography of the temporomandibular joint. Am J Radiol 134:995–1003, 1980.
103. Farrar, W. B., and McCarty, W. L. Inferior joint space arthrography and characteristics of condylar paths in internal derangements of the TMJ. J Prosth Dent 41(5):548–551, 1979.
104. Westesson, P. L., Omnell, K. A., and Roblin, M. I. Double contrast tomography of the temporomandibular joint: A new technique based on autopsy examination. Acta Radiol 21:777–784, 1980.
105. Doyle, T. Arthrography of the temporomandibular joint. A simple technique. Clin Radiol 34:147, 1983.
106. Bell, K. A., and Walters, P. J. Videofluoroscopy during arthrography of the temporomandibular joint. Radiology 147:879, 1983.
107. Manzione, J. V., Katzberg, R. W., Brodsky, G. L., et al. Internal derangements of the temporomandibular joints: Diagnosis by direct sagittal computed tomography. Radiology 150:111–115, 1984.
108. Moaddab, M. B., Dumas, A. L., Chavoor, A. G., et al. Temporomandibular joint: Computed tomographic three-dimensional reconstruction. Am J Orthod 8:342–352, 1985.

109. Kursunoglu, S., Kaplan, P., Resnick, L. D., et al. Three-dimensional computed tomography analysis of the normal temporomandibular joint. J Oral Maxillofac Surg 44:257–259, 1986.
110. Katzberg, R. W., Schenck, J., Roberts, D., et al. Magnetic resonance imaging of the temporomandibular joint meniscus. Oral Surg 59:322–375, 1985.
111. Roberts, D., Schenck, J., Joseph, P., et al. Temporomandibular joint: Magnetic resonance imaging. Radiology 155:829–830, 1985.
112. Schelhas, K. P., Wilkes, C. H., Heithoff, K. D., et al. Temporomandibular joint: Diagnosis of internal derangements using magnetic resonance imaging. Minn Med 69:516–519, 1986.
113. New, F. J., Rosen, B. R., Brady, T. J., et al. Potential hazards and artifacts of ferromagnetic and non-ferromagnetic surgical and dental materials in nuclear magnetic resonance imaging. Radiology 147:139–148, 1983.
114. Weijs, W. A. Biomechanical models and the analysis of form: A study of the mammalian masticatory apparatus. Am Zoology 20:707–719, 1980.
115. Hannam, A. G., DeCou, R. E., Scott, J. D., et al. The relationship between dental occlusion, muscle activity and association jaw movement in man. Arch Oral Biol 22:25, 1977.
116. Ramfjord, S., and Ash, M. M. Occlusion: Signs and symptoms of chronic joint arthritis and recurrent muscle pain. Philadelphia, W. B. Saunders Co., 1971.
117. Eversole, L. R., and Machado, L. Temporomandibular joint internal derangements and associated neuromuscular disorders. J Am Dent Assoc 110:69–79, 1985.
118. Bush, F. M. Malocclusion, masticatory muscle, and temporomandibular joint tenderness. J Dent Res 64(2):129–133, 1985.
119. Jarabak, J. R. An electromyographic analysis of muscular and temporomandibular joint disturbances due to imbalances in occlusion. Angle Orthodont 26:170–190, 1956.
120. Schwartz, L. Disorders of the Temporomandibular Joint. Philadelphia, W. B. Saunders Co., 1959.
121. Laskin, D. M. Etiology of the pain dysfunction syndrome. J Am Dent Assoc 79:144, 1969.
122. Arlen, H. The otomandibular syndrome: A new concept. Ear Nose Throat J 56:61, 1977.
123. Lerman, M. D. A unifying concept of the TMJ pain dysfunction syndrome. J Am Dent Assoc 86:833–841, 1973.
124. Howe, G. L. Disorders of the masticatory apparatus. Br Dent J 155:405, 1983.
125. Costen, J. B. A syndrome of ear and sinus symptoms dependent upon disturbed function of the temporomandibular joint. Ann Otol Rhinol Laryngol 43:1–5, 1934.
126. Kelly, H. T., and Goodfriend, D. J. Vertigo attributable to dental and TMJ causes. J Prosth Dent 14:159–173, 1969.
127. MacDonald, J. W. C., and Hannam, A. G. Relationship between occlusal contacts and jaw closing muscle activity during teeth clenching. Part II. J Prosth Dent 52(6):862–867, 1984.
128. Shapiro, H. H. The muscles of mastication. Int J Orthodont 20:12–17, 1934.
129. Perry, H. J., and Harris, S. C. The role of the neuromuscular system in functional activity of the mandible. J Am Dent Assoc 48:665–673, 1954.
130. Schwartz, L. L. A temporomandibular joint pain dysfunction syndrome. J Chron Dis 3(3):284–293, 1956.
131. Dolowitz, D., et al. The role of muscular incoordination in the pathogenesis of the temporomandibular joint dysfunction. Laryngoscope 74:790–801, 1964.

132. Ramfjord, S. P. Dysfunctional temporomandibular joint and muscle pain. J Prosth Dent 11:353–374, 1982.
133. Jankelson, B., Hoffman, G. M., and Hendron, J. A., Jr. Physiology of the stomatognathic system. J Am Dent Assoc 46:373–386, 1953.
134. Jankelson, B. Neuromuscular aspects of occlusion: Effects of occlusal position on the physiology and dysfunction of the mandibular musculature. Dent Clin North Am 23:157–168, 1979.
135. Posselt, V. The temporomandibular joint syndrome and occlusion. J Prosth Dent 25:432, 1971.
136. Rocabado, M. Arthrokinematics of the temporomandibular joint. Dent Clin North Am 27(3):573–594, 1983.
137. Klineberg, I. J., Greenfield, B. E., and Wyke, B. D. Stimulus-response characteristics of temporomandibular articular mechanoreceptors. International Association for Dental Research 48th General Meeting, Abstract 626, 1970.
138. Wyke, B. D. Neurophysiological aspects of joint function with particular reference to the temporomandibular joint. J Bone Joint Surg (Br) 43:396–397, 1961.
139. Cooper, B., and Rabuzzi, D. Myofacial pain dysfunction: A clinical study of asymptomatic subjects. Laryngoscope 94:68–75, 1984.
140. Newton, A. V. Predisposing causes for temporomandibular joint dysfunction. J Prosth Dent 22:647, 1969.
141. McNeil, C., et al. Craniomandibular (TMJ) disorders: The state of the art. J Prosth Dent 44(4):434–437, 1980.
142. Riise, C., and Sheikholeslam, A. Influence of experimental interfering occlusal contacts on the activity of the anterior temporal and masseter muscles during mastication. J Oral Rehab 11:325–333, 1984.
143. Ramfjord, S. P. Dysfunctional temporomandibular joint and muscle pain. J Prosth Dent 11(2):353–374, 1961.
144. Greene, C., et al. Psychological factors in the etiology, progression, and treatment of MPD syndrome. J Am Dent Assoc 105:443–447, 1982.
145. Rugh, J. D., and Solberg, W. K. Psychological implications in temporomandibular pain and dysfunction. Oral Sci Rev 7:3–30, 1976.
146. Funakoshi, M., Fujita, N., and Takehana, S. Relations between occlusal interference and jaw muscle activities in response to changes in head position. J Dent Res 55:684, 1976.
147. Rieder, C. E. The incidence of some occlusal habits and headaches/neckaches in an initial survey population. J Prosth Dent 35:445, 1976.
148. Rugh, J. D., and Robins, W. Oral habit disorders. In Ingersall, B. (ed.). Behavioral Aspects in Dentistry. New York, Appleton-Century-Crofts, 1981, pp. 179–202.
149. Darnell, M. W. A proposed chronology of events for forward head posture. J Craniomandibular Pract 1(4):49–54, 1983.
150. Ramfjord, S. P. Bruxism—a clinical and electromyographic study. J Am Dent Assoc 62:35–58, 1961.
151. Kinnie, B. H. From the outside, looking in. Presented to the American Academy of Dental Radiology, Atlanta, October 19, 1984.
152. Bellinger, D. H. Arthritis of temporomandibular joint: Diagnosis and management. J South Calif Dent Assoc 23:19, 1955.
153. Moffett, B. Clinical biology of the craniofacial articulations. In Coy, R. E. (ed.). Compendium, Vol 15. American Equilibration Society, 1980, pp. 420–443.

154. Ogus, H. Degenerative disease of the temporomandibular joint and pain dysfunction syndrome. J R Soc Med (Lond) 71:748–754, 1978.
155. Toller, P. A. Osteoarthrosis of the mandibular condyle. Br Dent J 134:223–231, 1973.
156. Farrar, W. B., McCarty, W. L. The TMJ dilemma. J Alabama Dent Assoc 63:19–26, 1979.
157. Granados, J. I. The influence of the loss of teeth and attrition on the articular eminence. J Prosth Dent 42(1):78–85, 1979.
158. Bonica, J. J. Management of myofascial pain syndromes in general practice. JAMA 164(7):732–738, 1957.
159. Kraus, H. Muscle pain: Noninvasive therapy, Part I. Medical Times, September, 1982.
160. Travell, J. G., and Simons, D. G. Myofascial pain and dysfunction. Trigger Point Manual, Vol 1. Baltimore, Williams & Wilkins, 1983.
161. Rocabado, M. Physical therapy and dentistry: An overview. J Craniomandibular Pract 1(1):47–49, 1982–1983.
162. Hargreaves, A. S., and Wardle, J. J. M. The use of physiotherapy in the treatment of temporomandibular disorders. Br Dent J 155:121–124, 1983.
163. Fox, C. W., Abrams, B. L., Williams, B., et al. Protrusive positioners. J Prosth Dent 54(2):258, 1985.
164. Goharian, R. K., and Neff, P. A. Effect of occlusal retainers on temporomandibular joint and facial pain. J Prosth Dent 44(4):206–208, 1980.
165. Clark, G. T. A critical evaluation of orthopedic interocclusal appliance therapy: Design, theory and overall effectiveness. J Am Dent Assoc 108:359–364, 1984.
166. Kawazoe, Y., et al. Effect of occlusal splints on the electromyographic activities of masseter muscles during maximum clenching in patients with myofascial pain dysfunction syndrome. J Prosth Dent 43:578–580, 1980.
167. Green, C. S., and Laskin, D. M. Splint therapy for the myofascial pain dysfunction (MPD) syndrome: A comparative study. J Am Dent Assoc 84:624, 1972.
168. Christiansen, L. V. Effects of an occlusal splint on integrated electromyography of masseter muscle in experimental tooth clenching in man. J Oral Rehabil 7:281, 1980.
169. Kovaleski, W. C., and DeBoever, J. Influence of occlusal splint on jaw position and musculature in patients with temporomandibular joint dysfunction. J Prosth Dent 33:321, 1975.
170. Agerberg, G., and Carlsson, G. E. Late results of treatment of functional disorders of the masticatory system. J Oral Rehabil 1:309–316, 1974.
171. Carraro, J. J., and Caffesse, R. G. Effect of occlusal splints on TMJ symptomotology. J Prosth Dent 40:563–566, 1978.
172. Magnusson, T., and Carlsson, G. E. Treatment of patients with functional disturbances in the masticatory system. A survey of 80 consecutive patients. Swed Dent J 4:145–153, 1980.
173. Farrar, W. B. Differentiation of temporomandibular joint dysfunction to simplify treatment. J Prosth Dent 28:629–636, 1972.
174. Toller, P. Non-surgical treatment of dysfunctions of the temporomandibular joint. Oral Sci Rev 7:70–85, 1976.
175. Isberg, A. Disk displacement of TMJ and subsequent conditions. American Equilibration Society Meeting, Chicago, Illinois, February, 1986.
176. Isacsson, G. Pathological findings of the TMJ dysfunction. American Equilibration Society Meeting, Chicago, Illinois, February, 1986.

177. Guichet, N. F. Clinical management of occlusally related orofacial pain and TMJ dysfunction. J Craniomandibular Pract 1:60–73, 1980.
178. Scapino, R. P. Histopathology associated with malposition of the human temporomandibular joint disc. Oral Surg 55:382–397, 1983.
179. Solberg, W. K. Temporomandibular disorders: Clinical significance of TMJ changes. Br Dent J 160:231–236, 1986.
180. McCarty, W. L., Jr., and Farrar, W. B. Surgery for internal derangements of the temporomandibular joint. J Prosth Dent 42(2):191–196, 1979.
181. Rugh, J. D. Psychophysiologic concepts. American Association of Oral and Maxillofacial Surgeons' Conference on a Multidisciplinary Approach to TMJ Dysfunction. Philadelphia, March, 1982.
182. Dolwick, M. F., et al. Criteria for TMJ meniscus surgery. Presented at the Ad Hoc Study Group of TMJ Meniscus Surgery of the American Association of Oral and Maxillofacial Surgeons, Chicago, November, 1984, p. 20.
183. Kellaway, P. The part played by electric fish in early history of bioelectricity and electrotherapy. The William Osler Medal Essay. McGill University, Montreal, Spring, 1946.
184. Melzack, R., and Wall, P. D. Pain mechanisms: A new theory. Science 150:971–973, 1965.
185. Shealy, C. N., Mortimer, J. T., and Reswick, J. B. Electrical inhibition of pain by stimulation of the dorsal columns: Preliminary clinical report. Anesth Analg 46:489–491, 1967.
186. Shealy, C. N. Transcutaneous electrical stimulation for the control of pain. Clin Neurosurg 21:269–277, 1974.
187. Sweet, W. H., and Wepsic, J. G. Treatment of chronic pain by stimulation of fibers of primary afferent neurons. Trans Am Neurol Assoc 93:103–105, 1968.
188. Andersson, S. A., and Holmgren, E. On acupuncture analgesia and the mechanism of pain. Am J Clin Med 3:311–334, 1975.
189. Andersson, S. A. Pain control by sensory stimulation. In Bonnica, J. J., et al. (eds.). Advances in Pain Research and Therapy, Vol 3. New York, Raven Press, 1979.
190. Eriksson, M. B., Sjolund, B. H., and Nielzen, S. Long-term results of peripheral conditioning stimulation as an analgesic measure in chronic pain. Pain 6:335–347, 1979.
191. Dixon, H. H., O'Hara, M., and Peterson, R. D. Fatigue contracture of skeletal muscle. Northwest Med 66:813, 1967.
192. Yavelow, I., Forster, I., and Wininger, M. Mandibular relearning. Oral Surg 36:632, 1973.
193. Kovacs, R. Electrotherapy and Light Therapy, 4th ed. Philadelphia, Lea & Febiger, 1942.
194. Shaber, P. Skeletal muscle: Anatomy, physiology and pathophysiology. Dent Clin North Am 27(3):435–443, 1983.
195. Kawazoe, Y., Kotani, H., Metani, T., et al. The slopes of the fatigued muscle voltage tension curves decreased to a greater degree with percutaneous stimulation than by rest alone. Arch Oral Biol 26:795–801, 1981.
196. Trott, P. H., and Goss, A. H. Physiotherapy in diagnosis and treatment of myofascial pain dysfunction syndrome. Int J Oral Surg 7:360, 1978.
197. Melzack, R. Prolonged relief of pain by brief, intense transcutaneous somatic stimulation. Pain 1:357–373, 1975.
198. Inhalalnen, V., and Perkki, K. The effect of transcutaneous nerve stimulation (TNS) on chronic facial pain. Proc Finn Dent Soc 74:86–90, 1979.

199. Long, D. M., and Hagfors, N. Electrical stimulation in the nervous system: The current status of electrical stimulation of the nervous system for relief of pain. Pain 1:109–123, 1975.
200. Terezhalmy, G. T., et al. Transcutaneous electrical nerve stimulation treatment of TMJ-MPDS patients. Ear Nose Throat J 61(12):22–24, 1982.
201. Dubner, R. Neurophysiology of pain. Dent Clin North Am 22:11, 1978.
202. Chapman, C. R., Wilson, M. E., and Gehrig, J. D. Comparative effects of acupuncture and TENS on the perception of painful dental stimulation. Pain 2:265, 1976.
203. Piper, H. Elecktrophysiologe menschlicher Muskeln. Verlag von Berlin, Springer, 1912.
204. Clark, G. T., Beemsterboer, P. L., and Jacobsen, R. The effect of sustained submaximal clenching on maximum bite force in myofascial pain dysfunction patients. J Oral Rehabil 11:387–391, 1984.
205. Viitasalo, J. H., and Komi, P. V. Signal characteristic of EMG during fatigue. Eur J Appl Physiol 37:111–121, 1977.
206. Hughes, J. Isolation of endogenous compound from the brain with the pharmacologic properties similar to morphine. Brain Res 88:295–308, 1975.
207. Hughes, J., Smith, T. W., and Kosterlitz, H. W. Identification of two related pentapeptides from the brain with potential opiate agonist activity. Nature 258:577, 1975.
208. Chapman, C. R., and Benedetti, C. Analgesia following transcutaneous electrical stimulation and its partial reversal by a narcotic antagonist. Life Sciences 21:1645–1648, 1976.
209. Pomeranz, B., and Chiu, L. D. Nalaxone blockade of acupuncture analgesia: Endorphin implicated. Life Sciences 19:1757–1762, 1976.
210. O'Neil, R. Relief of chronic facial pain by transcutaneous electrical nerve stimulation. Br J Oral Surg 19:112–115, 1981.
211. Sjolund, B., Terrenius, L., and Eriksson, M. Increased cerebrospinal fluid levels of endorphins after electro-acupuncture. Acta Physiol Scand 100:382–384, 1977.
212. Sjolund, B., and Eriksson, M. Electro-acupuncture and endogenous morphines. Lancet 11:1085, 1976.
213. Cheng, R. S. S., and Pomeranz, B. Electroacupuncture analgesia could be mediated by at least two pain relieving mechanisms: Endorphin and non-endorphin systems. Life Science 25:1957, 1979.
214. Mayer, D. M., Price, D., and Rafii, A. Antagonism of acupuncture analgesia in man by narcotic antagonist naloxone. Brain Res 121:368–372, 1977.
215. Thomas, N. R. Spectral analysis in the pre and post TENS condition. Presented at the 5th convocation of the International College of Craniomandibular Orthopedics. Honolulu, Hawaii, March, 1987.
216. DeBoever, J., and McCall, W. D. Physiological aspects of masticatory muscle stimulation: The myomonitor. Quintescence Int 3:57, 1972.
217. Jankelson, B., and Swain, C. W. Physiological aspects of masticatory muscle stimulation: The myomonitor. Periodont Oral Hyg 12:Dec. 1972.
218. Jankelson, B., and Radke, J. C. The myomonitor: Its use and abuse. Quintescence Int Dent Dig 9:35–39, 47–52, 1978.
219. Jankelson, B., Sparks, S., Crane, P., and Radke, J. C., Neural conduction of the myomonitor stimulus: A quantitative analysis. J Prosth Dent 34:3, 245–253, 1975.
220. Fujii, H., and Mitani, H. Reflex response of the masseter and temporalis muscles in man. J Dent Res 52:1046–1051, 1973.

221. Choi, B. B., and Mitani, H. On the mandibular position regulated by myomonitor stimulation. J Jap Prosth Soc 17:79–96, 1973.
222. Konchak, P. A., Thomas, N. R., et al. Vertical dimension and freeway space: A kinesiographic study. Angle Orthodont April:145–154, 1987.
223. Rugh, J. D., and Drago, C. J. Vertical dimension: A study of clinical rest position and jaw muscle activity. J Prosth Dent 45:670, 1981.
224. Rugh, J. D., Drago, C. J., and Barghi, N. Comparison of electromyographic and phonetic measurements of vertical rest position. J Dent Res 58 (special issue A):316, Abstr. No. 899, 1979.
225. Mohl, N. D. Neuromuscular mechanisms in mandibular function. Dent Clin North Am 22(1):63–71, 1978.
226. Dinham, G. Myocentric—a clinical appraisal. Angle Orthodont 54(3):211–217, 1984.
227. Jankelson, B. Research Findings and Resultant Management of Craniomandibular (TMJ) Symptom Cluster Syndrome. Proceedings of the 2nd International Prosthetic Congress. St. Louis, C. V. Mosby Co., 1979, pp. 291–294.
228. Wood, W. W., and Tobias, D. L. EMG response to alteration of tooth contact on occlusal splints during maximal clenching. J Prosth Dent 51(3):394–396, 1984.
229. Guyton, A. C. Textbook of Medical Physiology, 6th ed. Philadelphia, W. B. Saunders Co., 1981, p. 137.
230. Mannas, A., Miralles, R., and Guerrero, F. The changes in electrical activity of the postural muscles of the mandible upon varying the vertical dimension. J Prosth Dent 45(4):438–445, 1981.
231. Kawamura, Y. Neurophysiologic background of occlusion. Periodontics 5:175, 1967.
232. Carlsoo, S. An electromyographic study of the activity of certain suprahyoid muscles (mainly the anterior belly of the digastric muscle) and the reciprocal innervation of the elevators and depressor musculature of the mandible. Acta Anat (Basel) 26:81, 1956.
233. Jarabak, J. R. Electromyographic analysis of muscular behavior in mandibular movements from rest position. J Prosth Dent 7:682, 1957.
234. Garnick, J., and Ramfjord, S. P. Rest position—an electromyographic and clinical investigation. J Prosth Dent 12:895, 1962.
235. Manns, M., Miralles, R., and Pallazzi, C. EMG, bite force and elongation of the masseter muscle under isometric voluntary contractions and variation of vertical dimension. J Prosth Dent 42:674, 1979.
236. Lund, J. P. Sensoriomotor integration in the control of mastication. In Klineborg, I., and Sessle, B. (eds.). Oral-Facial Pain and Neuromuscular Dysfunction. New York, Pergamon Press, 1985, Chap. 13.
237. Wessberg, G. A., Carroll, W. L., Dinham, R., et al. Transcutaneous electrical stimulation as an adjunct in the management of myofascial pain dysfunction syndrome. J Prosth Dent 45(3):307–314, 1981.
238. Shore, N. Occlusal Equilibration and Temporomandibular Joint Dysfunction. Philadelphia, J. B. Lippincott, 1959.
239. Magnusson, T., and Carlsson, G. E. Occlusal adjustment in patients with residual or recurrent signs of mandibular dysfunction. J Prosth Dent 49(5):706–710, 1983.
240. Neff, P., Binderman, I., and Arcan, M. The diagram of contact intensities: A basic characteristic of occlusion. J Prosth Dent 53(5):697, 1985.
241. Jankelson, B. A technique for obtaining optimum functional relationships for the natural dentitions. Dent Clin North Am 4:132–134, 1960.

242. Jankelson, B. Coronoplasty technique (video). Seattle, Washington, Myotronics, 1981.
243. McGowan, P., McKinney, J., Chase, D., et al. Treatment of anterior disc displacement with Jankelson Myosplint: Retrospective study. J Dent Res 62:1216, 1983 (Abstr. No. 12).
244. Hamada, T., et al. Effect of occlusal splints on the EMG activity in masseter and temporal muscles in bruxism with clinical symptoms. J Oral Rehabil 9:119–123, 1982.
245. Holmgren, K., and Sheikholeslam, A. A long-term study of the effect of an occlusal splint in patients with parafunctional disorders. J Dent Res 57 (special issue A):341, 1978.
246. Clark, G. T., et al. Nocturnal electromyographic evaluation of myofacial pain dysfunction in patients undergong occlusal splint therapy. J Am Dent Assoc 99(4):607–611, 1979.
247. Solberg, W. K., Clark, G. T., and Rugh, J. D. Nocturnal electromyographic evaluation of bruxism patients undergoing short-term splint therapy. J Oral Rehabil 2:215, 1975.
248. Calendar, J. M. Orthodontic application of the mandibular kinesiograph. Part I, J Clin Orthodont 18:10, 1984. Part II, J Clin Orthod 18:11, 1984.
249. Moffet, B. J., Johnston, L.C., McCabe, J. B., et al. Articular remodeling in the adult temporomandibular joint. Am J Anat 115:119–141, 1964.
250. Mongini, F. Condylar remodeling after occlusal therapy. J Prosth Dent 43:568–577, 1980.
251. Danzig, W. N., and VanDyke, A. R. Physical therapy as an adjunct to temporomandibular joint therapy. J Prosth Dent 49(1):96, 1983.
252. Carkhuff, R. R., and Berenson, B. G. Beyond Counseling and Therapy. New York, Holt, Rinehart and Winston, 1967.
253. Siegel, B., Love, Medicine and Miracles. New York, Harper & Row, 1986.

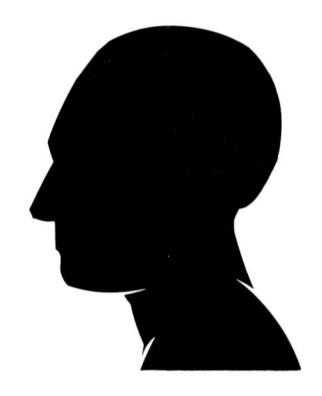

Chapter 9
Rehabilitation Management of Neck Pain

Thirumoorthi V. Seshan

Patients presenting with neck and arm pain pose an extraordinary challenge to the physician's skills in diagnosis and management. A wide range of clinical syndromes affects the cervical spine and its associated structures. This chapter will deal with the anatomy of the cervical spine and the structures closely related to it, clinical syndromes of this region, differential diagnosis, and rehabilitation management of these syndromes.

The cervical spine consists of vertebrae, intervertebral disks, and supporting ligaments. The cervical spine, while permitting considerable mobility, protects the spinal cord, nerve roots, and blood vessels. The intervertebral disk, paired joints of Luschka, and paired facet joints form the five-joint complex that extends from C2 to C7.

Anatomy of Cervical Spine

Vertebrae

There are seven cervical vertebrae. The first cervical (atlas) vertebra articulates with the occiput and the odontoid process of the second cervical (axis) vertebra. These articulations function as one unit, whereas the third through the sixth also function as one unit. The seventh cervical vertebra functions like a thoracic vertebra. There are five joints in the cervical spine (Fig. 9–1). Two adjoining vertebrae articulate with each other, and an intervertebral disk and two projections from the posterolateral part of the

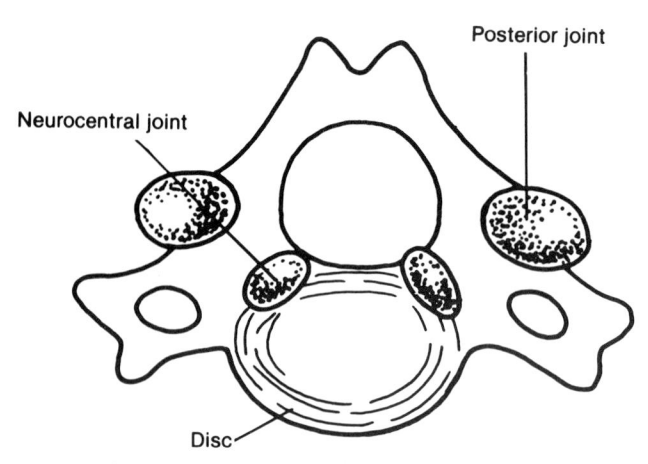

FIGURE 9–1. Cervical vertebra. (From MacNab, I. Symptoms in cervical disc degeneration. In Cervical Spine Research Society. The Cervical Spine. Philadelphia, J. B. Lippincott, 1983.)

vertebral body form a pair of joints of Luschka and a pair of facet joints posteriorly.

INTERVERTEBRAL DISK

The intervertebral disk consists of an outer lamellated fibrocartilaginous annulus fibrosus and an inner soft, gelatinous nucleus pulposus. The intervertebral disks are strong up to the second decade of life and can be damaged only by fractures through the vertebral body. The inferior and superior surfaces of the disks are made up of cartilaginous vertebral endplates. After the second decade the disks undergo degenerative changes, resulting in necrosis and sequestration of the nucleus pulposus as well as softening and weakening of the annulus fibrosus. Often minor strain may cause an eccentric displacement of the nucleus pulposus, resulting in sudden onset of neck pain, or the nucleus pulposus may actually rupture through the annulus fibrosus, causing a posterolateral or central herniation.

FACET JOINTS

The facet joints from C2 to C7 are synovial joints. They are covered with lax fibrous joint capsules that allow a gliding motion of the vertebrae above and below.

JOINTS OF LUSCHKA

In the posterolateral portions of the body of the vertebra there is a pair of hooklike, upward projections from the lower vertebra that form a pseudoarthrosis with the convex surfaces of the upper vertebra. These are referred to variously as the uncovertebral joints, the joints of Luschka, or the neurocentral joints. They are in close proximity with the pedicles, the neural foramina, and the nerve roots.

Periosteum

The periosteum covering the vertebral bodies is extremely pain-sensitive, and therefore fractures, lesions of the vertebral body, and traction on the periosteum by ligaments, tendons, and muscles produce segmental neck pain.

Ligaments

ANTERIOR LONGITUDINAL LIGAMENTS
The anterior longitudinal ligament is a strong band of longitudinally oriented fibers that runs the entire length of the vertebral column anteriorly from atlanto-occipital membrane; it is attached to the vertebral bodies and intervertebral disks at each level.

POSTERIOR LONGITUDINAL LIGAMENT
Located within the spinal canal and originating at the posterior portions of the body of the axis vertebra, the posterior longitudinal ligament attaches to the posterior margins of the vertebrae and the intervertebral disks. It is broad and strong in the upper cervical spine and somewhat narrower in the lower.

INTERSPINOUS LIGAMENTS
These ligaments are poorly developed, membranous structures that connect the adjoining vertebrae as well as the ligamenta flava in front and the supraspinous ligament in back.

LIGAMENTA FLAVA
The ligamenta flava are broad but thin, paired ligaments composed of yellowish elastic tissue that connect the laminae of the adjacent vertebrae. They permit controlled flexion of the spine in which the laminae of the adjacent vertebrae separate, and a gradual elastic recoil results in the return of the neck to the original position. They blend with the capsule of the facet joints anteriorly.

Spinal Cord

The spinal cord is covered by three membranes, termed the *dura mater*, the *arachnoid*, and the *pia mater*, which are separated from each other by two spaces, the subdural space and the subarachnoid space. The spinal cord is protected by its suspension from the dentate ligaments, which are lateral extensions of the pia mater in the subarachnoid space containing cerebrospinal fluid. The cervical enlargement of the spinal cord extends from the third cervical to the second thoracic level, corresponding to the attachments of the cervical and thoracic nerve roots to the upper extremities. It is widest at the level of the sixth cervical vertebra.

Nerve Roots

The cervical nerve roots are formed by ventral and dorsal roots that arise from the spinal cord. The ventral root carries the axons from the anterior (alpha and gamma) motor neurons and lateral horn (autonomic) cells. The dorsal root carries the sensory fibers to the dorsal horn of the spinal cord. The dorsal root ganglion is located at the level of the intervertebral foramina and contains the cell bodies of the sensory axons. Each dorsal root gives rise to a sinuvertebral nerve, which reenters the intervertebral foramen to provide the sensory supply for the vertebrae, ligaments, blood vessels of the spinal cord, and its meninges. Just distal to this, ventral and dorsal roots unite to form the mixed cervical root located at the level of the intervertebral foramen, which then divides into anterior and posterior primary rami. The anterior primary ramus receives a gray ramus communicans from the corresponding ganglion of the sympathetic trunk. The anterior primary rami of C4 to T2 form the brachial plexus. The posterior primary ramus supplies the posterior paravertebral muscles as well as the skin of the posterior cervical area.

Vertebral Artery

This artery arises from the subclavian artery, passes between the longus colli and scalenus anterior, and then passes through the transverse process of the upper six cervical vertebrae. It passes behind the lateral mass of the atlas, entering the skull through the foramen magnum. At this point the vertebral arteries join to form the basilar artery. In the neck they give off radicular (segmental spinal) arteries and muscular branches. Radicular arteries supply the cervical nerve roots and the vertebral body. At their termination the vertebral arteries give off an anterior spinal artery, which descends along the anterior median fissure of the spinal cord, supplying the anterior two-thirds of the spinal cord. The paired posterior spinal arteries usually arise from the posterior inferior cerebellar artery but may also arise from the vertebral artery itself; they supply the posterior third of the spinal cord.

Clinical Symptoms of Cervical Spine Lesions

Pain

Posterior neck pain is the most common presenting complaint of patients with a variety of lesions of the cervical spine. The pain may either radiate or be referred to the head, one or both upper extremities, interscapular area, medial border of the scapula, or the chest wall. Although there is some degree of overlap in pain patterns, they vary somewhat with lesions of different structures (Table 1). The pain that is perceived may be segmental, such as that seen in cervical radiculopathy, or it may be referred

TABLE 9-1. Pain-Sensitive Structures

Cervical spine	Ligaments
Vertebrae	Anterior longitudinal
Facet joints	Posterior longitudinal
Neurocentral joints	Interspinous
Periosteum	Spinal cord
Intervertebral discs	Nerve roots
Annulus fibrosus	Brachial plexus

Data from Cailliet, R. Neck and Arm Pain. Philadelphia, F. A. Davis, 1964.

in both segmental and extrasegmental distributions, as occurs when the dura mater is affected. Cyriax believes that there is no difference in the nature or extent of pain in either root pain or referred pain but merely a difference in the movements that evoke it.[2] A root lesion is suggested by the presence of paresthesia, sensory and motor deficits, and depressed or absent deep tendon reflexes. Lesions of the muscle and tendon cause pain on active and resisted motion as well as on passive stretching of the involved muscle.

Lesions of the ligament, joint capsule, bursa, fascia, nerve root, and dura mater cause pain at the extreme active or, more importantly, at the extreme passive range of motion.

Pain following a flexion-hyperextension (whiplash) type of injury (Fig. 9-2) is common in motor vehicle accidents. The severity, location, and nature of neck pain depend on the structures involved, the severity of trauma, and associated injuries. When only ligaments and muscles are involved (sprains and strains), patients notice mild stiffness with a progressive

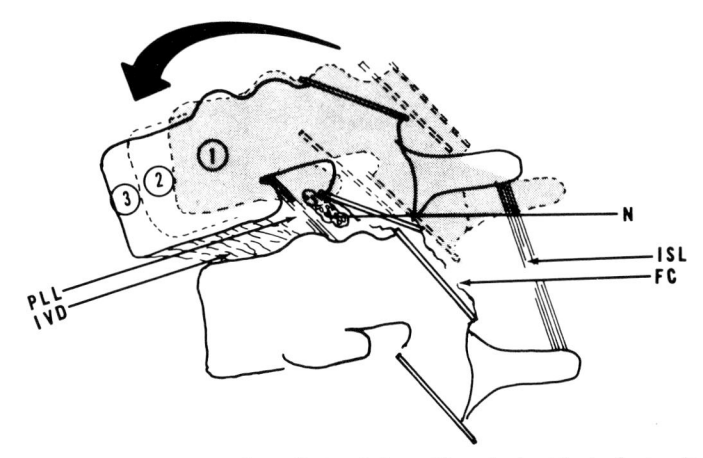

FIGURE 9-2. Hyperextension-hyperflexion Injury. Normal physiologic flexion (1 to 2) is possible with no soft tissue damage. When motion is exceeded (3), the intervertebral disk (IVD) is pathologically deformed and the posterior longitudinal ligament (PLL) strained or torn; the nerve (N) is acutely entrapped; the facet capsule (FC) is torn or stretched; and the interspinous ligament (ISL) is damaged. (From Caliet, R., Soft Tissue Pain and Disability. Philadelphia, F.A. Davis Co., 1977.)

increase in the intensity of neck pain in a few hours to days. This pain may be accompanied by swelling, tenderness in the anterior aspect of the neck, and increasing stiffness of the neck. Swelling and pain in the anterior aspect of the neck suggest a fracture of the vertebral body or anterior longitudinal ligament sprain with bleeding in the prevertebral space. This pain is usually central but may be bilateral and is somewhat relieved by slight forward flexion. However, in severe injuries the disk, nerve roots, vertebrae, cervical sympathetics, and vertebral artery may be involved, resulting in pain, tenderness, and spasm of the posterior paravertebral muscles and upper trapezius, headache, dizziness, and visual disturbances.

Pain in cervical intervertebral disk herniation is rare because of the strong posterior longitudinal ligament and the protection offered by the joints of Luschka posteriorly. Pain caused by disk herniation results from irritation due to traction on the posterior longitudinal ligament, strain on the "five-joint complex," or compression of the nerve root and or the spinal cord. Patients are usually in their third or fourth decades. There is sudden onset of unilateral neck pain, scapular pain, and torticollis in which the head is turned away from the side of the pain due to severe spasm of the ipsilateral sternocleidomastoid muscle. The pain may radiate to the upper extremity corresponding to the nerve root that may be affected. Neurologic examination of the affected extremity helps to differentiate this type of pain from that due to involvement of the articular structures of the spine in which the active, passive, and resisted range of motion reproduce or increase the symptoms.

Pain in Cervical Spondylosis. The term *cervical spondylosis* refers to degenerative changes in intervertebral disks. The pain in the early stages of cervical spondylosis is due to the effect on the posterior longitudinal ligament and the facet joints. With progressive loss of disk height posteriorly, the vertically oriented bony prominences of the joints of Luschka come in contact with each other, resulting in formation of osteophytes (Fig. 9–3). These osteophytes then encroach on the neural foramina and the spinal canal, compressing the nerve root or the spinal cord, or both (Figs. 9–4 to 9–6). The pain due to compression of the nerve root (radiculopathy) may then radiate to the occiput, upper thorax, scapular area, and those areas of the upper extremity innervated by that particular root. This pain may be accompanied by weakness, sensory impairment, and depressed or absent deep tendon reflexes in the distribution of that root. If there is compression on the dura, the pain may be referred to the head, thoracolumbar spine, or both lower extremities. Compression of the vertebral artery (Fig. 9–7) during its course through the foramina in the transverse processes may result in vertebrobasilar insufficiency. If the radicular arteries that accompany the cervical roots are compressed by the degenerated disk or the osteophyte, the result may be not only ischemic root pain but also impairment of the circulation to the spinal cord, because these arteries contribute to the segmental supply of the anterior spinal artery.

Compression of the cervical spinal cord results in cervical myelopathy. This results in a lower motor neuron type of paralysis at the level of the

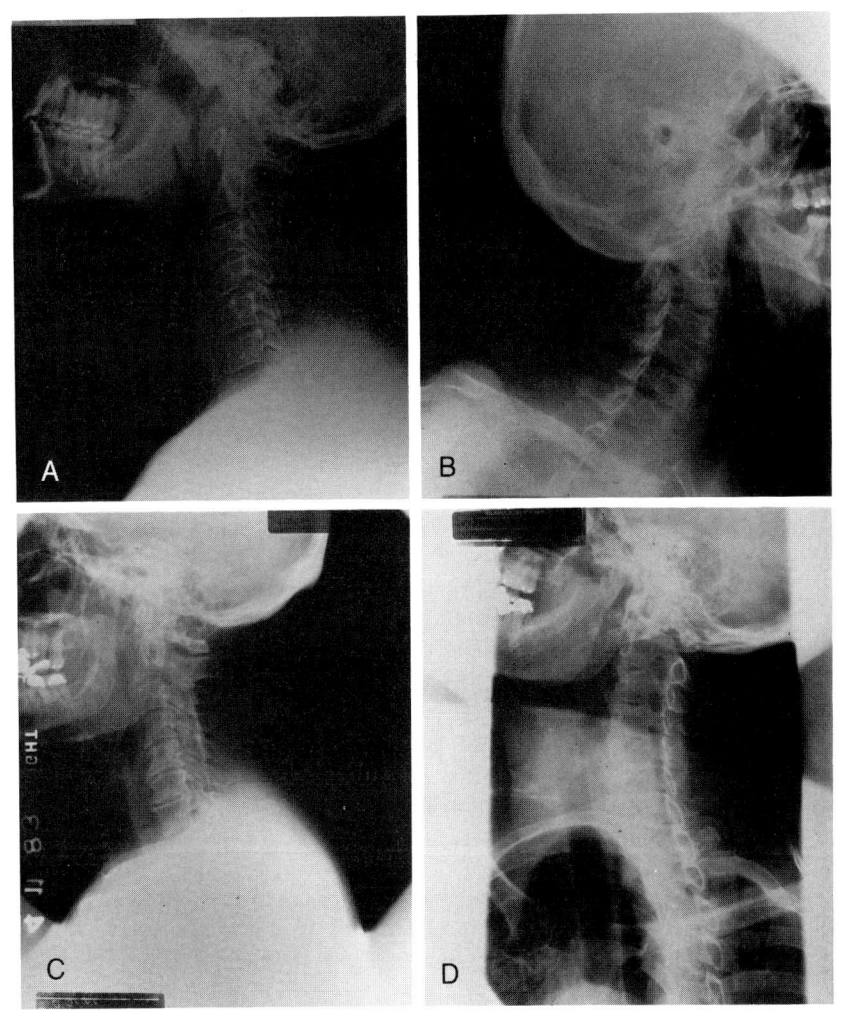

FIGURE 9–3. A, Radiograph of normal cervical spine, lateral view. B, Radiograph of normal cervical spine, oblique view showing normal foramina. C, Radiograph of cervical spondylosis, lateral view. D, Radiograph of cervical spondylosis, oblique view. Foraminal narrowing of C4–5, C5–7.

lesion and an upper motor neuron type of paralysis below the lesion. Concomitant root and spinal cord lesions are termed *myeloradiculopathy*.

Pain in Spinal Cord Injury. These patients may complain of a "dural" type of pain (see above under discussion of cervical spondylosis) or may suffer from radicular pain. Phantom pain is also described by patients who complain of pain in areas where there is no sensory or motor function. These patients may respond to reassurance and treatment with antidepressants. The pain may also be due to associated lesions of structures other than the spinal cord.

Pain in Cervical Radiculopathy. This type of pain is often a radiating, shooting pain that occurs along the dermatome or the myotome of the

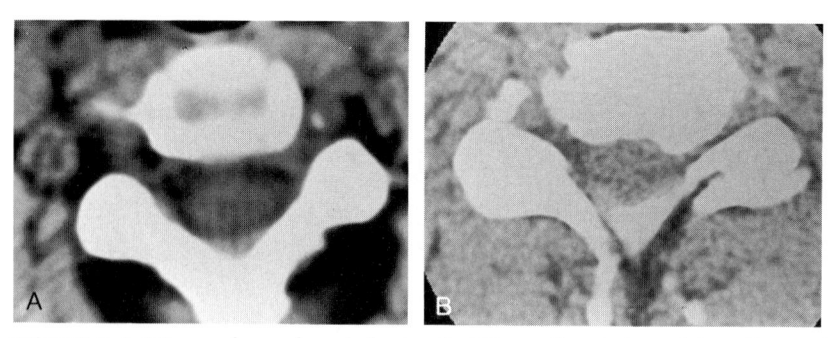

FIGURE 9-4. CT scan of normal cervical spine. B, CT scan of cervical spondylosis; foraminal narrowing, left C5-6.

affected root. Weakness or paresthesia accompanying the pain usually suggests that the pain is of radicular or spinal cord origin (Figs. 9-8 and 9-9). The ventral and dorsal rami of the upper four cervical roots form the anterior and posterior cervical plexus respectively. The C1 nerve root usually does not contain sensory fibers. In lesions of the C2-C3 nerve roots pain radiates to the posterior and lateral aspects of the neck, causing parieto-occipital and temporal headache, pain behind the eyes, and weakness of the trapezius and sternocleidomastoid muscles.[2] Lesions of the C4 root cause diffuse posterolateral neck pain, pain in the supraclavicular area, and partial paralysis of the ipsilateral diaphragm. Lesions of the C5 root produce pain in the lateral aspect of the shoulder and the upper arm, weakness of shoulder girdle movements, and depressed biceps jerk. Lesions of the C6 root result in pain in the radial aspect of the forearm, paresthesia

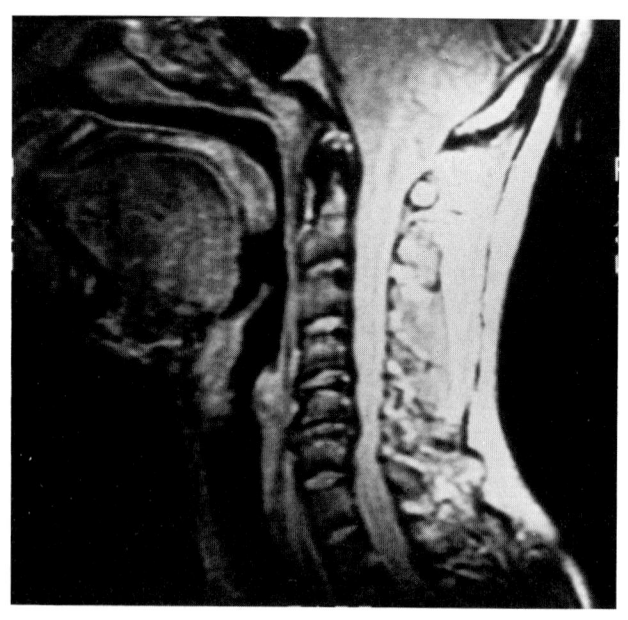

FIGURE 9-5. Spinal cord compression.

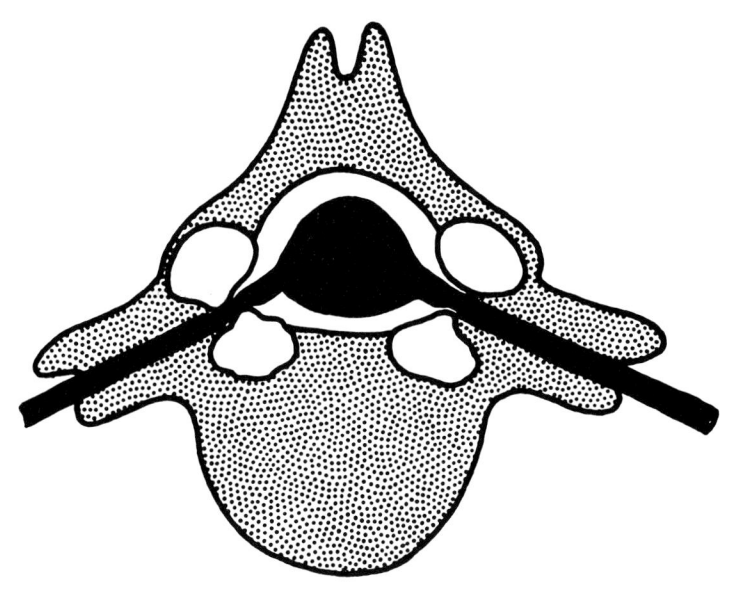

FIGURE 9-6. Neurocentral joints and cervical disk protrusion. (From MacNab, I. Symptoms in cervical disc degeneration. In Cervical Spine Research Society. The Cervical Spine. Philadelphia, J. B. Lippincott, 1983.)

in the thumb and index fingers, weakness of the elbow flexors, and depressed brachioradialis reflex. Lesions of the C7 root cause radiating pain along the posterior forearm, paresthesia in the middle finger, weakness of the elbow extensors, wrist flexors, finger extensors and depressed triceps jerk. Lesions of the C8 root result in radiating pain in the ulnar aspect of

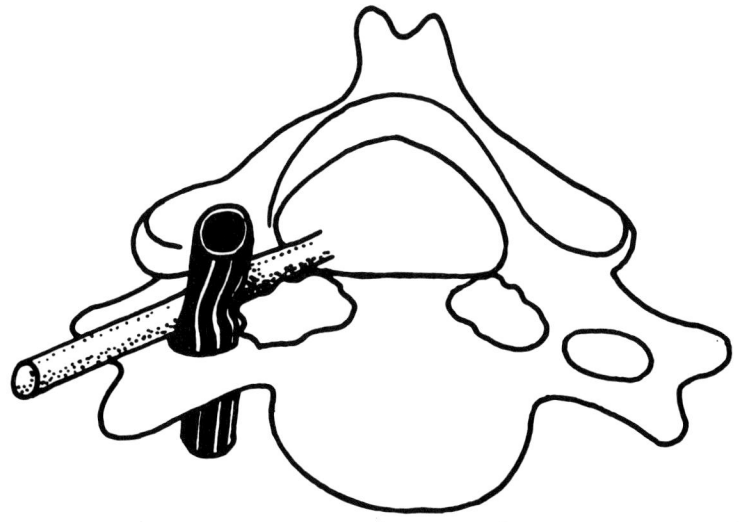

FIGURE 9-7. Vertebral artery compression. (From MacNab, I. Symptoms in cervical disc degeneration. In Cervical Spine Research Society. The Cervical Spine. Philadelphia, J. B. Lippincott, 1983.)

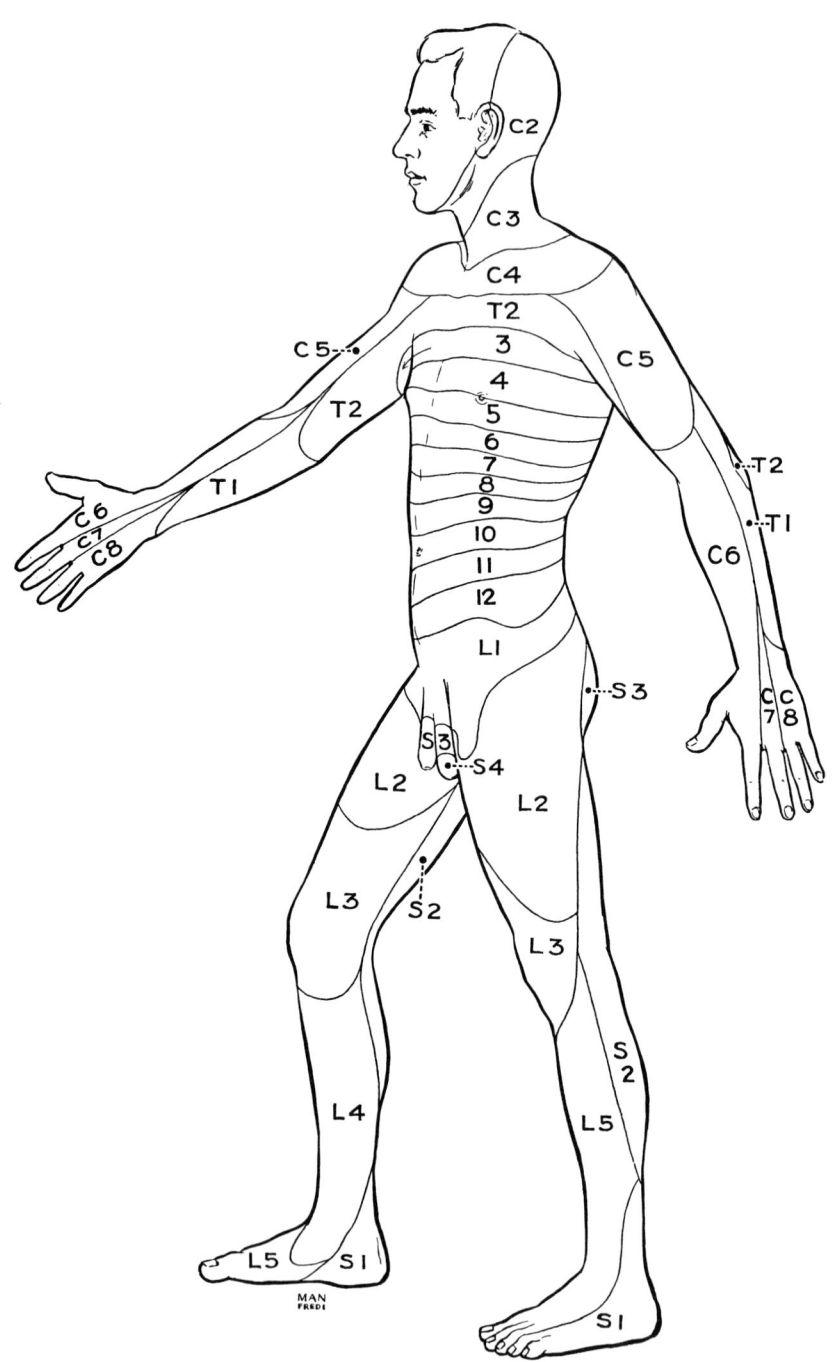

FIGURE 9–8. Dermatome chart, side view. (From Haymaker, W., and Woodhall, B. Peripheral Nerve Injuries, 2nd ed. Philadelphia, W. B. Saunders, 1953.)

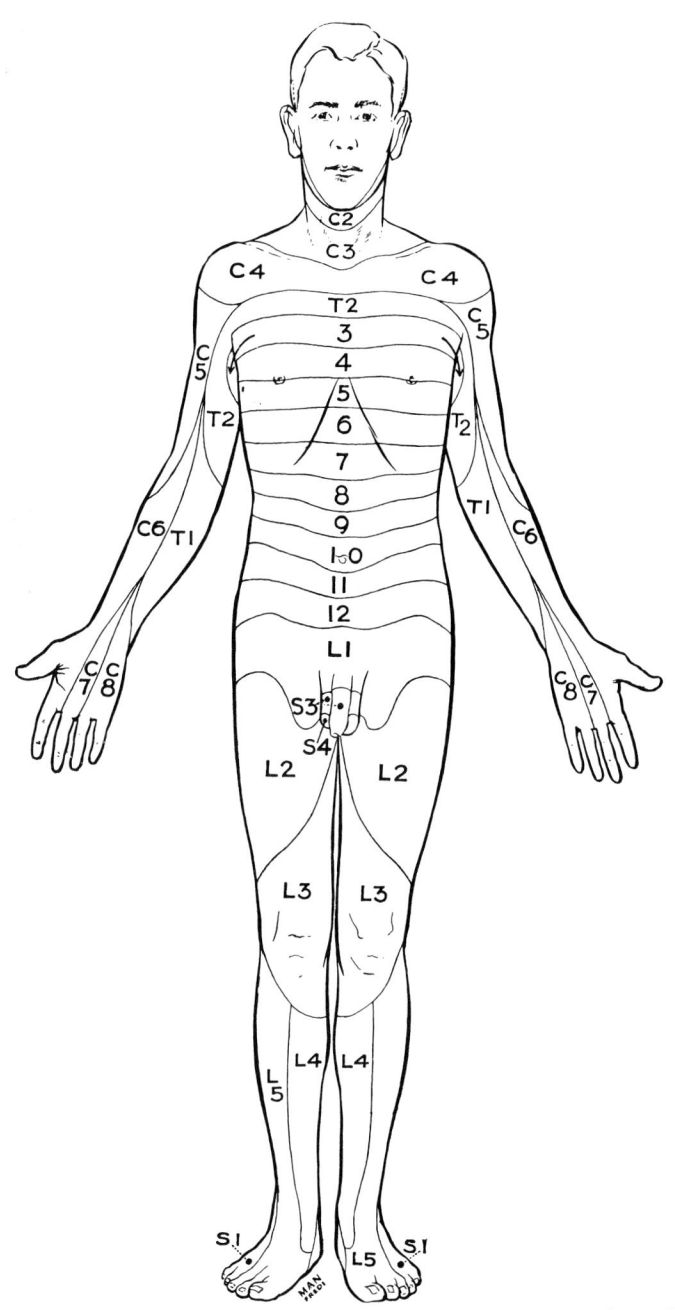

FIGURE 9–9. Dermatome chart, anterior view. (From Haymaker, W., and Woodhall, B. Peripheral Nerve Injuries, 2nd ed. Philadelphia, W. B. Saunders, 1953.)

the forearm, paresthesia in the ulnar aspect of the little finger, weakness of the finger flexors, and Horner's syndrome due to involvement of the cervical sympathetics. Radiculopathies affecting the mixed spinal nerves may be differentiated from anterior horn cell involvement by the presence of sensory signs and symptoms in the former. Radiculopathies may be differentiated from plexopathies either by the characteristic distribution of signs and symptoms or by electrodiagnostic studies.

Pain in Vertebral Artery Compromise. Although occlusion of the vertebral artery may result in various neurologic syndromes, the usual presentation is most likely caused by a lesion of the sympathetic fibers that accompany the artery, resulting in vertigo, tinnitus, retro-ocular pain, and blurred vision. Severe compromise may result in ischemia of the brainstem and spinal cord with development of Wallenberg's syndrome. This syndrome is characterized by dysphagia, dysphonia, dysarthria, ipsilateral anesthesia of the face, ipsilateral ataxia of the trunk and extremities, Horner's syndrome, and contralateral hemianesthesia of the extremities and trunk. In his experimental work Seleki noted that after 30 degrees of rotation the contralateral vertebral artery kinks and stretches. As rotation increases, the ipsilateral vertebral artery also kinks. In elderly patients with atherosclerosis of the vertebral arteries, extreme movements of the neck may induce ischemic events in the distribution of these arteries. The vertebral artery may also be compressed by degenerative changes in the joints of Luschka.

Pain in Facet Joint Arthropathy. Although there are patients with incidental radiologic findings of facet joint arthropathy and a restricted range of motion of the cervical spine, many are asymptomatic.[3] However, some patients do complain of dull, aching, unilateral neck pain that is aggravated by passive range of motion. In acute flare-ups there may be concomitant muscle spasm. Unless there are osteophytes that compress the adjacent structures, the limited passive range of motion and tenderness over the facet joints are the only signs.

Upper Extremity Weakness

Next to pain and paresthesia, weakness in the upper extremity is the most common complaint. The weakness may be of either the upper motor neuron or lower motor neuron type. Lower motor neuron lesions are caused by lesions of the anterior horn cells or the cervical roots. Lesions of the C2–C3 nerve roots cause weakness of shoulder shrug and rotation of the neck due to paralysis of the trapezius and sternocleidomastoid muscles. Lesions of the C4 root cause partial paralysis of the ipsilateral diaphragm. Lesions of the C5 root produce weakness of shoulder girdle movements and a depressed biceps jerk. Lesions of the C6 root result in weakness of the elbow flexors, wrist extensors, and a depressed brachioradialis reflex. Lesions of the C7 root cause weakness of elbow extension, wrist flexion, and finger extension and a depressed triceps jerk. Lesions of the C8 root result in weakness of the finger flexors and Horner's syndrome owing to involvement of the cervical sympathetics. Lesions of the T1 root result in weakness of the intrinsic hand muscles and Horner's syndrome. Weakness of the posterior paravertebral muscles are uncommon because there is overlapping innervation from the other segments.

Lower Extremity Weakness

Weakness or even complete paralysis of the lower extremities is due to a partial or complete spinal cord lesion. Symptoms include spasticity, hyperreflexia, pathologic reflexes, bowel and bladder incontinence, long tract sensory impairment, and ataxia. These may develop gradually in patients with cervical spondylosis or may be acute in cases of sudden and violent trauma to the cervical spine. The syndrome of cervical myeloradiculopathy resembles the motor neuron disease. In the latter, there is no history of significant neck pain, no sensory impairment, and normal bowel and bladder function, but there may be coexisting bulbar signs. It should be noted, however, that bulbar signs may be seen in vertebral artery compression due to cervical spondylosis, making this condition further difficult to distinguish. Somatosensory evoked potentials are normal in the motor neuron disease but may be absent or abnormal in cervical myeloradiculopathy.

Traumatic cervical spine injuries are most common, particularly in motor vehicle accidents. The initial history should include the type of trauma involved, such as a motor vehicle accident, a work-related accident, or other trauma. Details of a motor vehicle accident such as the type of collision, whether the patient anticipated the accident (stiffening the neck) in the preceding moments, history of unconsciousness, and the type of care received by the patient following the accident should be investigated. The type of collision, such as rear end, front end, side, or other, is important in determining the direction of force causing the cervical spine injury. Details of work-related accidents such as the type of the work, nature of the accident, history of prior accidents, and the type of care received should be investigated.

Physical Examination

Posture

The normal cervical spine has a slight lordotic posture, in which the head is held directly above the center of gravity. Changes in this posture may be due to familial, habitual, or pathologic reasons. Deliberate trunk rotation rather than rotation of the head and neck is usually seen in acute injuries to the cervical spine owing to the splinting effect and muscle spasm. Patients may present with torticollis, "straightening of the spine," or loss of normal lordosis, increased lordosis, or reversal of lordosis, the latter two having far more serious implications. Increase in cervical lordosis suggests a hyperextension injury resulting in rupture of the disks, stretching of the anterior longitudinal ligament, narrowing of the spinal canal, or compression fractures of the posterior elements of the spine. Reversal of lordosis suggests an anterior compression fracture, fracture dislocations, disk herniation, severe posterior ligamentous sprain with or without interlocking facet joints, or narrowing of the spinal canal due to hyperflexion injuries.[4] Patients with cervical spondylosis present with considerable forward flexion at the neck, mostly due to restricted range of motion. Patients with increased thoracic kyphosis or scoliosis show a compensatory increase in cervical lordosis or scoliosis. These postural changes, if they persist, may contribute to degenerative changes in the five-joint complex, resulting in neurovascular lesions.

Torticollis

Torticollis, in which the head is turned away from the side of the pain due to severe spasm of the ipsilateral sternocleidomastoid muscle, is commonly noted following subluxation of the C1–C2 vertebrae or cervical disk herniation causing compression of the nerve root or the spinal cord.

Loss of Lordosis

Although loss of normal cervical lordosis is one of the most common clinical and radiologic findings, the specific mechanism causing it is not very clear. It is thought to be due to "spasm" of the posterior paravertebral muscles. Gore et al reported in a 10-year follow-up study that the presence or severity of "pain" was not related to the presence of degenerative changes, the sagittal diameter of the spinal canal, the degree of cervical lordosis, or to any changes in these measurements during the evaluation period.[3]

Passive Range of Motion

CERVICAL SPINE

Passive range of motion testing using a goniometer or visual judgment provides only a gross estimate of the capability of movements in the head and neck.[5] Accurate measurement requires radiographic methods.[6] However, one should be aware that in testing the movements of the head and neck, there are three distinct segments to be noted (Table 9–2).[7,8] The first segment is the Occipitoatlantal (C1) articulation, which permits moderate flexion-extension (nodding), minimal lateral flexion, and no rotation. The second segment is the atlantoaxial (C1–C2) articulation, which controls half of the total rotation capability of the cervical spine, moderate flexion-extension, and minimal lateral flexion. The third segment consists of articulations of C2–C7, which permit all motions, particularly the greatest amount of flexion-extension followed by lateral flexion and rotation. Blanchard et al., in a study of male students 15–29 years of age, noted that as age increases, the range of motion in the cervical spine decreases.[9] Lysell

TABLE 9-2. Segmental Motion of Cervical Spine in Degrees

MOVEMENT	OCCIPUT-C1	C1–C2	C2–C7
Flexion	10	5	45
Extension	25	10	45
Lateral flexion—right	5	5	30
Lateral flexion—left	5	5	30
Rotation—right	0	45	30
Rotation—left	0	45	30

noted that lateral rotation is associated with lateral flexion in C2–C7 vertebrae.[10] Excess of passive range of motion may lead to facet joint dislocations. It is, however, important to remember that in any history or suspicion of serious head and neck injury testing the passive range of motion should be deferred. The range of motion may be limited owing to reluctance on the part of the patient, muscle spasm, cervical spondylosis, arthritis, fractures, dislocation, or congenital deformity such as Klippel-Feil syndrome.

Compression-Extension Maneuver

Axial compression of the head combined with extension of the neck causes narrowing of the intervertebral foramina. In patients with compromise of the foraminal space by a protruding disk, osteophytes, or other space-occupying lesions, this maneuver causes reproduction or exacerbation of radicular symptoms. This maneuver should be avoided in patients with recent acute head and neck trauma.

Distraction-Flexion Maneuver

The distraction-flexion maneuver relieves pressure on the cervical root by opening the intervertebral foramina and increasing the spinal canal diameter.

Joints

Examination of the joints of the extremities and spine for evidence of rheumatoid arthritis, osteoarthritis, or spondyloarthropathies is essential in assessing the generalized nature of the problem. Patients with rheumatoid arthritis are prone to instability of the cervical spine, most notably at C1–C2 articulation. They are therefore prone to cervical myeloradiculopathy. Manipulations of the spine in such patients should be avoided.

Neurologic Examination

Complete initial neurologic examination and periodic reassessment are essential in almost all patients with lesions of the cervical spine. Anatomic localization of the lesion and its severity will be of the utmost value in planning further diagnostic tests, treatment, and prognosis. In patients with severe pain or who are unconscious due to associated head trauma, the examination is often limited initially to recording the patient's mental status, ability to move the extremities on command, ability to perceive various sensations, and control of the bowel and bladder. In a patient with acute trauma the neurologic examination ideally should be carried out after adequate immobilization of the cervical spine.

Inspection

Atrophy of the muscles suggests lower motor neuron involvement. Atrophy of the muscles may follow a radicular pattern in lesions of a specific nerve root, such as atrophy of the shoulder girdle muscles and elbow flexors with C5–C6 lesions. If atrophy is diffuse and distal, it suggests advanced peripheral polyneuropathy. If atrophy is confined to the distribution of a single peripheral nerve, mononeuritis or focal entrapment neuropathy is the most likely cause. In lesions of a single nerve root, atrophy may not be prominent because of the overlapping innervation of different segments. Fasciculations may be seen in old or chronic radiculopathies, slowly progressing myeloradiculopathies, and motor neuron disease. Trophic skin changes are seen in chronic denervation and in sympathetic lesions. Muscle spasm is a nonspecific finding and may be due to almost any lesion of the spine or nerve root, or to sprains. Muscle spasm contributes to immobility, which may have a protective effect in the immediate postinjury phase. However, muscle spasm also contributes to persistent headache and neck pain due to irritation of the nerve endings in and around the contracting muscle and traction on the periosteum of the spine and skull where the muscles are attached.

Tenderness over the brachial plexus and peripheral nerves may be elicited in patients with radiculopathies and myofascial pain syndrome. Tenderness of the skin is usually noted in causalgia and reflex sympathetic dystrophy.

Tone

Flaccid paralysis may be due to any lower motor neuron lesion such as lesions of the nerve root, anterior horn cells, plexus, or peripheral nerves as well as primary muscle disease. Patients with cervical spine lesions may present with flaccid paralysis due to a significant lesion of the nerve root or multiple nerve roots. It is rare to see significant flaccid paralysis or atrophy in a single nerve root lesion because almost all skeletal muscles are innervated by more than one nerve root. Patients with spinal cord injuries may present with flaccid paralysis during the "spinal shock" phase.

Spasticity is a sign of an upper motor neuron lesion and is defined as an increased muscular resistance to a passive stretch. It is seen in patients with spinal cord injuries, brainstem lesions due to vertebral artery compromise, and similar conditions. If spasticity is noted in the shoulder girdle muscles the lesion is at least rostral to the C5 spinal cord segment. Mixed lower motor neuron lesions in the upper extremities and upper motor neuron lesions in the lower extremities suggest cervical myeloradiculopathy or motor neuron disease.

Strength

Testing of muscle strength should include testing the muscles of the neck and both upper and lower extremities. Muscle strength testing is often unreliable in patients who are not cooperative or in pain, who have upper motor neuron lesions, or who are malingerers or hysterics. In such patients, observation of functional activities, such as dressing and ambulation, gives an estimate of the strength of the muscles. Muscle strength testing is graded and recorded. The pattern of muscle weakness and the rest of the examination suggest the anatomic diagnosis. Again, it is important to note that skeletal muscles are usually innervated by more than one cervical nerve root, and some nerve roots contribute more to one muscle than others (dominant innervation); for instance, the C7 nerve root is dominant in the innervation of the triceps brachii.

Sensibility

Sensory examination for pain, temperature, joint position, and vibration should be performed in patients with isolated nerve root lesions. The sensory examination may be entirely normal because of overlapping innervation from other nerve roots. If the spinal cord sensory pathways are affected by lesions of the cervical spine, specific sensory abnormalities may be dependent on which direction such lesions approach the spinal cord. Slowly progressing lesions of the posterior elements of the spine such as osteophytes from the facet joint lamina may compress the posterior columns of the spinal cord, causing abnormalities in joint position sense and vibration in the upper and lower extremities. In patients with lesions of the cervical nerve roots, sensibility may be impaired in the dermatomal pattern for that root.

Reflexes

Deep tendon reflexes of both upper and lower extremities are recorded in patients with lesions of the nerve roots. Specific reflexes may be decreased or absent. In a lesion of the C7 nerve root, triceps brachii reflex may be diminished or absent. In spinal cord or other central nervous system lesions the reflexes are hyperactive with or without overflow to the other segments. Babinski's sign may also be noted.

Cranial nerve lesions, particularly those of cranial nerves V, IX, X, and XI, are noted in patients with vertebral artery insufficiency. The fifth cranial nerve is tested by asking the patient to open the mouth and clench the teeth and by sensory testing of the face and head; the corneal reflex is also tested. The ninth and tenth cranial nerves are tested by asking the patient to swallow and by noting the hoarseness of the voice and gag reflex. The eleventh cranial nerve is tested by checking for weakness in the sternocleidomastoid and trapezius muscles.

Functional State

Careful assessment of the patient's neurologic and musculoskeletal function and disability should be followed by evaluation of his or her ability to perform activities of daily living including ambulation. Patients with spinal cord injury and patients with vertebral artery insufficiency may be dependent in some or all of these activities. Patients with cervical radiculopathies seldom have significant or lasting disability and may be able to perform daily activities independently. In some patients with significant cervical spine lesions such as fractures or disk herniation, activities may be restricted owing to required immobilization and rest even if they have little or no neurologic compromise. Details of the patient's occupational history are important in determining the patient's ability to return to work.

Other Diagnostic Studies

The history and physical examination give some clues to the anatomic diagnosis and perhaps even the etiology of the lesion. Further studies may be necessary to arrive at a more precise diagnosis. These include radiologic and electrodiagnostic studies.

Radiologic Studies

After adequate immobilization, patients with acute head and neck trauma should have plain radiographs taken of the cervical spine. These films should consist of at least a good lateral view that includes C7 vertebra and permits visualization of the vertebral bodies, the overall alignment of the spine, the disk spaces, spinal canal, and, to some extent, the soft tissues. The lateral view usually identifies several unstable lesions of the spine by showing disruption of the normal curvature of the spine and therefore the potential for spinal cord damage. Widening of the prevertebral space in the lateral view by soft tissue swelling caused by hematoma suggests significant lesions of the anterior longitudinal ligament, avulsion fractures of the vertebral body, or osteophytes. If the lateral view suggests abnormalities, further views are necessary to identify lesions such as interlocking facets and compression fractures of the vertebral body. The anteroposterior view is best suited for visualizing the joints of Luschka, interlocking facets, and fractures of C1 and C2 vertebrae. Oblique views are ideal for visualizing the intervertebral foramina. An open mouth view permits visualizing the C1–C2 joint and any possible lateral instability.

Computed tomography (CT) is now widely employed for diagnosing lesions of the cervical spine (see Fig. 9–4). The CT scan provides better resolution of the vertebrae and soft tissues than plain radiographs. It also provides excellent cross-sectional views of the bony structures of the spine and the spinal canal. Some lesions such as compression fractures, congenital deformities, and bony fusion that are visible in plain radiographs may not be visible in CT scans. Visualization of the spinal cord often requires injection of a contrast material such as metrizamide.

Magnetic resonance imaging provides outstanding resolution of the spine, spinal canal, and spinal cord (see Fig. 9–5). It is gaining in popularity for diagnosis of various lesions.

Electrodiagnostic Testing

Electrodiagnostic studies are a logical extension of the clinical examination of the patient. They are helpful in establishing an anatomic diagnosis, in detecting the pathophysiology of the neurologic lesion, and to some extent, in determining the prognosis. Electrodiagnostic studies consist of motor and sensory nerve conduction studies of selected nerves of the upper extremities, F-wave latency, electromyographic examination of selected muscles of the upper extremities and paravertebral muscles, and somatosensory evoked potential studies of selected nerves of the upper and lower extremities. The parameters used in electrodiagnostic studies are as follows:

1. In motor and sensory conduction studies
    a. Latency
    b. Amplitude
    c. Duration
    d. Conduction velocity
2. In electromyographic examination
    a. Activity of the muscle at rest (normally silent)
    b. Spontaneous response of the muscle to needle movement
    c. Motor unit action potential shape
    d. Motor unit action potential amplitude
    e. Motor unit action potential recruitment patterns
3. In somatosensory action potentials
    a. Absolute latency
    b. Interpeak latency
    c. Central conduction time
    d. Amplitude
    e. Side-to-side difference of the above

Latency is the recording of conduction time along a segment of peripheral nerve from the site of stimulus to the site of recording of the nerve or muscle action potential (Fig. 9–10). It is usually dependent on the fastest (large myelinated) axons. Segmental lesions causing demyelination produce slowing of conduction time along these axons, and therefore latency is delayed. As a rule, proximal lesions of the peripheral nerve plexus, nerve root, and anterior horn cells do not cause a delay in the latency of the more distal parts of the peripheral nerve unless there is a significant reduction in number of the faster conducting axons.

The amplitude measurement gives an estimate of the number of functioning axons. A more precise estimate of the number of functioning nerve axons is made by calculating the area under the curve of an action potential. In motor nerve conduction studies, the amplitude of the compound muscle action potential from a muscle recorded by a surface electrode by stimulation of the mixed or motor nerve to that muscle provides an estimate of the number of functioning muscle fibers and therefore the number of functioning axons. Amplitude is measured in millivolts for measuring compound muscle action potentials and in microvolts for measuring sensory nerve action potentials. The duration of the action potential gives an estimate of the distribution of the population of axons that conduct at different speeds. The conduction velocity measures the speed of conduction along a segment of the nerve and is expressed in meters per second.

MOTOR NERVE CONDUCTION STUDIES

In the upper extremity, a motor nerve conduction study consists of stimulating the median and ulnar nerves at the wrist, elbow, and other proximal sites and recording a series of compound muscle action potentials from the intrinsic hand muscles. The motor nerve conduction study is helpful in differentiating lesions of the peripheral nerves from those of the plexus and roots by demonstrating focal slowing or absence of conduction in peripheral nerve segments. Demonstration of normal peripheral nerve conduction is helpful in differentiating peripheral neuropathies and focal entrapment syndromes such as carpal tunnel syndrome and cubital tunnel syndrome, which often mimic cervical radiculopathies. Normal peripheral nerve conduction velocity with reduced amplitude suggests a more proximal lesion because the number of axons, and therefore the number of muscle fibers, is reduced. Recording the latency of the F wave in such cases may identify more proximal lesions such as cervical radiculopathy or brachial plexopathy. Such a diagnosis can be further confirmed when a focal slowing of conduction is demonstrated by stimulating various cervical nerve roots in the posterior neck and recording the response from the corresponding muscles.

SENSORY NERVE CONDUCTION STUDIES

Sensory nerve conduction studies are performed by stimulating mixed or sensory nerves and recording the sensory nerve action potential. Again, the latency, amplitude, duration, and conduction velocity of the action

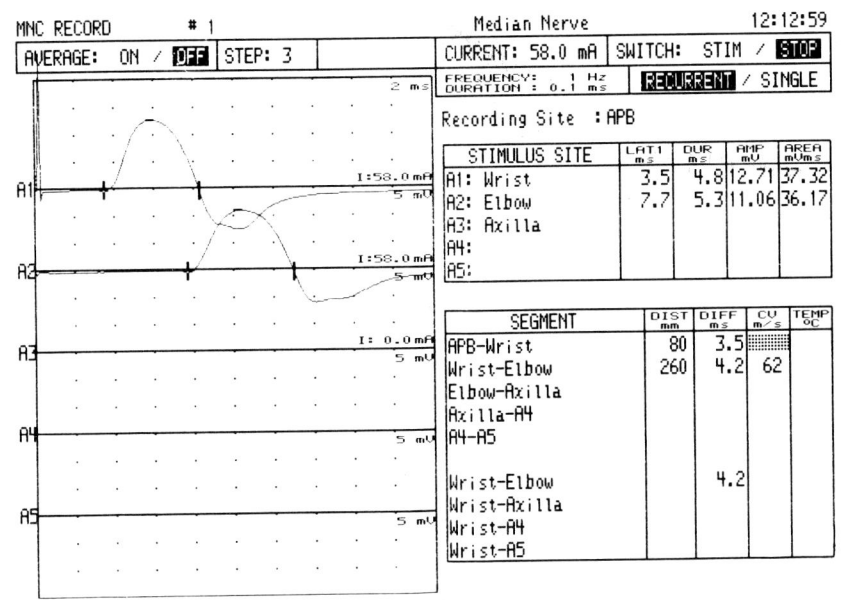

FIGURE 9–10. Electrodiagnostic study: measurement of latency, amplitude, and conduction velocity of median (motor) nerve.

potentials of the fastest fibers are recorded. The dermatomal sensory nerve root innervation of the individual fingers (see Figs. 9–8 and 9–9) is different for different fingers. The thumb and index fingers are innervated by C6, the middle finger by C7, and the ring and little finger by C8 nerve roots. In a patient with clinical evidence of C6 radiculopathy, for example, peripheral sensory nerve conduction to the thumb and index fingers may be normal but the amplitude may be reduced or absent. Studies of sensory nerve conduction usually show the earliest abnormalities in focal entrapment neuropathies and peripheral polyneuropathies. Sensory nerve conduction is normal and is of considerable help in the diagnosis of cervical root avulsion, in which the parent sensory cell bodies in the dorsal root ganglion are intact even though the patient has complete anesthesia and motor paralysis (abnormal motor nerve conduction and electromyographic results) in the distribution of that root.

ELECTROMYOGRAPHY

Electromyographic examination consists of recording the electrical activity of a muscle at rest, its response to needle insertion, and the amplitude, shape, and recruitment of the motor units in response to minimal and maximal voluntary contractions.

A Teflon-coated monopolar needle electrode or a stainless steel concentric needle electrode is used to record the electrical activity from a muscle. These activities are amplified and displayed in an oscilloscope and through loudspeakers. A normal muscle is electrically silent. On needle movement some "insertional" activity is normally seen. A denervated muscle exhibits "spontaneous activity" at rest. These are sometimes termed *denervation potentials*. They indicate axonal degeneration and denervation of muscle fibers. In a completely denervated muscle no motor unit action potentials are noted on attempted voluntary movement. In a partially denervated muscle there is a reduced number of motor unit action potentials, which are often "polyphasic" and are of longer duration. In patients with radiculopathies these findings are confined to a set of muscles innervated by a common nerve root in the upper extremity and often in the related posterior paravertebral muscles, which are innervated by the posterior primary rami. In lesions of the brachial plexus and peripheral nerves, electromyographic abnormalities are confined to the appendicular muscles innervated by the anterior primary rami that form the plexus and the peripheral nerves. In isolated lesions of the anterior horn cells the electromyographic findings may be abnormal, but the sensory nerve amplitudes are normal. Thus the distribution of electromyographic abnormalities coupled with other electrodiagnostic studies helps to localize the site of the lesion.

SOMATOSENSORY EVOKED POTENTIALS

Somatosensory evoked potentials are used to diagnose lesions of the somatosensory pathways of the sensory receptors, sensory or mixed peripheral nerves, plexus, nerve roots, spinal cord, brainstem, and thalamocortical areas. Segmental localization of the lesions of sensory pathways is possible by stimulating the sensory or mixed peripheral nerves and recording the ascending sensory volley from the different areas of the neuraxis. The potentials recorded consist of extremely small negative (N or upgoing) and positive (P or down going) peaks and require the use of an averaging computer. These peaks are labeled by their polarity and the usual latencies at which they occur.

Stimulation of a mixed peripheral nerve at the wrist gives rise to an initial negative peak that occurs at approximately 9 msec (N9) while recording from the skin over the brachial plexus. This potential is therefore felt to represent the brachial plexus potential. Likewise, negative potentials are recorded by an electrode placed at the C2 or C7 vertebra, representing activity at the cervical spinal cord (N11) and at the lower brainstem (N13). Electrodes placed over the scalp record thalamocortical activity (N19) and possibly activity at the somatosensory cortex (P22). The interpeak latencies provide an estimate of the conduction time between two sites in the neuraxis; absence of a particular waveform or a significant delay in either the absolute or the interpeak latency period (mean + 3SD [standard deviation]) compared to normal values or compared to the other side indicates the presence of pathology. The study is for the most part noninvasive. Demonstration of an isolated delay in the proximal segments (recording from the brachial plexus and the cervical spine) suggests that the lesion is in the roots or the spinal cord.

Management

Initial management depends on such factors as the etiology and severity of the neck pain. Cervical spine and other associated injuries requiring surgical intervention should be referred to the appropriate specialists. Management of lesions requiring no surgical intervention consists of immobilization with cervical orthoses, use of anti-inflammatory drugs, rest, and physical therapy.

Rest

Bed rest at home for 2 to 5 days is indicated in patients with acute neck and arm pain. When the cervical sympathetic nerves are involved, with signs of dizziness and visual and auditory disturbances, longer periods of immobilization may be necessary.

Immobilization

In addition to systemic rest, resting the painful neck by means of an appropriate cervical orthosis may be necessary for a few days to a few weeks. Cervical orthoses are used to immobilize the spine in some or all ranges to prevent further damage to the neurovascular structures, support the weight of the head, thereby providing some distraction, and permit healing. There are several types of cervical orthoses. Frequently they are referred to by the place of their design or the name of the designer. Different cervical orthoses provide varying degrees of restriction of cervical spine motion and should be prescribed accordingly[11, 12] (Fig. 9–11). Halo devices provide excellent restriction of all motions of the cervical spine and are used in unstable fractures of C1 and C2 as well as for fractures to the lower cervical spine. Application and adjustments of the halo devices are best left to well-trained spinal surgeons and neurosurgeons. The Yale cervicothoracic orthosis provides good flexion-extension and lateral rotation control and fair lateral flexion control. The four-poster orthosis permits a little more flexion-extension and rotation movement than the Yale device. The SOMI (Sterno-Occipital-Mandibular-Immobilizer) controls flexion of

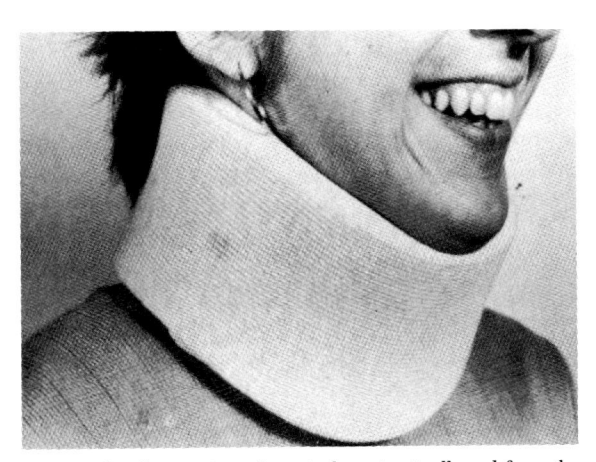

FIGURE 9–11. Cervical orthosis. Normal cervical motion is allowed from the occiput to the first thoracic vertebra. (From Johnson, R. M., Hart, D. L., Simmons, E. F., et al. Cervical orthosis: A study comparing their effectiveness in restricting cervical motion in normal subjects. J Bone Joint Surg 59A:332, 1977.)

the upper cervical spine and is therefore useful in some fractures of C2 to C5 vertebrae. This orthosis is easy to apply and adjust.

The Philadelphia collar is made of soft Plastizote and is almost as comfortable as a "soft collar." It comes in two easily removable pieces that are fastened by Velcro tabs, and it provides good control of flexion-extension, fair lateral rotation, and lateral flexion control. It is prefabricated and comes in several different sizes to allow for various widths and heights of the neck.

The familiar soft collar does not restrict cervical spine motion significantly and when used, serves mostly as a reminder to the patient. It is therefore preferable to use the Philadelphia collar for most cases of cervical sprains and strains.

The most serious injuries, such as fractures, dislocations, and severe lesions of the posterior ligaments, require the use of a cervical orthosis until satisfactory healing or surgical intervention occurs. In mild to moderate sprains and strains the patient is advised to use the collar initially night and day for up to 10 days and then wear it less often during the next few weeks. In these patients early active and passive range of motion exercises are started to avoid stiffness.

Anti-Inflammatory Drugs

Nonsteroidal anti-inflammatory drugs (NSAIDs) may be useful when the patient's symptoms are due to inflammation. They are particularly indicated for the management of rheumatic diseases such as osteoarthritis, rheumatoid arthritis, and spondyloarthropathies. Their anti-inflammatory and analgesic effects are most likely due to their inhibition of prostaglandin synthesis. The dosage required for anti-inflammatory action is generally higher than that needed for analgesic actions. The selection of a specific drug from the large number of these drugs depends on the efficacy, side effects, and convenience of dosages of each.

Muscle Relaxants

Spasm of the posterior paravertebral muscles is a common finding in patients with cervical spine lesions. Such spasms are involuntary and may aggravate the patient's symptoms. Although muscle spasms serve as an internal splint to protect the tissues from further trauma, sometimes they may last longer, requiring therapeutic intervention. Most minor strains and sprains that cause muscle spasm respond to rest, immobilization, and anti-inflammatory drugs. Patients with severe muscle spasm due to strains, sprains, or radiculopathy may require treatment with muscle relaxants, which provide adjunctive pain relief. Most commonly prescribed muscle relaxants are central skeletal muscle relaxants, which probably act by depressing the spinal and brainstem polysynaptic reflexes. A common side effect is sedation, which may help in relief of spasm. Patients should be advised to avoid potentially dangerous machinery during treatment with muscle relaxants. Long-term use of these drugs should be avoided because of the potential for dependency in some patients. Most commonly prescribed central skeletal muscle relaxants include cytobenzaprine, methocarbamol, chlorzoxazone, diazepam, and carisoprodol.

Referral to a Specialist

A primary care physician managing a patient with neck pain may choose to refer the patient to other specialists for a more detailed workup and management. Most minor cervical strains and sprains can be managed by rest, immobilization, anti-inflammatory drugs, and muscle relaxants until the patient is pain free and has regained full mobility of the cervical spine. Clues to the seriousness of the injury may come from the nature of the trauma, if any, and the associated neurologic or vascular symptoms, signs, and radiologic findings. Patients with associated head trauma or symptoms suggestive of cerebrovascular insufficiency may be referred to a neurologist or a neurosurgeon. Patients suspected of having severe sprains, fractures, dislocations, or disk herniation or degeneration may be referred to an orthopedic spine specialist. Several cervical spine lesions may require a team effort by different specialists and the primary care physician. Patients who require conservative nonsurgical management are referred to specialists in physical medicine and rehabilitation (physiatrists), who will assist in the diagnosis of neuromusculoskeletal lesions and prescribe and supervise appropriate physical and occupational therapy. Referral to a pain clinic may be necessary in patients with chronic neck pain, headaches for which there is little organic basis. These patients may undergo behavioral changes that in turn contribute to pain and related disability. The comprehensive pain clinics offer a multidisciplinary approach to diagnosis and management of these patients. Patients may be managed on an outpatient or an inpatient basis depending on the need for invasive procedures.

Nerve Blocks

Nerve blocks are discussed in detail in Chapter 11.

Physical Therapy

Physical therapy is prescribed after a careful history, physical examination, and workup have been done. Goals of therapy should be clearly defined to the patient as well as in the prescription to the therapist. Even though patients focus their attention on pain relief, impairment of their joint mobility, strength, and overall function should be identified and discussed with the patient and the family and appropriate therapy prescribed. In patients with acute pain, the initial goals of therapy may indeed be pain relief and treatment of specific conditions. In chronic pain patients, functional and behavioral changes need to be addressed in addition to the pain itself. Control of pain is achieved with various modalities such as superficial heat, deep heat, cryotherapy, traction, massage, electrical stimulation, active, passive, and relaxation exercises, and so on. Therapeutic techniques may need to be modified depending on the patient's response. During and after treatments, the focus should be shifted to not just reduction in pain but also restoration of function.

Heat

Application of heat is a time-honored remedy for relief of pain, spasm, and stiffness. The effect of heat is achieved both generally and locally. General effects of heat are elevated body temperature and sedation. Local effects are usually produced by direct action of heat on the underlying tissues. Heat promotes flexibility of collagen tissue, relieves muscle spasms by decreasing muscle spindle activity, increases the conduction velocity of nerve fibers, and increases local blood flow. Heat should be applied with caution. It is contraindicated over anesthetic areas, in unconscious patients, applied directly over malignant tumors, and in patients with vascular insufficiency.

SUPERFICIAL HEAT

Heat application may be superficial or deep. Examples of superficial heat are hydrocollator packs, hydrotherapy, paraffin baths, and fluidotherapy. For patients with neck and arm pain requiring superficial heat, the hydrocollator pack, which provides moist heat, is applied over the area of pain and spasm for 20 to 30 minutes prior to any other treatment. Application of heat to the areas of referred pain in the extremities is generally ineffective unless there are associated problems such as arthritis, which is best treated with paraffin baths, hydrotherapy, or fluidotherapy.

ULTRASOUND

Ultrasound is the modality of choice in heating the deepest structures such as joints and the surrounding tissues. The ultrasound device is equipped with a transducer in which the high-frequency current is converted to acoustic vibrations (ultrasound) by a quartz crystal. Ultrasound is also used in the technique of phonophoresis, in which ultrasonic energy is used to drive some drugs such as steroids deep into the tissues. It is considered more effective than iontophoresis.

SHORTWAVE DIATHERMY

Heating of deeper tissues is achieved with shortwave and microwave diathermies and ultrasound. In shortwave diathermy, high-frequency electrical currents are converted to heat at tissue interfaces. This method is useful in heating subcutaneous fat, superficial layers of muscles, and the fat-muscle interface.

MICROWAVE DIATHERMY

In microwave diathermy, electromagnetic wave forms are converted to heat in the tissue interfaces, including most of the skeletal muscle.

Cryotherapy

Therapeutic cold application is used for reduction of muscle spasm and spasticity, acute but minor trauma, and pain relief. Cold application by lowering muscle spindle activity and temperature reduces muscle spasm or spasticity in upper motor neuron lesions. Cold is applied to the body by means of ice packs, ice massage, ice water immersion, and vapocoolant spray. Treatment lasts about 10 to 20 minutes depending on the size of the individual. The effects of treatment may last several hours after discontinuation of therapy. Following acute trauma, cold application causes local vasoconstriction, which controls local bleeding and swelling. Pain relief probably occurs owing to reduced nerve conduction velocity, relief of muscle spasm, and counterirritant effect. Vapocoolant sprays such as fluorimethane or ethyl chloride are often used to treat myofascial pain syndrome and are followed by slow stretching of the muscle. These sprays act as a counterirritant when sprayed on the skin.[13]

Traction

Cervical traction is used to distract the cervical spine to achieve reduction and alignment in spinal fractures and dislocations, separation of intervertebral disk spaces and intervertebral foramina, stretching of the muscles and ligaments, and separation of the articular surfaces of facet joints. Traction therefore is one of the most accepted and widely used treatment modalities in dealing with various cervical spine lesions, and the goals and techniques of traction therefore differ somewhat.

Traction may be manual or mechanical and may also be intermittent, static, or positional. Manual traction has the advantage of controlling both the traction force and the angle of pull and fine-tuning to achieve desirable effects. Mechanical traction devices are usually prescribed for home use. In their simplest form they consist of a head halter connected to a rope and weights controlled by a pulley. They provide continuous traction in the desired angle and are easy to use. Motorized traction units are found in physical therapy units. Their advantage lies in the fact that they are easily applied and adjusted to suit a wide range of conditions and patients. They may be intermittent or static and have a programmable on-off cycle, weight amount, and angle of pull.

Traction is contraindicated in patients with primary or secondary malignant disease of the spine, and in those with clinical evidence of real or potential spinal cord compression, osteoporosis, or rheumatoid arthritis, and in elderly patients.

Traction is not used in the acute stages of sprains and strains. In subacute or chronic stages, when the mobility of the cervical spine is limited, traction is useful in stretching the scarred and contracted ligaments and muscles in conjunction with superficial or deep heat. It is used in intervertebral disk protrusions to achieve reduction of the protrusion. There are differing study results and recommendations for type, amount, angle, and duration of traction by different investigators. Jackson, in his study of cervical intermittent traction by cineradiography, noted that 10 pounds of tractive force was needed to lift just the weight of the head, and 20 to 25 pounds were necessary to achieve visible distraction of the vertebrae and an increase in the size of the intervertebral foramina.[14] Colachis and Strohm noted significantly more anterior and posterior separation of the vertebrae when 50 pounds of traction were used compared to 30 pounds.[15] They also noted that the posterior intervertebral space opened five times more than the anterior space. However, about 20 minutes after discontinuation of traction, residual effect on the posterior intervertebral space was no longer seen, although some effect was seen anteriorly. Hinterbuchner noted that this result may be due to a relatively inelastic anterior longitudinal ligament, which, when stretched, may take longer to return to normal.[16]

Judovich recommended 25 pounds as the minimal amount of traction required for pain relief in intervertebral disk herniation.[17] Crue reported that when traction was applied with 20 to 30 degrees of flexion, 10 of 20 patients showed relief of pain compared to no relief when traction was applied in the supine position.[18] Hinterbuchner stated that relief of pain may be achieved by flexion of the neck alone when pain is due to compression of the root as it passes through the intervertebral foramina.[16]

The most widely accepted parameter for cervical traction for relief of neck and arm pain is supine or sitting traction (intermittent, static, or positional). The neck is flexed to about 20 degrees, and an initial force of 8 to 15 pounds is applied, gradually increasing to about 20 to 25 pounds applied for 10 to 20 minutes.

Electrical Stimulation

Electrical stimulation has been used for relief of pain for several decades. Barcalow, in 1919, introduced a battery-operated stimulator for pain relief.[19] In 1965, Melzack and Wall proposed the landmark gate control theory of pain.[20] Shealy and Mortimer developed the dorsal column stimulator in 1967 based on this theory.[21] This was later followed by development of the transcutaneous electrical nerve stimulator, which has been widely used in the treatment of pain since the early 1970s.

TRANSCUTANEOUS ELECTRICAL NERVE STIMULATION

The rationale for transcutaneous electrical nerve stimulation (TENS) is based on the gate control theory of pain and the endogenous opiate theory. Melzack and Wall proposed that "control of pain may be achieved by selectively influencing the large, rapidly conducting fibers and that the 'gate' may be closed by decreasing the small fiber input and also by enhancing the large fiber input."[20] The endogenous opiate theory suggests that endorphins and enkephalins are released in response to specific types of electrical stimuli and acupuncture.[22, 23]

There are four commonly used TENS modes: the conventional, acupuncturelike, burst, and brief intense. These are believed to control different nerve fibers and various qualities of pain. Therefore, in a patient who has experienced no pain relief, an adequate trial of TENS should include all these modes; selection of the appropriate electrode placement and length of treatment are also important variables.

TENS units are usually small and portable and are battery operated. They are easy to learn to use and are therefore widely used by ambulatory patients at home and at work. The electrodes commonly used are carbon-silicone, self-adhesive karaya gum, or agaphore. The carbon silicone electrodes require the use of conductive gel and adhesive tape to hold them in place.

The stimulus parameters can be adjusted to produce varying amplitude (mA), rate of stimulation (Hz), and width of the pulse (us). The rate, amplitude, and width of the wave form can be varied (modulated) to provide different intensities of stimulation that change periodically. The amplitude and width of the pulse determine the intensity. In conventional mode, the rate of stimulation is set between 50 and 100 Hz; the width of the pulse, if adjustable, is usually between 30 and 75 us. The amplitude is adjusted to provide persistent electrical paresthesia. This type of stimulation is effective in patients with a wide range of pain syndromes. This low-intensity, high-rate mode apparently works by the gate control mechanism.

The acupuncturelike TENS mode increases the release of endorphins and enkephalins. It is effective for deep aching and chronic pain. The parameters selected are wide pulse duration (150 to 250 us), low rate (1 to 4 Hz), and an amplitude adjusted to produce slow, rhythmic muscle contractions. This stimulus mode excites the afferent sensory fibers including the pain fibers and alpha motor neurons.

In the burst mode, a train of high frequency impulses can be delivered in "bursts" or interrupted at preset intervals. This stimulus can be delivered in a high-intensity mode for treatment of deep aching or chronic pain. The burst mode in low-intensity stimulation is useful in the treatment of superficial or acute pain.

The brief intense mode is used less frequently for pain relief because of the higher intensity of stimulation and the shorter duration of post-stimulus analgesia. The parameters are adjusted to provide a very high rate (>100 Hz) and wider pulse duration (150 to 250 us) and an amplitude that produces strong tetanic muscle contractions or electrical paresthesia.

The only absolute contraindication for use of TENS is the presence of the demand-type of cardiac pacemakers. However, caution should be used not to stimulate the areas close to the carotid sinus, heart, and bony prominences.

HIGH-VOLTAGE GALVANIC STIMULATION

High-voltage galvanic (electrical) stimulation, either alone or in combination with ultrasound, is used to treat pain and muscle spasm, to reduce edema, and to increase joint mobility. The stimulator produces currents of over 150 volts. Its effectiveness is due to the production of high peak current that is of short duration, resulting in low average current. Because of these stimulus characteristics, pain relief is achieved by selective stimulation of large-diameter fibers. This type of stimulation also can reach the deeper layers of muscles and is therefore useful in relief of muscle spasm.

IONTOPHORESIS

In iontophoresis direct current is utilized to transfer ions of some drugs across the skin. Iontophoresis has some disadvantages, such as poor depth of penetration of drug, erratic dosage, and the possibility of local surface burns if precautions are not taken.

Range of Motion Exercises

Patients with acute neck pain require adequate pain relief prior to commencing any exercise program. The goals of the exercise program vary, depending on the pathology and the time of onset of the patient's symptoms. The most important goal after pain relief is to achieve adequate range of motion of the cervical spine and then stengthen the weakened muscles. Most patients with neck pain can begin with isometric exercise for the posterior paravertebral muscles and can perform them at home. Range of motion exercises are started only after the stability of the cervical spine is ensured. Passive range of motion (no joint movement) exercises are started as early as possible to maintain or increase mobility. Active assistive and active range of motion exercises are performed at first in a pain-limited arc that progresses to full range of movement. Resistive exercises such as isotonic and isokinetic exercises are started when the patient complains of little or no pain and when passive range of motion is normal. These exercises strengthen the muscles weakened either by immobility or by a neurologic lesion.

General Conditioning Exercises

Patients recovering from various cervical spine disorders become relatively immobile and decondition rapidly. They can be started on a program of walking, stationary bicycling, or swimming for 20 to 30 minutes three to five times a week. Such exercise improves their general physical condition and permits early return to work and resumption of other activities.

Occupational Therapy

Patients with neurologic lesions involving the spinal cord, nerve roots, or brainstem require assistance in some or all activities of daily living such as bathing, dressing, feeding, and transfers to and from a bed or a chair. These patients are taught to increase their independence in self-care through the use of specific exercises, retraining other muscle groups, and adaptive equipment. Patients who recover from some of these disabilities may need evaluation and training to be able to return to their previous employment. Physiatrists and occupational therapists can evaluate specific disabilities and devise appropriate therapy programs.

Return to Work

Patients are permitted to return to work if and when they achieve significant pain relief, which can vary with individuals, and when they have a stable cervical spine and adequate function in the extremities.

Vocational Counseling

If patients suffer from a long-term or permanent disability, they are referred to an office of vocational rehabilitation, where they may undergo evaluation and retraining for another type of employment.

References

1. Cailliet, R. Neck and Arm Pain. Philadelphia, F. A. Davis, 1964.
2. Cyriax, J. Cervical intervertebral disc lesions. In Textbook of Orthopedic Medicine, 7th ed. Vol. 1. London, Bailliere Tindal, 1979.
3. Gore, D. R., Sepic, S. B., Gardner, G. M., et al. Neck pain: A long-term follow-up of 205 patients. Spine 12(1):1–5, 1987.
4. Penning, L. Radiological evaluation of the cervical spine. In Cervical Spine Research Society. The Cervical Spine. Philadelphia, J. B. Lippincott, 1983.
5. Kottkee, F. J., and Mondale, M. O. Range of mobility of the cervical spine. Arch Phys Med 40:379, 1959.
6. Fielding, J. W. Cinematography of the normal cervical spine. J Bone Joint Surg 39A:1280–1281, 1957.
7. Werne, S. The possibilities of movement in the craniovertebral joints. Acta Orthop Scand 28:165–173, 1959.
8. Werne, S. Studies in spontaneous atlas dislocation. Acta Orthop Scand 23(Suppl), 1957.
9. Blanchard, R. S., and Kottke, F. J. The study of degenerative changes of the cervical spine in relation to age. Bull Univ Minn Hosp 24:470, 1953.
10. Lysell, E. Motion in the cervical spine. Acta Orthop Scand 123 (Suppl), 1969.
11. Johnson, R. M., Hart, D. L., Simmons, E. F., et al. Cervical orthoses: A study comparing their effectiveness in restricting cervical motion in normal subjects. J Bone Joint Surg 59A:332, 1977.
12. Johnson, R. M., Owen, J. R., Hart, D. L., et al. Cervical orthoses: A guide to their selection and use. Clin Orthoped 54:34, 1981.
13. Lehmann, J. F., and De Lateur, B. J. Diathermy and superficial heat and cold therapy. In Kottke, F. J., et al. (eds.). Krusen's Handbook of Physical Medicine and Rehabilitation, 3rd ed. Philadelphia, W. B. Saunders, 1982, pp. 328–332.
14. Jackson, R. The Cervical Syndrome, 2nd ed. Springfield, Ill., Charles C Thomas, 1958.
15. Colachis, S. C., Jr., and Strohm, B. R. Cervical traction: Relationship of time to varied tractive force with constant angle of pull. Arch Phys Med Rehabil 46:815–819, 1965.

16. Hinterbuchner, C. Traction. In Rogoff, J. B. (ed.) Manipulation, Traction and Massage, 2nd ed. Baltimore, Williams & Wilkins, 1980.
17. Judovich, B. D. Herniated cervical disk: A new form of traction therapy. Am J Surg 84:646–656, 1952.
18. Crue, B. L. Importance of flexion in cervical traction for radiculitis. U.S. Air Force Med J 8:374–380, 1957.
19. Barcalow, D. R. Electreat Relieves Pain. Product Literature, Electreat Manufacturing Co., Peoria, Illinois, 1919.
20. Melzack, R., and Wall, P. Pain mechanisms: A new theory. Science 150:971, 1965.
21. Shealy, C. N., Mortimer, J. T., and Reswick, J. B. Electrical inhibition of pain by stimulation of dorsal column: Preliminary clinical report. Anesth Analg 45:489, 1967
22. Mannheimer, J. S., and Lampe, G. N. Clinical Transcutaneous Electrical Nerve Stimulation. Philadelphia, F. A. Davis, 1984.
23. Sjolund, B., and Erickson, M. Endorphins and analgesia produced by peripheral conditioning stimulation. In Bonica, J. J., et al. (eds.). Advances in Pain Research and Therapy. Vol. 3. New York, Raven Press, 1979.

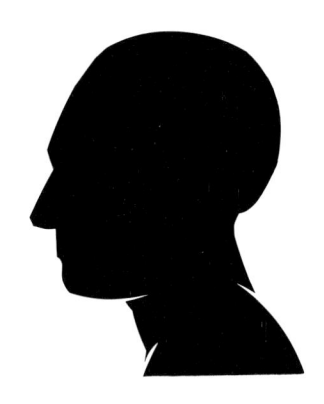

Chapter 10
The Psychiatric Aspects of Head, Neck, and Facial Pain

David A. Shapiro

This chapter deals with the psychiatric aspects of evaluation, assessment, and treatment of head, neck, and facial pain. It is important to note at the outset that the great majority of these patients never seek psychiatric intervention, and when they do it is only after many other treatments have been tried and failed. Usually the psychiatrist is not concerned with patients in whom the condition is self-limited or simply resolved. When a clear structural or physiologic diagnosis is made and there are no secondary psychiatric sequelae, no psychiatric intervention is necessary.

Although many psychiatrists have a passing awareness of the psychiatric vicissitudes of these pain syndromes, there have been few systematic psychiatric studies of these patients. Attempts have been made, however, to correlate temporomandibular joint dysfunction and some mental phenomena.[1-5] In sharp contrast, much attention has been given to the headache syndromes, which are not in the purview of this chapter.

Historical Perspective

Historically, the field of psychiatry that has focused on physical illness was called psychosomatic medicine. In the 1950s Franz Alexander suggested that specific psychological conflicts activate a specific disease through sustained autonomic activity—the so-called specificity theory.[6] Following his theory, many psychoanalytically oriented psychiatrists studied and pursued theory-building covering a wide range of physical illnesses including duodenal ulcer, ulcerative colitis, ileitis, asthma, and many others. Weiner and associates, for example, conducted a predictive study of duodenal ulcers in army recruits.[7] They tied psychoanalytical conflict theory to certain physical variables. They helped establish the necessary elements in future research in psychosomatic medicine—that is, biologic predisposition, personality vulnerability, and psychosocial stress. These concepts were bold and innovative attempts to bridge the mind–body gap and should be seen in that context. Many hypotheses have been proposed, and most have been discarded in current psychiatric thinking. In regard to head, neck, and facial pain syndromes there is no known causality linking psychic conflict and symptom formation.

The emerging fields of consultation and liaison psychiatry and behavioral medicine take a much more complex and comprehensive view of the interaction between mind and body. Genetic and constitutional factors are taken into account as well as psychosocial variables in the lives of the patients and their families.

The Psychiatric Referral

The timing and tact needed in making a psychiatric referral for these patients is of the utmost importance. The selection of the psychiatrist is also an important part of that decision. A psychiatrist who is familiar with biologic medicine and its various manifestations is preferable. The consultant should be willing to work within a medical–dental team approach. The psychiatrist should have a wide range of understanding and not be wedded to one ideologic approach. He or she should have a varied, flexible, and wide-ranging armamentarium that includes somatic, pharmacologic, and psychosocial treatments.[7–11]

Many physicians and dentists, when unable to find the cause of a patient's pain or treat it effectively, say, "There is nothing wrong with you, it is all in your mind." In modern medicine this is an outrageous statement. It is equivalent to saying to a patient, "Your mind is nothing," or, "If I cannot see it or treat it, it really doesn't exist," or, "You are crazy." This attitude is unfortunately all too common. It is arrogant and contemptuous of patients and their families. It drives patients to seek quacks and esoteric practitioners and healers. Above all, it is bad medicine.

A more rational, systematic, and humane approach to a psychiatric referral is necessary. It is never too soon to consider a psychiatric referral. A psychiatric evaluation or treatment is compatible with any other treatment. The referring physician or dentist should view the psychiatrist as a helpful participant in what may become a team approach. On the other hand, a referral made too late in the course of the problem may be perceived by the patient as a device undertaken by a physician or dentist who is frustrated and giving up. The patient then may refuse the consultation or see it as negative and threatening, or he may experience it as an attempt to get rid of him. The following statement is an appropriate way to recommend a psychiatric consultation to a patient:

> I know you have been suffering for a long time, and so far we have not been able to treat your pain effectively. This is in itself depressing to you and your family. I think that you should see Doctor Smith, who is a psychiatrist interested in the treatment of pain. He may be able to help us understand what is causing your pain and suggest some ways to help you.

This statement (as an example) is empathic, tactful, and encouraging. It fosters a good working alliance with the patient and the family. It encourages the patient to become an important agent and active participant in his or her own therapy. Above all, it is good medicine and good psychiatry.

Goals of a Psychiatric Consultation

The psychiatrist should aim:

1. To take a thorough history of the pain as well as a complete psychiatric history and mental status examination. This should elucidate any contributing psychological or psychosocial factors influencing the patient's problem. It should also establish the presence or absence of any major psychiatric disorder.

2. To assess the secondary effects of the "pain syndrome" on the patient and the family. The psychiatric consultation should identify any obstacles or compliance problems with the already ongoing treatments instituted by other specialists.

3. To recommend, design, and implement a psychiatric treatment when indicated and to consult with the other treating specialists on ways to implement or change their treatments.

A discussion of these three goals as well as clinical case material will follow.

History and Diagnosis

The most obvious clinical situation in which there is linkage to temporomandibular joint pain and myofacial pain disorder occurs in patients with generalized anxiety or depression with stress phenomena such as jaw clenching and nocturnal teeth grinding. Treatment of the underlying states can lead to relief of the pain symptoms.

Case A

A middle-aged physician consulted his dentist for temporomandibular joint pain that was increasing in frequency and severity. A careful history revealed that the pain was worse on certain days and seemed to be associated with a tendonitis of the right elbow. The patient played tennis twice weekly and described his tenseness during the competitive play with accompanying tensing of his jaw and facial muscles. With this realization, he paid attention to his behavior during the tennis matches, and his symptoms were easily reversed. This is an instance in which quick recognition of a tension state in a sophisticated and compliant patient led to an uncomplicated and quick result. Most cases are not this simple.

Patients with major psychiatric disorders frequently present pain as part of their clinical picture. Often they first appear in pain clinics or in the offices of medical and dental specialists and do not consult psychiatrists.

Patients with schizophrenic disorders frequently have body image distortions, somatic delusions, or some specific physical ritual that may be causing dysfunction and pain. Although these patients are psychotic, it may not be readily apparent to a nonpsychiatric observer. They may be highly intelligent and articulate and may present their physical complaints in a very sophisticated manner. These patients often go from doctor to doctor and may become vulnerable to iatrogenicity. Paranoid schizophrenics frequently are litigious. Physicians and dentists should be alert to this possibility.

Case B

A man in his middle thirties, after many years of seeking medical and surgical intervention, finally was admitted to a psychiatric hospital, where a diagnosis of paranoid schizophrenia was made. For many years he complained of pain and vague discomfort around the front of his face and mouth. He believed that this caused him to have a permanent scowl. He called this his "persona" and believed that it caused people to dislike and avoid him. He visited surgeons and dentists with requests for dental and surgical procedures to change his "persona." Most of the physicians he consulted refused surgery, knowing intuitively that the situation was bizarre. Some, however, tried plastic surgical procedures. By the time he was admitted the patient had had several surgical procedures, had seen about 20 doctors and dentists, and was severely suicidal and despairing.

This is a very severe and dramatic case, especially in hindsight. There are many patients who insist on invasive treatments. A high index of suspicion regarding the underlying psychiatric condition may help the physician or dentist avoid these tragic situations.

Case C

A 30-year-old single woman was referred by her dermatologist, from whom she sought relief from facial pain that was incapacitating and, according to the patient, resulted from a previous dermatologic procedure that she sought to deal with some minor blemishes. The pain was temperature-sensitive and necessitated staying indoors, which interfered severely with both work and social life. The pain became the only focus of this attractive young woman's life. She felt doomed, attacked, abused, and hopeless. At the time of the evaluation she was suicidal. Psychiatric history and evaluation revealed a longstanding personal and family history of bizarre behavior. There was child abuse and child neglect in her background, as well as parental alcoholism and suicide. A diagnosis of a borderline personality disorder was made, and supportive psychotherapy was undertaken. The symptom of facial pain did not disappear totally but became a minor factor in this woman's life.

MAJOR AFFECTIVE DISORDERS

It is well known in general medicine that patients with major depressions often present physical symptoms and complaints. These complaints range from generalized weakness, lethargy, and insomnia to specific localized pains. All systems may be involved, including the head, neck, and face. Less commonly, the somatic components of the manic phase of the bipolar disorders may be seen. It is especially rewarding to make this diagnosis because treatment with lithium carbonate is so highly specific and effective.

Case D

A woman in her twenties, an opera singer, with a well-documented history of bipolar illness (manic-depressive), also has a diagnosis of temporomandibular joint pain and is currently being treated in a dental clinic specializing in this condition. She has had the temporomandibular joint symptoms intermittently for the last 5 years, approximately the same length of time that she has been symptomatically bioplar. She feels grateful to the dentist and believes he has helped her. She likes him so much that she was ashamed to tell him about her mental problems. This patient's hypomanic symptoms and temporomandibular joint symptoms seem to be coincidental but not necessarily causal. Her response to lithium carbonate was therapeutic for both syndromes. This patient's case history makes a strong case for close cooperation between psychiatrist and dentist.

CHARACTER DISORDERS

Pain syndromes may be present in patients with any of the character disorders: compulsive personality disorder, hysterical personality disorder, borderline personality disorder, and narcissistic disorders. These are complex clinical pictures, and I will not go into the phenomonology of these disorders here. More should be said, however, about the masochistic personality disorder. This disorder generally does not include masochistic perversions but refers primarily to "moral masochism." These patients frequently present with pain and suffering. They seek out physicians frequently, usually to no avail. For these patients, suffering is their raison d'etre. Indeed, it may be said that they have an unconscious agenda to suffer and to defeat anyone who tries to help them. They are frustrating patients to their physicians and dentists and often induce veiled sadistic attacks from their physicians. Their response to psychiatric treatment is often no better than that to other treatments. If a masochistic disorder is suspected, consultation should be sought quickly. It is wise to remember the Hippocratic injunction with these patients—"Above all do no harm."

Assessment of the Secondary Effects of the Pain Syndromes

It is well known to physicians and dentists who are involved in the treatment of chronic illness and pain that patients frequently complain that they feel "depressed," "frustrated," and "hopeless." They also experience disruptions in both love and work. Sleep disturbances, difficulties in concentration, and decreased libido are often present. In these cases the primary treating physician is in the best position to intervene and help. A willingness to listen empathically and an encouraging attitude are required. The role of the psychiatrist here is less clear. It depends on the knowledge of the primary physician of the indications for and use of psychotropic medication. It will also depend on the patient's interest in seeing a psychiatrist. A team effort here is of utmost importance.[12–17]

Case E

Mrs. Z. is a married woman in her middle forties. She has one child who is about to graduate from college. She is a bright and attractive woman, and she and her husband are successful both socially and economically. She was referred by an orthopedic surgeon following 6 months of neck pain and vague complaints of weakness and dizziness. During that period she consulted a neurologist and an ear, nose, and throat specialist. Many diagnostic tests were done including a CT scan and magnetic resonance imaging (MRI). Various symptomatic treatments were tried with only limited success. Mrs. Z. despaired and felt hopeless. She wondered whether she would be well enough to attend her daughter's graduation. She worried that she had a degenerative disease (multiple sclerosis), since one of the physicians mentioned this possibility based on a nonspecific finding on the MRI. At this point the patient herself requested a psychiatric referral. She was tearful and depressed and dreaded the possibility of never recovering. Psychiatric history revealed a similar episode 10 years earlier that responded well to brief supportive psychotherapy. Within 6 weeks of psychotherapy and continued physical therapy most of the patient's symptoms were gone. Six months later there were no depressive symptoms and no evidence of any degenerative disease. Her daughter graduated, and she was able to attend. Mrs. Z. is now in intensive psychotherapy dealing with longstanding characterologic issues, which could help preclude a recurrence.

Frequently the secondary effects of physical illness interfere with the life of family members. When this is the case, spouses and children should be included in the evaluation process. By including family members the patient is also relieved and unburdened. The family can be enlisted in the implementation of a treatment program.

Recommendation for and Implementation of Treatment

At the outset of any discussion about treatment it is important to remember that a recommendation for no further treatment is a legitimate recommendation if the physician believes that no treatment is indicated at that time. This recommendation is especially true in psychiatry, when patients sometimes seek out therapy with magical expectations. It is certainly not good medicine nor is it good psychiatry to raise false hopes that will lead only to disappointments.

On the other hand, some patients seeking treatment with magical expectations have outstanding results. The so-called "transference cures" and "flights into health" are well known to experienced psychiatric clinicians. It is important to remember that such cures may be short-lived and transient or lasting and substantive.

It is important for all physicians and dentists to be aware of the powerful forces at work in the patient–doctor relationship. Psychiatrists accept and understand these forces and often use them in the treatment process. A great deal of skill, wisdom, and integrity is required to make the most of the doctor–patient relationship. There are also risks involved in this process. There is the ever-present danger of regression and excessive dependency, as well as the exploitation of patients by unethical physicians.

For the purposes of this chapter I will divide psychiatric treatments into two categories—somatic treatments and psychosocial treatments. This division does not imply that these treatments are mutually exclusive. In fact, combined therapy is frequently used, and there is significant evidence, especially in the treatment of depression, that psychotherapy and antidepressant medication are synergistic. A good treatment plan for a specific patient should be carefully designed from a broad range of possibilities. Treatment should not simply be related to a particular ideology of the psychiatrist. It should be flexible and adaptive and address both constitutional and biologic factors as well as psychosocial issues. A well-designed treatment should engage the patient in the treatment process, not exclude him from it. Whatever else psychiatric treatment is, it is a collaborative enterprise.

PSYCHOSOCIAL TREATMENTS

Psychosocial treatments are a group of psychiatric treatments in which talking within the context of an interpersonal relationship is the therapeutic modality. These are sometimes called the "talking therapies." There are many types of psychosocial therapies. Their characteristics can only be highlighted and described briefly here as they apply to patients with the pain syndromes.

Therapies Defined by the Content of the Interchange
Psychodynamic-Psychoanalytic Therapy. These therapies are modern derivatives of Freud's innovations and those of the early psychoanalysts. They have a conflict-based therapy model that relies heavily on the use of the "transference" experience as a therapeutic tool. Few pain patients will benefit from these treatments because they are more change oriented than symptom-relief oriented.

Behavior Therapy. The content of this therapy is always related to behavior modification in the service of symptom relief and improvement. Various relaxation techniques and biofeedback systems have been tried extensively with patients who suffer chronic pain. This type of therapy has been used particularly in headache, temporomandibular joint pain, and myofacial pain dysfunction patients. The results have been mixed. Patient selection here is of the utmost importance.

Cognitive Therapy. These therapies, employing models from learning and cognition theory, are growing in popularity. Unlike the psychodynamic psychotherapies, they are concerned more with short-term behavioral change and symptom relief. They are less concerned with past experience and conflict than they are with "relearning" and changing unadaptive patterns of behavior. They are suitable for crisis intervention and short-term treatment. In experienced hands, cognitive therapy is a good treatment for the management of the secondary effects of chronic pain.

Therapies Defined by Their Length
In the last 15 years psychiatric therapeutic practice has moved more and more toward time-limited psychotherapies. In large part this movement has been a response to mental health manpower and economic considerations. However, setting time limits on psychotherapy has heuristic value and seems quite suitable for many of the syndromes that appear in the mental health field. These therapies may be dynamic, behavioral, or cognitive. Some authors recommend a specific number of sessions, and others are less rigid about the number. Some authors are "focal" oriented, and others are more symptom-relief oriented. The time-limited or "brief" psychotherapies seem eminently suitable for the "pain patients" that we are concerned about here. These therapies eschew "chronic patienthood."

Therapies Defined by the Number of Participants
The expanding interest in psychotherapy has been innovative not only in the ways described above but also in the number of people participating in the therapeutic situation. Today there are therapies that are dyadic (one on one), triadic (couples therapy), groups, and, in some rare instances, entire social networks (network therapies). They can be dynamic, behavioral, cognitive, or supportive. Time limits may be set, or open-endedness may be the format.

Chronic pain patients are difficult to treat in a vacuum. It is frequently both necessary and desirable to include spouses and other family members, depending on the age of the patient and his or her social situation. Group therapies can be designed on a homogeneous, symptom-related basis, or they may be more randomly selected. Patients with chronic physical illness or pain tend to regress less in group therapy settings than they do in individual therapy. This is especially true of patients with hypochondriasis.

Finally, the selection of a psychotherapeutic modality for any given patient is an important and complex decision. It is a decision that should be made with the patient and the referring physician or dentist. The selection of modality may change along the way, depending on the therapeutic outcome.

SOMATIC THERAPIES
The somatic therapies that pertain to the treatment of head, neck, and facial pain patients are predominantly psychopharmacologic. Biofeedback techniques have been mentioned in connection with behavior therapy and relaxation techniques. Electric shock therapy (electroconvulsive therapy [ECT]), although still a useful treatment in psychiatry, is usually reserved for severe depressive disorders, especially if they have been refractory to antidepressant medication. There are many psychotropic drugs; however, only a few of them are useful in the treatment of pain disorders and in the underlying psychiatric conditions associated with them. The broad categories will be mentioned here, and the most used drugs in each category will be specifically covered.

ANTIPSYCHOTIC AGENTS
The antipsychotic agents are generally used in the treatment of patients with acute and chronic schizophrenia and other acute psychotic and agitated states. They are complex and powerful drugs and should be prescribed by an experienced clinician. They have many adverse side effects and sometimes have paradoxical reactions.

In the case of the phenothiazines, parkinsonlike syndromes may occur and should be treated immediately with antiparkinson agents. Tardive dyskinesia is a serious, irreversible side effect of long-term phenothiazine therapy. These drugs, especially at high doses, will rarely be required in patients with chronic pain.

Phenothiazine

1. Thorazine (chlorpromazine hydrochloride) 30 to 75 mg/day in divided doses can be used for nonpsychotic anxiety, tension, and agitation. If used in pain patients the appearance of dystonia or akasthesia should cause prompt discontinuation and a switch to another neuroleptic. Thorazine in continued administration can be depressogenic.

2. Stelazine (trifluoperazine hydrochloride) 1 to 2 mg/day in divided doses can be given for nonpsychotic anxiety. The same side effects and precautions that apply to thoraxine apply here.

3. Mellaril (thioridazine hydrochloride) 20 to 40 mg/day in divided doses can be given for nonpsychotic anxiety. The same precautions that apply to

other phenothiazines apply here. Mellaril is less depressogenic and has a lower incidence of parkinsonlike side effects. Orthostatic hypotension, galactorrhea, and retrograde ejaculation have been reported. They are rare and reversible.

Lithium Carbonate

It should be mentioned here that when one of the pain syndromes coexists with a bipolar disease (manic-depressive illness), lithium carbonate is the treatment of choice. Lithium carbonate requires careful monitoring of blood levels and should always be prescribed by a psychiatrist experienced in its use.

Antianxiety Agents

The antianxiety agents (minor tranquilizers) are in common use and can be useful in the management of patients with pain syndromes. They can be used for acute stress or anxiety states that are secondary to chronic pain. They can be used to facilitate sleep and muscle relaxation. In patients with "panic disorder" associated with chronic pain, tranquilizers can help in treating acute panic. There drugs are addictive in high doses over long periods. Generally, in low to moderate doses for brief periods these drugs are very helpful. Listed below are some of the antianxiety agents most frequently prescribed.

Benzodiazepines

1. Ativan (lorazepam): 2 to 10 mg/day in divided doses with a larger dose at bedtime.
2. Librium (chlordiazepoxide hydrochloride): 15 to 75 mg/day in divided doses.
3. Valium (diazepam): 5 to 30 mg/day in divided doses, and 5 to 10 mg at bedtime for sleep.
4. Xanax (alprazolam): 0.25 to 4 mg/day in divided doses.

The benzodiazepines are central nervous system depressants and should be given with caution to patients who take other central nervous system depressants including alcohol. The clinician is well advised to become familiar with one or two of these drugs rather than to prescribe those with which he or she is less familiar.

Nonbenzodiazepines

1. Atarax (hydroxyzine hydrochloride): 50 to 100 mg/day in divided doses.
2. Miltown (meprobamate): 1200 to 1600 mg/day in divided doses.

The same precautions apply to this group of drugs as apply to the benzodiazepines.

Antidepressants

The antidepressants that are generally used for the treatment of chronic pain and the depressive syndromes are the tricyclic antidepressants (TCAs). Other antidepressants such as monoamine oxidase inhibitors (MAOIs) should be used only when TCAs have failed and a major depressive illness is present. MAOIs should be prescribed only by a psychiatrist experienced in their use.

TCAs can be used in low doses for pain and have demonstrated benefits in the treatment of chronic pain. Their use in the treatment of depression or dysthymia usually requires high doses, 150 mg/day or as much as 300 mg/day. At these doses blood levels should be monitored. It is very important for the clinician prescribing TCAs to know their adverse effects. Such knowledge will greatly improve patient compliance. Most of the side effects of TCAs are minor, transient, and reversible. Initial drowsiness, blurred vision, and dry mouth are common and are usually transient. These are anticholinergic effects. Alerting patients to these symptoms and assuring them of their transient nature are helpful. TCAs should be given with caution to patients with bladder neck obstruction, narrow-angle glaucoma, and cardiac arrhythmias. In vulnerable patients acute urinary obstruction can occur and is reversible.

It is important to tell the patient taking a TCA that the actual antidepressant effect of the drug begins only after 10 days to 2 weeks. Even though some benefit might appear sooner, this is usually the result of some sedation or a placebo effect.

TCAs include:

1. Elavil (amitriptyline hydrochloride): 30 mg/day at bedtime for minor pain, or 150 to 300 mg/day either divided or in one dose for major depression or dysthymic disorder.

2. Norpramin (desipramine hydrochloride): Same dosage recommendation as above.

3. Tofranil (imipramine hydrochloride): Same dosage recommendation as above.

Summary

Chronic head, neck, and facial pain as well as the pain associated with the temporomandibular joint and myofacial pain dysfunction is more common than many physicians and dentists realize. The pain itself as well as the disruptive effect that it has on patient's lives causes great suffering. It is important to keep in mind that chronic pain is multidetermined and that a broad and multisymptom approach to treatment is desirable.

The role of the psychiatrist has been described and outlined above. The psychiatrist may be either a minor participant in the treatment team or the primary therapist. Above all, a total approach to the patient is required, which includes both biologic and psychosocial variables.

References

1. Marbach, J. J. and Lipton, J. A. Biopsychosocial factors of the temporomandibular pain dysfunction syndrome. Dent Clin North Am 31(3): 1987.
2. Reich, J. and Tupin, J. P. Psychiatric diagnosis of chronic pain patients. Am J Psychiat 140:1495–1498, 1983.

3. Remick, R. A., Blasberg, B., Campos, P. E., et al. Psychiatric disorders associated with atypical facial pain. Clin J Psychiat 28:175–181, 1983.
4. Rugh, J. D. and Solberg, W. K. Psychological implications in temporomandibular joint pain and dysfunction. Oral Sci Rev 7:3–30, 1976.
5. Salter, M., et al. Is the temporomandibular pain and dysfunction syndrome a disorder of the mind? Pain 17:151–166, 1983.
6. Alexander, F. Psychosomatic Medicine: Its Principles and Applications. New York, W. W. Norton, 1950.
7. Weiner, H. Psychobiology and Human Disease. New York, Elsevier North-Holland, 1977.
8. Keefe, F. J. Behavioral assessment and treatment of chronic pain: Current status and future directions. J Consulting Clin Psychol 50:896, 1982.
9. Bonica, J. J. Neurophysiologic and pathologic aspects of acute and chronic pain. Arch Surg 112:750–761, 1977.
10. Sternbach, R. A. Clinical Aspects of Pain: The Psychology of Pain. New York, Raven Press, 1978, pp. 241–264.
11. Engel, G. L. Psychogenic pain and the pain prone patient. Am J Med 26:899–918, 1959.
12. Bonica, J. J., Chapman, C. R. and Pilowsky, I. Pain, depression, and illness behavior in a pain clinic population. Pain 4:183–192, 1977.
13. Kramlinger, K. G., Swanson, D. W. and Maruta, T. Are patients with chronic pain depressed? Am J Psychiat 140:747–749, 1983.
14. Bassett, D. L. and Pilowsky, I. Pain and depression. Br J Psychiat 141:30–36, 1982.
15. Cavenar J., Jr., and Michels, R. Psychiatry. New York, Basic Books, 1986.
16. Bradley, J. J. Severe localized pain associated with the depressive syndrome. Br J Psychiat 109:741–745, 1963.
17. Lund, P. and Marbach, J. J. Depression, anhedonia, and anxiety in temporomandibular joint and other facial pain syndromes. Pain 11:73–84, 1981.
18. Clarkin, J. F., Frances, A. and Perry, S. Differential Therapeutics In Psychiatry: The Art and Science of Treatment Selection. New York, Brunner/Hazel, 1984.
19. Chessick, R. and Kohut, H. The Technique and Practice of Intensive Psychotherapy. New York, Jason Aronson, 1974.
20. Wolpe, J. Psychotherapy By Reciprocal Inhibition. Stanford, Stanford University Press, 1958.
21. Bandura, A. Principles of Behavior Modification. New York, Holt, Rinehart & Winston, 1969.
22. Beck, A. T. Cognitive Therapy and the Emotional Disorders. New York International University Press, 1976.
23. Meichenbaum, D. Cognitive Behavior Approach: An Integrative Approach. New York, Plenum Press, 1977.
24. Malan, D. H. A Study of Brief Psychotherapy. New York, Plenum Press, 1963.
25. Mann, J. Time Limited Psychotherapy. Cambridge, Harvard University Press, 1973.
26. Sifneds, P. E. Short Term Psychotherapy and Emotional Crisis. Cambridge, Harvard University Press, 1972.
27. Davfloo, H. Basic Principles and Techniques in Short Term Dynamic Psychotherapy. New York, Spectrum Books, 1978.
28. Kocher, R. The use of psychotropic drugs in the treatment of chronic severe pains. Eur Neurol 14:458–464, 1976.
29. Ellinwood, E. H., France, R. D. and Houpt, J. L. Therapeutic effects of antidepressants in chronic pain. Gen Hosp Psychiat 6:55–63, 1984.

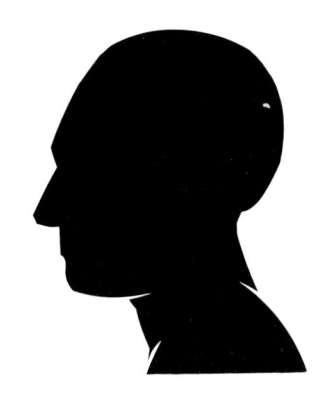

Chapter 11
Management of Chronic Pain of the Head and Neck: An Anesthesiologist's Perspective

Mathew Lefkowitz, Sheldon Goldstein, and Allen Lebovits

Chronic pain takes a major toll on our society. Billions of dollars are spent each year on medical fees, payments for compensation or litigation, and work days lost. Orofacial pain as well as neuralgic, visceral, and vascular pain accounts for approximately $4.1 billion lost per year to the American economy due to work days lost and health care.[1] The amount of patient suffering endured and the enormous financial burden on society emphasize the importance of proper evaluation and treatment of patients with chronic pain.

The Nuprin Pain Report, published in 1985, is a national survey that provides a broadly based, systematic study of the frequency, severity, and cost associated with pain. It showed headache to be the most common cause of chronic pain, followed by backache and general musculoskeletal pain (Table 11–1). In 1979, the estimated cost of chronic pain states to the American economy was approximately $55 billion.[2]

Pain is the most frequent medical symptom brought to the attention of physicians. As defined by the Internal Association for the Study of Pain, pain is "an unpleasant sensory and emotional experience associated with actual or potential tissue damage or described in terms of such damage."[3] This definition recognizes that pain perception is not exclusively reliant on tissue damage or organic dysfunction. Research and clinical experience demonstrate that pain perception is strongly influenced by psychological,

TABLE 11–1. Economic Cost of Pain in the United States, 1985

	PERCENT OF ADULTS WITH PAIN > 1 DAY PER YEAR (PERCENT)	LOST WORK DAYS FOR TOTAL U.S. ADULT POPULATION
Headache	73	637.9 million
Backache	56	1,307.8 million
Muscle pain	53	617.3 million
Joint pain	51	961.3 million
Stomach pain	46	394.1 million
Premenstrual or menstrual pain	40	74.3 million
Dental pain	27	70.3 million
Other	6	Not available
		4,063.0 million

societal, and cultural factors. Persistent pain refractory to medical interventions, along with functional disability that supersedes organic pathology, underscores the complex nature of chronic pain management.

Not all pain is indicative of its cause. Chronic pain may not be associated with a specific etiology. It is frequently refractory to therapy. Chronic pain syndromes require extensive evaluation to determine etiology and treatment strategy. The subjective nature of pain makes it difficult to assess. Objective signs such as tachycardia, diaphoresis, hidrosis, facial expressions, and hypertension that may help to indicate the intensity and severity of the pain are often absent.

There has been a surge of knowledge in the area of chronic pain management in the past decade. The objective of this review is to summarize the diagnosis and management of chronic pain in the head and neck.

Acute and Chronic Pain

It is important to note that inappropriate application of acute pain therapies in patients with chronic pain often leads to failure because illness behavior patterns are perpetuated. For example, the use of narcotic analgesics is appropriate for acute pain but contraindicated in the chronic pain patient, in whom the potential for addiction is significant.

Chronic pain can persist after the inciting injury has healed, and frequently it cannot be related to a specific injury. It may or may not have a well-defined onset and has typically not responded to treatment. It is often associated with personality or life-style changes, depression, hopelessness, weight gain, loss of sexual desire, and abnormal patterns of sleep. Patients with chronic pain may learn to overreact to their symptoms and limit their activities more than required by their pain, thus resulting in serious and inappropriate disability. This can lead to the chronic pain syndrome, which is manifested by the patient who withdraws to the point where he is essentially homebound. When he does venture outside, it is to seek one doctor after another, looking for the magical quick "cure" and approaching each with a preconceived notion that he will not be helped.[4]

The Pain Clinic

Since chronic pain syndromes require a multifaceted evaluation, the need to establish pain clinics to serve as specialized centers in the treatment of chronic pain cannot be overemphasized. There are over 1200 multidisciplinary pain clinics in the United States today.[5] Anesthesiologists are in an excellent position to make a major contribution to pain clinics. Their original entree to the role of chronic pain specialist arose from their ability to perform nerve blocks. In addition, they have in-depth knowledge of the pharmacology of analgesics, including local anesthetics and non-narcotic and narcotic medications, as well as the expertise in airway management necessary to manage possible toxic and anaphylactic reactions. In fact, more pain clinics are directed by anesthesiologists than by all other specialists combined (Table 11-2).[6]

Typically, a multidisciplinary pain clinic is composed of a group of specialists who coordinate their knowledge and skills to alleviate or manage chronic pain syndromes. The multidisciplinary staff deals with both the medical and psychological aspects of chronic pain as well as research and teaching programs. The clinical staff of pain clinics often includes an anesthesiologist, neurologist, orthopedic surgeon, psychologist or psychiatrist, and social worker. Consultation relationships also exist with internists, neurosurgeons, and general surgeons.[7]

Typically, a patient is referred to the Pain Management Service of the SUNY Health Science Center at Brooklyn by his primary care provider. A history is elicited, noting not only the location, severity, and characteristics of the pain but also the events surrounding the initial pain period as well as the past medical and surgical therapies. A physical examination is performed, followed by a psychological interview. Social work interviews

TABLE 11-2. Directorship of Pain Clinics by Specialty

	PERCENT
Anesthesiology	61
Neurology/neurosurgery	11
Psychiatry/psychology	7
Physical medicine	4
Orthopedics	4
Dental	3
Internal medicine	1
Combinations or other	9

are used to identify the action of family and environmental factors that contribute to the pain. Often the patient is instructed to keep a pain diary, which can provide insight into illness behavior. Appropriate consultations are arranged.

The above information is evaluated and reviewed at a clinical conference. A preliminary diagnosis is formulated, and recommendations are made for therapy. A primary manager, responsible for coordinating treatment, may be the anesthesiologist, psychologist, neurologist, resident, physical therapist, or social worker. The choice of the manager depends on the patient's diagnosis.

Anatomy and Physiology of Pain Transmission

In the adult the spinal cord occupies the upper two thirds of the vertebral canal, extending from the foramen magnum to the L1–L2 junction. Each side contains pairs of nerves, composed of dorsal and ventral roots. Small unmyelinated C fibers and myelinated A-delta fibers are the afferent sensory nerves that carry pain information from the periphery to the spinal cord. This information enters the spinal cord through the dorsal roots and is significantly modified in the dorsal horn.

The dorsal horn is divided into nine laminae. Laminae I through V play an important role in nociception, and it is here that pain transmission is altered by neurotransmitters, enkephalin and opioid receptors, ascending systems, and descending modulation systems.[8,9] Pain information is transmitted centrally through the large myelinated fibers of the anterolateral system, which is composed of two major divisions, the anterior spinothalamic and the lateral spinothalamic tracts. The fibers of the lateral spinothalamic tract transmit impulses associated with pain and temperature. The fibers cross within one spinal segment to the opposite side of the cord. They then project directly to the thalamic nuclei and send collaterals to the reticular formation. The anterior spinothalamic tract fibers carry signals associated with pain and light touch. The fibers at the level of the spinal cord cross over several spinal segments and ascend contralaterally. The tract relays to the reticular formation the periaqueductal gray matter and the thalamus.[8]

From the thalamus the pain signals are transmitted to the somatosensory cortex, the reticular nuclei of the brainstem, the medulla, the intralaminar nuclei of the thalamus, and the periaqueductal gray matter.[10,11] It is believed that the thalamus and the associated basal regions of the brain play the dominant role in pain sensation. The brain can focus its attention on different areas of the sensory system, presumably by facilitating or inhibiting the cortical receptive areas, possibly as directed by signals from the thalamus.[12,13]

The descending pain modulation system is made up of fibers from the raphe-spinal tract. This system modulates and inhibits nociceptive transmission at the level of the laminae. Cortificugal signals originate in the cortex, periaqueductal gray matter, thalamus, and nucleus raphe magnus in the brainstem, and descend to the dorsal horn laminae to mediate transmission of noxious stimuli.

At the level of the spinal cord, opiate receptors and neurotransmitters such as serotonin, glycine, gamma-amino-butyric acid (GABA), and dopamine play an important role in analgesia, whereas substance P, norepinephrine, and glutamic acid inhibit analgesia. Opiatelike peptides such as enkephalins and endorphins, which are found throughout the central nervous system (CNS), bind to receptors in the periaqueductal gray matter to activate the raphe-spinal system and to receptors in the dorsal horn to inhibit nociceptive transmissions.[14] The binding of enkephalin to specific receptors suppresses the release of substance P, and pain transmission to higher centers is prevented. In fact, acupuncture, biofeedback, relaxation techniques, and transcutaneous electrical neural stimulation (TENS) are thought to produce analgesia partially through the release of endorphins at the level of the spinal cord.

The Gate Control Theory

The gate control theory, first proposed by Melzack and Wall in 1965, provides a model for the processing of pain at the level of the spinal cord.[15] The gate theory permits higher cerebral and brainstem centers to influence the volume of pain stimuli that reaches conscious levels by turning the gate on or off at the spinal cord level. Painful stimuli must pass through a gate located in the dorsal horn. Target cells located in several laminae of the dorsal horn allow transmission of pain stimuli to higher centers in the brain, whereas the cells of the substantia gelatinosa, located in laminae II and III, inhibit transmission.[16] Nociception is therefore controlled by the excitatory and inhibitory interplay of these cells. Their firing patterns are controlled by the afferent nociceptive stimulus of the small-diameter, slowly conducting A-delta and C fibers, afferent large myelinated fiber barrage, descending central modulating system, and neurotransmitters.[16]

A-delta and C fibers suppress the output of the cells of the substantia gelatinosa, allowing pain stimuli to be transmitted centrally. Large-diameter, rapidly conducting myelinated fibers, which transmit proprioception, activate the cells of the substantia gelatinosa, causing inhibition of the target cells and prevention of pain transmission. This theory would, for example, explain why the pain in an injured toe is lessened if the toe is grasped—i.e., proprioceptive input enters the same level of the spinal cord that is processing pain information from the injured toe to prevent its transmission. The gate theory permits higher cerebral and brainstem centers to influence the volume of pain stimuli that reaches conscious levels by turning the gate on or off at the spinal cord level. This theory also explains many aspects of causalgia. Since most nerve lesions shift the balance of impulse transmission to the smaller fibers, overactivity of the target cells results, and pain transmission continues. This theory is presently the most widely accepted explanation of the pain mechanism. It accounts for both the sensory and emotional aspects of pain perception.

Spinal Reflexes and Pain of Sympathetic Origin

Causalgia and reflex sympathetic dystrophy are two painful syndromes that create spinal reflexes that contribute to chronic pain.[17] Causalgia refers to the pain syndrome, autonomic dysfunction, and tissue changes resulting from injury following nerve damage (Fig. 11–1).[18] It occurs in 2 to 5 percent of all patients with nerve injuries.[19] Reflex sympathetic dystrophy arises with less severe trauma, surgery, fractures, or soft tissue injuries.

Injury elicits increased activity of sympathetic efferent fibers that does not subside, causing continued firing of afferent somatic fibers and giving rise to a vicious cycle of pain.[20] The environment of peripheral nociceptors is changed by this continued sympathetic response because of the resultant vasoconstriction and ischemia as well as sensitization by locally released substances such as kinins, prostaglandins, and norepinephrine, which further contribute to this state of persistent pain.

The pain of reflex sympathetic dystrophy is described as a constant ache with burning and hyperesthetic components. The pain is exacerbated by movement, cutaneous stimulation, and stress. Signs of sympathetic nervous

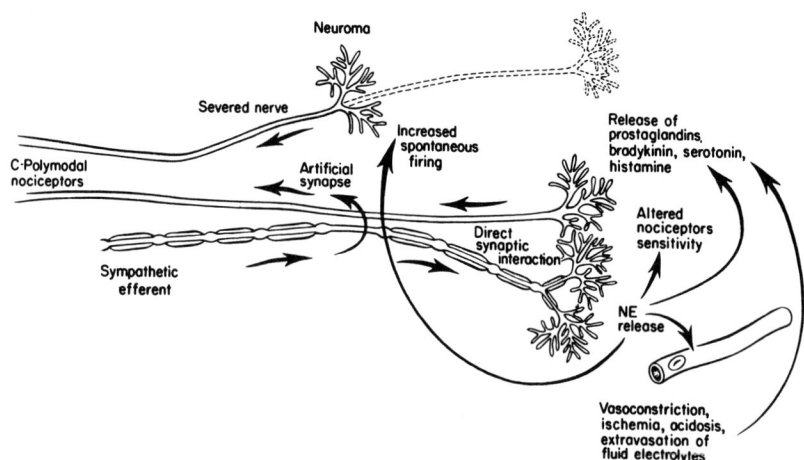

FIGURE 11–1. Some proposed mechanisms of interaction between sympathetic efferent and nociceptive afferent fibers in causalgia. (From Bonica, J. Causalgia and other reflex sympathetic dystrophies. In Bonica, J., et al. Advances in Pain Research and Therapy. Vol. 3. New York, Raven Press, 1979.)

system activity, including hyperhidrosis, cyanosis, and edema, are evident.[21] The skin is most often cool to the touch, although at times it may be warm. Dysesthesia may be so severe that the touch of a bedsheet may cause excruciating pain. If appropriate treatment is not instituted early, dystrophic changes and Sudek's atrophy can occur. These changes include bone demineralization, muscle atrophy, and joint stiffness as well as trophic skin changes such as smooth, shiny skin, curved nails, and altered patterns of hair growth.[18, 22]

Early treatment is believed to prevent this vicious cycle of pain by blocking sympathetic activity. This is accomplished by sympathetic blocks such as a stellate ganglion block for reflex sympathetic dystrophy of the head, neck, arm, and chest, and lumbar sympathetic or epidural sympathetic block for reflex sympathetic dystrophy of the legs.

Therapeutic Modalities

The various modalities of treatment in a pain clinic are, in order of frequency:*

Nerve blocks	75 percent
TENS	30 percent
Psychotherapeutic intervention	60 percent
Pharmacological management (as sole treatment)	25 percent

Nerve Blocks

Nerve blocks are the most common treatment modality in the pain clinic. They can be divided into three different categories. As diagnostic procedures they differentiate the neurologic pathways involved, such as peripheral nerves, spinal roots, central, or sympathetic. *Prognostic blocks* are performed to predict the outcome of more permanent procedures such as chemical or surgical neuroablation. *Therapeutic blocks*, performed singly or in a series, may provide long-lasting relief that can in many cases outlast the duration of a local anesthetic. This is accomplished by interrupting the painful spinal reflex arc and restoring function and mobility to the affected part. Common injected substances include local anesthetics, steroids, and neurolytic agents such as alcohol or phenol. The specific blocks pertaining to chronic pain of the head and neck will be discussed later in this chapter.

---

*Based on 1987 data from the Pain Management Service of SUNY Health Science Center at Brooklyn.

Pharmacotherapy

Before examining the specific classes of drugs, it is important to review some important concepts. Effective pharmacologic management cannot be achieved unless the problem of addiction and polypharmacy is controlled. A pattern of maladaptive drug ingestion that is reinforcing or perpetrating chronic illness behavior must be identified. Narcotics and CNS depressants should be reduced by gradually diminishing the doses. One should prescribe analgesics only on a fixed time and fixed dosage schedule, not on an "as needed" basis. It has been clearly shown that patients will actually use less of a drug if it is not given on a p.r.n. basis. Swings in plasma levels with p.r.n. medications result in troughs in which the patient has minimal or no pain relief and peaks of overmedication in which the higher plasma level produces significant side effects such as dysphoria, confusion, or sedation. Patients actually require less medication when the dosing schedule is constant. They report better and more continuous pain relief because steady blood levels are achieved. The ideal properties of a drug for long-term therapy include availability of the oral form, minimal sedative and sensorimotor side effects, nonaddiction potential, and low cost. Medications to treat chronic pain of the head and neck are most often employed on an outpatient basis. Therefore, this discussion will concentrate on agents that are effective orally. When choosing an agent it is important to remember that the patient may be using this drug for months or even years. Narcotics should be avoided in patients with chronic benign pain, and medications should be restricted to nonsteroidal anti-inflammatory drugs (NSAIDs), aspirin, and acetaminophen. Antidepressants are added for additional analgesia and to help regulate sleeping patterns.[23]

Nonsteroidal Anti-inflammatory Drugs

Aspirin is the prototype of the anti-inflammatory, analgesic, and antipyretic drugs (NSAIDs). Its therapeutic action is based on inhibition of the synthesis of prostaglandins. Prostaglandin 2 (PGE_2) sensitizes nociceptors of peripheral nerves to the pain-producing effect of mediators such as bradykinin, histamine, 5-hydroxytryptamine, chemotactic factors, bradykinin, and leukotrienes.[24] NSAIDs inhibit the enzyme cyclo-oxygenase, thereby preventing the formation of PGE_2. Since the cyclo-oxygenase enzyme in different tissues responds variably to these drugs, it is possible that there are several forms of the enzyme. It would then seem logical that one NSAID in this class may prove superior to others for treating a specific clinical syndrome and its associated pain.[25]

NSAIDs are usually effective for pain of mild to moderate severity. Chronic postoperative pain or pain secondary to inflammation or bone and joint trauma are fairly well controlled; however, pain from the hollow viscera usually is not. For severe pain, NSAIDs are not as effective as narcotics. However, they do not cause lethargy, respiratory depression, or the dependency states associated with the opioids.

On a milligram-for-milligram basis acetaminophen and aspirin have essentially equal analgesic potency.[26, 27] Numerous studies have documented the relative efficacy and safety of the analgesic antipyretics.[28] For patients with nonmalignant chronic pain syndromes of the head and neck, it seems prudent to choose a drug that offers a balance between analgesic effect and safety of long-term use. Although the new nonsteroidal agents have not been shown to be more effective than aspirin, they do have fewer side effects. Acute inflammatory disorders often respond better to the NSAIDS than to aspirin.[28]

Acute gastrointestinal bleeding or silent perforation is a potential and important side effect of the NSAIDs. Endoscopic studies evaluating gastric injury produced by aspirin and other NSAIDs consistently show aspirin to be more toxic and irritating to the gastric mucosa. It is important, however, to note that there is no correlation between toxic injury and efficacy of the drug. Acetaminophen, on the other hand, in therapeutic doses has neither the gastrointestinal toxicity nor the antiplatelet effects of nonsteroidals.[29]

NSAIDs can have significantly different responses between patients. Maximal therapeutic effect is usually present after 7 days. Therefore, if the clinical response is inadequate at that time, another nonsteroidal agent should be prescribed.[30] Table 11–3 compares the relative potencies of some

TABLE 11–3. Relative Potencies of Analgesics Employed Orally for Less Severe Pain, Expressed in Terms of Doses Approximately Equivalent in Total Effect to 650 mg of Aspirin

	P.O. (MG)	SALIENT FEATURES
Pentazocine (Talwin)	30	Weak narcotic, agonist-antagonist, high analgesic potential,[a] low addiction liability
Codeine	32	Weak narcotic, high analgesic potential, relatively low addiction liability
Meperidine (Demerol)	50	Narcotic, high analgesic potential, high addiction liability
Propoxyphene (Darvon)	65	Weak narcotic, low analgesic potential, low addiction liability
Aspirin (ASA)	650	Non-narcotic, anti-inflammatory, low analgesic potential, no addiction liability or tolerance
Acetaminophen (paracetamol)	650	Similar to phenacetin, less potential renal toxicity
Sodium salicylate	1000	Similar to aspirin

[a]Analgesic potential refers to level of analgesia attained by increasing the dose to the point of limiting side effects.

From Houde, R. W. Systemic analysis and related drugs: Narcotic analgesics. In Bonica, J. J., et al. (eds.). Advances in Pain Research and Therapy. Vol. 2. New York, Raven Press, 1979.

of the commonly used aspirinlike analgesics with those of the oral narcotics.[30] Table 11–4 reviews some of the commonly used NSAIDs.[30]

Narcotic Analgesics

Opium, first described in the third century B.C., was probably the earliest pharmacotherapeutic agent in history. The opioids are a group of drugs that have opium or morphinelike properties. They share some properties with the naturally occurring peptides such as the enkephalins, the endorphins, and the dynorphins. Identification of highly specific opiate receptors located in the periaqueductal and periventricular gray matter, spinal cord, and gastrointestinal tract has enhanced our understanding of this group of drugs. Receptors, when combined with opioids, change their configuration, and pain transmission is inhibited.[31] The four major receptors and the effects they mediate are summarized in Table 11–5.[32]

The opioids are effective analgesics and are useful for visceral pain or severe pain that has not responded to NSAIDs. They have major effects on the central nervous system, producing analgesia, drowsiness, mood changes, respiratory depression, and alteration of the autonomic nervous system. They decrease gastrointestinal motility and cause nausea and vomiting. The morphinelike drugs act preferentially at the mu receptors. They relieve pain without loss of consciousness. Touch, vibration, vision, and hearing are not depressed. Though dull continuous pain is relieved more predictably than intermittent sharp pain, adequate dosages will also relieve the latter. The most impressive advantage of the opioids is that they have strong analgesic effects yet the patient remains conscious. For example, equal amounts of analgesia by other classes of analgesics such as volatile anesthetics, sodium pentathol, or ketamine frequently result in loss of consciousness. The analgesia produced by placebos may be due to activation of such pathways based on prior experience with pain relief. The mechanism by which opioids produce euphoria has not been definitively determined.[33]

Opioids not only alter the sensation of pain but also change the effective response. The result is that the patient may be able to tolerate more pain even though his ability to perceive the stimulus is unaltered. Unfortunately, these same properties are what give these drugs their addictive potential. The relative potencies of some of the narcotic analgesics are reviewed in Table 11–6.[30, 34]

Adjuvant Analgesics

Tricyclic antidepressants have been used to treat chronic pain for more than 20 years. Their intrinsic analgesic properties are not fully understood because chronic pain and depressive symptoms overlap considerably. Low levels of serotonin in the brain are associated with both depression and chronic pain.[35] Tricyclic antidepressants may provide direct analgesic action by blocking re-uptake of serotonin and norepinephrine at CNS synapses and potentiating opiate analgesia.[36] Studies have shown that antidepressants

TABLE 11-4. Nonsteroidal Analgesic-Antipyretics (inhibit synthesis of prostaglandins)

COMMENTS	PROTEIN BINDING (%)	HALF-LIFE (HR)	ORAL DOSE (MG)	ONSET (MIN)	DURATION (HR)	METABOLISM	EXCRETION	SIDE EFFECTS
Acetaminophen paracetamol (Tylenol) 1909	Minimal	1-4	325-650	20 min	3-4	Liver	Renal	Not anti-inflammatory; large doses hepatotoxic; analgesic nephropathy (hematuria)
Aspirin 1899	65-95	0.25-0.33	325-650	15 min	4 min	Liver	Renal	Analgesic nephropathy (hematuria); overdose causes convulsions, hallucinations, deafness
Fenoprofen (Nalfon) 1976	99	3	300-600	Few days	6-8	Liver	Renal	Muscle weakness; tinnitus; constipation; nervousness, palpitations
Ibuprofen (Motrin) 1974	90	1.8-2	300-600	30 min	6-8	Liver	Renal	Skin rashes
Indomethacin (Indocin) 1976	90	4.5	25-50	120-240 min	6-12	Liver	Renal, Biliary	Headache; weight gain, depression; enterohepatic circulation
Naproxen (Naprosyn) 1976	99	13	250-500	60 min	12	Liver	Renal	Tinnitus, constipation
Phenylbutazone (Butazolidin) 1952	90	77	100-200	24-96 min	8	Liver	Renal, Biliary	Blood dyscrasias; fluid retention
Piroxicam (Feldene) 1973	90	50	10-20	240 min	12-14	Liver	Renal, Fecal	Hepatic and renal toxicity
Sulindac (Clinoril) 1978	93	7.8	150-200	1-1.5 days	12	Liver	Renal	Skin rashes; constipation, diarrhea; hepatic toxicity
Tolmetin (Tolectin) 1976	99	1	400	Few days	8	Liver	Renal	Diarrhea; muscle weakness, fluid retention

From Houde, R. W. Systemic analgesics and related drugs: Narcotic analgesics. In Bonica, J. J., et al. (eds.). Advances in Pain Research and Therapy. Vol. 2. New York, Raven Press, 1979.

TABLE 11–5. Effects of Opioid Receptors

Mu	Analgesia, respiratory depression, euphoria, physical dependence
Kappa	Spinal anesthesia, sedation, and pupillary constriction
Sigma	Tachycardia, tachypnea, pupillary dilatation, dysphoria
Delta	Modulation of mu receptors

From Ramadhyani M. Opioid and nonopioid analgesics. In Attia, R. R., Orogono, A. W., and Domer F. R. (eds.). Practical Anesthetic Pharmacology. Norwalk, Conn., Appleton-Century-Crofts, 1987.

relieve pain independent of their antidepressant effects.[37, 38, 39] The antidepressants most commonly used are amitriptyline, trazodene, desipramine, imipramine, doxepin, and nortriphyline. Before prescribing tricyclics one should be aware of their side effects, including orthostatic hypotension, arrhythmias, and adverse interactions with other drugs.[35] They have effects on the autonomic nervous system and in elderly patients can produce anticholinergic effects, sedation, constipation, and urinary retention. A baseline electrocardiogram (EKG) should be obtained.[41]

Phenothiazines do not produce analgesia and are used as antiemetics when using narcotics. Side effects include tardive dyskinesia, a movement disorder with no known therapy.[36]

Anticonvulsants are particularly useful in chronic neuralgias such as trigeminal, postherpetic, glossopharyngeal, and post-traumatic neuralgias.

Steroids have specific and nonspecific effects in managing acute and chronic cancer pain. They have been used to treat neuralgias, vascular headaches, and temporal arteritis.

Benzodiazepines do not have analgesic or co-analgesic properties. Anxiety is not usually manifested in the chronic pain syndrome. Therefore, the use of these drugs is limited in these patients.

Transcutaneous Electrical Nerve Stimulation

Transcutaneous electrical nerve stimulation (TENS) is a unique mode of pain therapy that is essentially free of systemic side effects. Numerous reports document the use of TENS for the treatment of acute and chronic pain.[42] The mechanism by which TENS produces pain relief is thought to be through stimulation of the large myelinated A-alpha fibers that inhibit nociceptive transmission by the unmyelinated C and A-delta fibers to the spinal cord. TENS also stimulates release of endogenous opioids at the level of the spinal cord, inhibiting ascending pain transmission.[43] Head and neck applications include pain secondary to carcinoma, postherpetic neuralgia, myofascial pain syndrome, and autonomic hyperreflexia. Patients

TABLE 11–6. Narcotic Analgesics: Relative Potencies of Analgesics Commonly Employed for Severe Pain, Expressed in Terms of the Intramuscular (IM) and Oral (PO) Doses Approximately Equivalent in Total Effect to a 10-mg IM Dose of Morphine

	IM (mg)	PO (mg)	MAJOR DIFFERENCES FROM MORPHINE
Oxymorphone (Numorphan)	1	6	None
Hydromorphone (Dilaudid)	1.5	7.5	Shorter-acting
Levorphanol (Levo-Dromoran)	2	4	Relatively high PO to IM potency
Heroin	4		Shorter-acting
Methadone (Dolophine)	10	20	Relatively high PO to IM potency
Morphine	10	60	
Oxycodone (contained in Percocet)	15	30	Shorter-acting Relatively high PO to IM potency
Pentazocine (Talwin)	60	180	Narcotic antagonist-analgesic
Meperidine (pethidine, Demerol)	75	300	None
Codeine	130	200	Relatively high PO to IM potency Relatively more toxic in higher doses
Dextroproxyphene (Darvon)	240		Similar to codeine but more toxic in high doses

From Houde, R. W. Systemic analgesics and related drugs: Narcotic analgesics. In Bonica, J. J., et al. (eds.). Advances in Pain Research and Therapy. Vol. 2. New York, Raven Press, 1979.

using TENS on a chronic basis need to be advised of the necessity of rest periods, which are important to prevent damage to the skin and to avoid tolerance.

Cryoanalgesia

Cryoanalgesia is the use of cold to provide pain relief. It is most familiar to the lay person as the use of ethyl chloride by professional athletes to relieve the pain of acute injuries. Cryoanalgesia can be used for prolonged blockade of accessible peripheral nerves. It may be used to treat postherpetic neuralgia, atypical facial neuralgia, tic douloureux, post-traumatic neuralgia, and cancer pain. A popular application is the intraoperative use of cryotherapy to control post-thoracotomy pain, in which it has been shown to decrease postoperative analgesic requirements by up to 50 per cent.[44] Cryoanalgesia can provide pain relief for up to several months. It is particularly useful for malignant pain secondary to metastatic disease when the involved nerve can be clearly identified.

The duration of relief is determined by the regeneration of the peripheral nerve. One major advantage of cryoanalgesia over the use of neurolytic blocks is the lack of subsequent neuralgias, presumably due to the fact that it causes less fibrous tissue rejection. It should be noted that the cryoprobe must be accurately placed or it may damage nearby healthy tissues. Proposed mechanisms of injury induced by cryoanalgesia include changes in endoneural fluid pressure and subsequent Wallerian degeneration.[45]

Psychological Aspects of Chronic Pain

Depression

The most prevalent psychological characteristic of chronic pain patients is depression.[46] In addition to the frequent exhibition of a pervasive mood state disturbance characterized by tearfulness and a sad affect, chronic pain patients also typically have some or all of the following hallmark features of a depressive disorder: appetite disturbance, sleep disturbance, inability to concentrate, lack of enjoyment, loss of libido, social withdrawal, and suicidal ideation. The coincident presentation of depression and chronic pain occurs so frequently that chronic pain syndrome has been described as a variant of depressive disorder.[47, 48, 49, 50]

Depression may occur both as a precipitating factor that contributes partially or fully to chronic pain or as a sequelae of chronic pain. Psychogenic pain disorder[51] is a psychiatric disorder in which the essential feature is the etiologic role of psychological factors and pain. Typically, an event such as a death or loss of a job that is related to a psychological conflict or need initiates or exacerbates pain. Depression also, however, occurs as a result of the state of being in chronic pain. The pervasive effect that chronic pain has on the patient's life-style can produce feelings of demoralization and learned helplessness.

Somatization Disorder

Chronic pain has also been viewed as a form of somatization disorder.[52] The standard characteristics of this type of disorder are "recurrent and multiple somatic complaints of several years' duration for which medical attention has been sought but which are apparently not due to any physical disorder."[51] Dramatic and vague descriptions of physical complaints, as part of a complicated and exhaustive medical history, are also common features of chronic pain syndromes and somatization disorder.

Secondary Gain

The issue of secondary gain is extremely important in identifying and treating patients in chronic pain. Chronic pain frequently allows an individual to avoid a noxious activity or obtain support from the environment that he or she might not otherwise get. Chronic pain and chronic pain behavior are often "reinforced" by sympathetic attention from family members, by avoidance of a conflict such as sex with a spouse, and by avoidance of work. Disability payments, in particular, workmen's compensation, have been considered to be among the strongest factors that maintain chronic pain behavior.[53] In fact, it is not uncommon for pain management programs to exclude patients from their program if they have litigation pending.[54, 55] Pain reduction interventions are considered useless or much less efficacious in light of the powerful support and maintenance of disability provided by litigation and workmen's compensation. The lack of responsiveness to treatment has been studied with regard to the treatment of back pain[56] and nerve block treatments.[57, 58] Dworkin et al. found that patients who were working at the time of their initial evaluation responded better to treatment than patients who were not working.[53]

Provider-Patient Interactions

Good communication between the practitioner and patient can have an important enhancing effect on the rate of compliance with prescribed treatment regimens.[59] Additionally, a good provider-patient relationship based on effective communication can strengthen placebo effects. This is particularly significant in chronic pain patients, in whom the placebo response can play such an integral role in treatment.[60, 61] Beecher reported that the placebo effect is present in 35 percent of cases.[60]

The patient presenting with chronic pain is, however, difficult to treat, not only because of the refractory nature of the pain but also because of the passive-aggressive, noncompliant, and manipulative behavior that is often displayed toward the doctor. This behavior is characterized by a hostile mode of interaction with the doctor. Lebovits and Richlin[62] recently reviewed this issue and supported their findings with an outline of four clinical case reports. The presence of a mental health specialist on the pain team therefore is very important. Evaluation and treatment of this abnormal mode of interacting may well have a beneficial effect on the chronic pain itself.

Personality Factors

Early research attempting to identify a constellation of personality traits that would predispose a person to experience chronic pain was not successful. It is now thought that different personality factors are related to different kinds of pain.[63] The most widely used measure of personality, the Minnesota Multiphasic Personality Inventory (MMPI)[64] has been used extensively with chronic pain patients. Chronic pain patients typically show elevated scores on three MMPI scales[65]—hypochondriasis (the tendency to be overly concerned about physical health), hysteria (high levels of emotionality and exaggeration of symptoms), and depression. This constellation of factors, the "neurotic triad," reflects three common psychological characteristics of chronic pain patients. Additional research[60, 66] suggests that patients who show elevation of additional parameters on the MMPI may have characterologic disturbances that predate the onset of pain.

Treatment Modalities

Psychological intervention in pain management centers most often occurs in the behavioral-cognitive realm of therapies. Frequently, a combined cognitive-behavioral approach is utilized.[67] This approach emphasizes the need for the patient to reconceptualize his or her hopeless view of life to one that is more adaptive and positive. Adaptation of activities and behaviors that deal effectively with problems is an essential component of this approach. For patients who are not working because of pain, one of the most effective pain-reducing behaviors is the return to work. Chronic pain programs have increasingly included this directive as part of their intervention. A significantly greater percentage of patients do return to work when instructed to do so compared with patients who are not so directed.[68]

Operant-conditioning, pain groups, biofeedback, hypnosis, and relaxation training are similar but very specific modalities of psychological intervention that are commonly used with chronic pain patients. Traditional individual psychotherapy is also utilized but is reserved in many instances for patients whose psychological conflicts are the predominant contributory factor to their pain.[69, 70, 71]

Psychological intervention appears to be enhanced when it is used as part of an overall multidisciplinary pain management approach.[62, 72] A team approach involving a mental health professional, an anesthesiologist, and other medically trained professionals can be particularly helpful to the patient.

Chronic Pain Syndromes of the Head and Neck

The prior discussions have reviewed the medical therapy, including specialized techniques, available for the treatment of chronic pain. We now turn to specific discussions of the chronic pain syndromes of the head and neck and appropriate therapies.

Occipital Headache

The patient suffering from occipital neuralgia complains of chronic recurring, usually bilateral headache. The pain varies in intensity and occurs in the occipital area, occasionally radiating to the frontotemporal area, eyes, and neck. Related findings include a decreased range of motion, stiff neck muscles, and tender trigger points over the affected musculoskeletal regions.[73]

A form of occipital headache that occurs much less frequently is caused by pressure, injury, or inflammation of the occipital nerves, upper cervical spinal roots, dorsal horn, or dorsal root ganglia. The pain is a continuous, nonthrobbing ache and may last indefinitely. Associated muscle contraction and tenderness is present. The patient complains of a tingling or pricking sensation and increased sensitivity to pain in the scalp and neck.

Occipital nerve block with local anesthetic affords varying relief to these patients. In early occipital nerve entrapment syndromes this block can be quite useful. Since these syndromes are associated with inflammation, injection of a mixture of local anesthetic and corticosteroid can produce significant and even permanent relief. Nerve blocks should be accompanied by instruction in relaxation techniques, biofeedback, or hypnosis.

OCCIPITAL NERVE BLOCK

The greater occipital nerve is situated halfway between the mastoid process and the greater occipital protuberance at the crest of the occipital bone. The adjacent occipital artery is palpated. The nerve is located by directing the needle in a cephalad direction until it contacts bone. After withdrawing the needle 1 or 2 mm, 3 to 5 ml of a local anesthetic is injected. An attempt to elicit a paresthesia with a 25-gauge 2-cm needle can be made.

The lesser occipital nerve can be blocked by inserting the needle lateral to the mastoid process and directing it in a cephalad direction until contact with bone is made. The needle is then pulled back slightly, and 3 to 4 ml of the local anesthetic is injected. These blocks can be performed bilaterally[74] and will produce analgesia from the occipital region to the vertex (Fig. 11–2).

Myofascial Pain Syndromes

These disorders have been called rheumatism, myositis, myalgia, fibrositis, fasciolitis, and muscular strain. They must be distinguished from arthritis, myopathy, and acute inflammation. Typically, patients complain of a constant dull ache that is aggravated by pressure in a specific area of the muscle or by movement. There is usually no sensory deficit or reflex changes, and the distribution of the pain does not follow a dermatomal pattern.[77]

The cause of myofascial syndromes is acute trauma to myofascial structures or chronic muscle fatigue, both of which result in regional overloading of the muscle fibrils and consequent injury. This injury causes release of

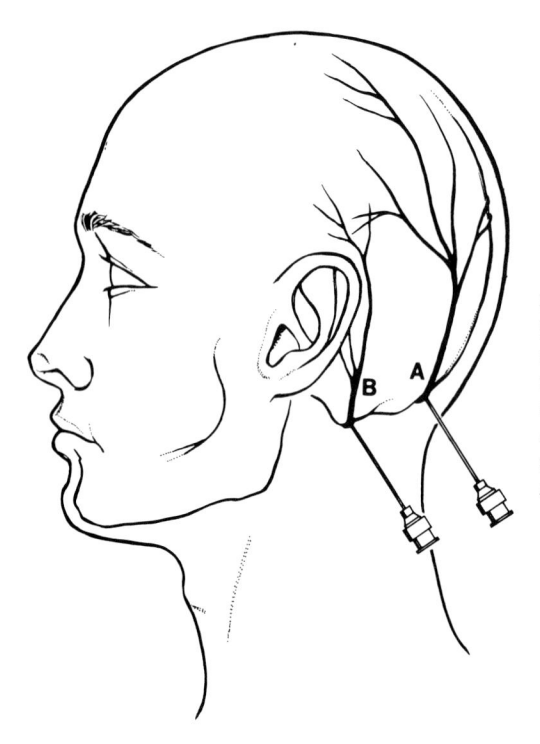

FIGURE 11-2. Occipital nerve block: Anatomic drawing showing relationships and distribution of the greater *(A)* and lesser *(B)* occipital nerves. (Modified from Carron, H. Control of pain in the head and neck. Otolaryngol Clin North Am 14(3): August 1981.)

ischemic metabolites and nerve-sensitizing substances, which eventually lead to development of a taut palpable band in the muscle. Myofascial syndromes may develop after mild injuries or repetitive microtrauma such as that associated with the use of typewriters[78, 79] (Fig. 11-3).

Four signs or criteria are used for the diagnosis of myofascial pain syndrome:[77]

1. The jump sign, in which palpation of the involved area causes the patient to jump.

2. The rope muscle sign, in which the muscles feel like ropes lying next to each other.

3. Dermographia, in which stroking the painful area results in blanching and hyperemia.

4. Elimination of the pain by treating the trigger area with an injection of a local anesthetic or by spraying it with a vapocoolant such as ethyl chloride.

Trigger areas develop at stressful sites such as the paravertebral muscles, levator scapulae, and trapezius muscle. To locate the trigger point, one meticulously palpates the entire area of the sensitive zone with a finger or the end of a pen. The patient is told to notify the physician when the point of maximal tenderness has been located. Palpation often reveals a distinct painful lesion within a taut band of muscle that can elicit referred somatic

Management of Chronic Pain of the Head and Neck

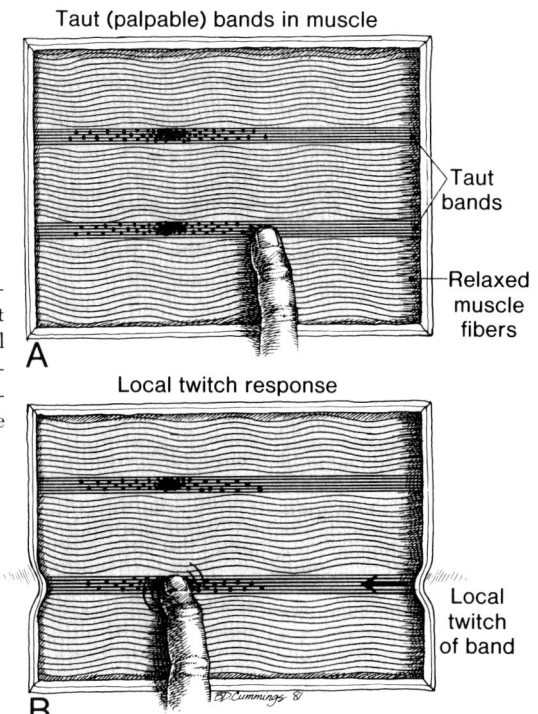

FIGURE 11-3. Method of palpating a flat muscle to elicit a taut band in the muscle (A) or a local twitch (B). (From Travell, J. Myofacial Pain and Dysfunction. Triggerpoint Manual. Baltimore, The Williams & Wilkins Co., 1983.)

pain. This referred pain usually has a dull, achy quality and varies from mild to severe. It is associated with tenderness and muscle spasm in the area of reference and subsequent weakness and limitation of motion.

Treatment involves interruption of the pain cycle at the trigger zone. This is accomplished most frequently and reliably by injection of a long-acting local anesthetic such as bupivacaine or etidocaine with or without steroid. The trigger point is palpated with two fingers and fixed. A 25-gauge 2-cm needle is inserted, and the patient is asked to identify the area of maximum pain. The anesthetic is forcefully injected in an attempt to break up the trigger point. Minutes after injection the pain will resolve, and mechanical stimulation should no longer cause referred pain. The associated referred tenderness, muscle spasm, decreased range of motion, and vasomotor disturbances may subside and may not return for hours or days after the local anesthetic action has worn off. Stretching of the muscle following injection is important. The patient should be forewarned that symptoms may be subsequently more pronounced and that a series of injections is often required. One injection may suffice for acute syndromes, but chronic syndromes often require repeated injections.[78]

Dry needling of the trigger point or spraying with ethyl chloride has resulted in cure but is probably not as effective as local anesthetic injections. The ethylchloride spray must usually be repeated 15 to 20 times to effect a cure. Often the muscle contractions caused by a high-amplitude and high-rate TENS will break up the trigger point. Acupuncture is also an alternative technique.[79]

Postherpetic Neuralgia

Acute herpes zoster infection is characterized by a vesicular rash and dermatomal pain of the sensory nerves that arise in the posterior root ganglia infected with the virus.[80] Apparently the virus can remain dormant in the spinal ganglia without symptoms and may be reactivated periodically. Although some patients have no underlying disease, the virus does tend to afflict those with depressed cellular immunity, including those with malignancies, Hodgkin's disease, or AIDS or those who have received immunosuppressive therapy.[81] The pain may range from mild to severe and may have a dull, sharp, or burning quality. The lesions begin as local redness and progress through papular, vesicular, pustular, and crusting stages. This acute pain is caused by inflammation, hemorrhage, or swelling in the affected dorsal root ganglion. The ganglion may eventually become completely replaced by scar tissue. In most patients healing in acute herpes zoster is complete within 3 weeks. In young patients, pain may persist for 1 to 2 weeks, and hypoesthesia or hyperesthesia may persist even longer. However, in patients over 60 years old, postherpetic neuralgia presents a significant problem, since more than 60 per cent have pain for more than 2 months despite the fact that the skin lesions have healed.[83] Pain in the distribution of the trigeminal nerve is caused by involvement of the trigeminal (gasserian) ganglion. Infection of the first division of the trigeminal nerve is associated with a higher incidence of postherpetic neuralgia than infection of the spinal segments.[80, 81]

Postherpetic neuralgia is often associated with a history of unilateral skin eruption, although this may be absent in some patients. There is often hyperpigmentation or scarring in the involved areas as well as sensory abnormalities. Patients complain of pain that is described as a constant aching or burning with superimposed shocks or stabs of pain. Dysesthesia causes even the slightest touch to be intolerable, although firm pressure may not cause as much discomfort. The pain most often involves an entire dermatome. Postherpetic neuralgia is often accompanied by anxiety, depression, and insomnia.

Various treatment modalities are advocated for the treatment of postherpetic neuralgia. The most therapeutic maneuver is prevention by early treatment of the acute herpes zoster infection. Nerve block treatments used include somatic nerve block, local infiltration, and sympathetic blocks. A somatic nerve block with local anesthetics can be used to predict a patient's response to a subsequent neurolytic block or surgical procedure; however, these procedures do not result in permanent relief. Local instillation of steroids and local anesthetic may relieve the symptoms in up to 75 per cent of patients. Epstein reported a decreased incidence of postherpetic neuralgia in patients with acute herpes zoster treated with triamcinolone-procaine injections.[84] There is some evidence that oral steroids may decrease the incidence of postherpetic neuralgia without increasing the risk of disseminated disease. However, the use of steroids is not recommended in patients known to have neoplasms or other underlying disease.[85, 86]

Tricyclic antidepressants such as amitriptyline or imipramine are frequently used and are especially effective for the burning component of the pain.[85] Their analgesic properties have been discussed earlier. Benzodiazepines can be added if anxiety is manifested. TENS, biofeedback, relaxation therapy, and cryotherapy are also useful.

In the Pain Management Service at the SUNY Health Science Center in Brooklyn, we prefer sympathetic nerve blocks or subcutaneous infiltration of a mixture of local anesthetic and steroid as the initial therapy. These blocks should be performed as early as possible. Mayne et al. found that if several instillations of triamcinolone and bupivacaine have not improved the symptoms, sympathetic blocks will not usually be helpful. However, if sympathetic nerve blocks are not initially helpful, subcutaneous infiltration of bupivacaine and triamcinolone should be attempted.[85]

For postherpetic neuralgia of the head and neck, a stellate ganglion block[88] can be performed (Fig. 11-4). The stellate ganglion is formed by the fusion of the inferior cervical and first thoracic ganglia. It is located in the prevertebral fascia anterior to the transverse process of C7. It lies deep to the subclavian artery near the origin of the vertebral artery.

There are several approaches to the stellate ganglion.[90] The most common is placement of the needle anterior to the C6 transverse process (Chassignac's tubercle) with instillation of 10 to 15 ml of local anesthetic into the prevertebral fascia that filters down to the ganglion. This block is performed by placing the patient in the supine position with the neck slightly extended. The physician palpates Chassignac's tubercle, which is located approximately at the level of the cricoid cartilage. The sternocleidomastoid muscle and the carotid sheath are retracted laterally. The needle is placed medial to the tip of the index finger and advanced perpendicularly in all places until it comes in contact with the tubercle.

Other approaches used to block the stellate ganglion have been described.[90] One advantage of the C6 approach is the low incidence of pneumothorax as a complication. Inadvertent vertebral artery injection may be manifest by loss of consciousness, apnea, seizures, hypotension, and resultant cardiac arrest. Due to the proximity of the subarachnoid space one must be concerned to avoid inadvertent injection resulting in total spinal anesthesia with its accompanying apnea and hypotension. Other possible complications include hematoma, neuritis, partial brachial plexus block, recurrent laryngeal nerve block, and phrenic nerve block.

Trigeminal Neuralgia

Trigeminal neuralgia, also known as tic douloureux, usually occurs in patients in the fifth and sixth decades; there is a 60 per cent prevalence in women.[91] It causes pain in the lips, gums, cheek, or chin and in the

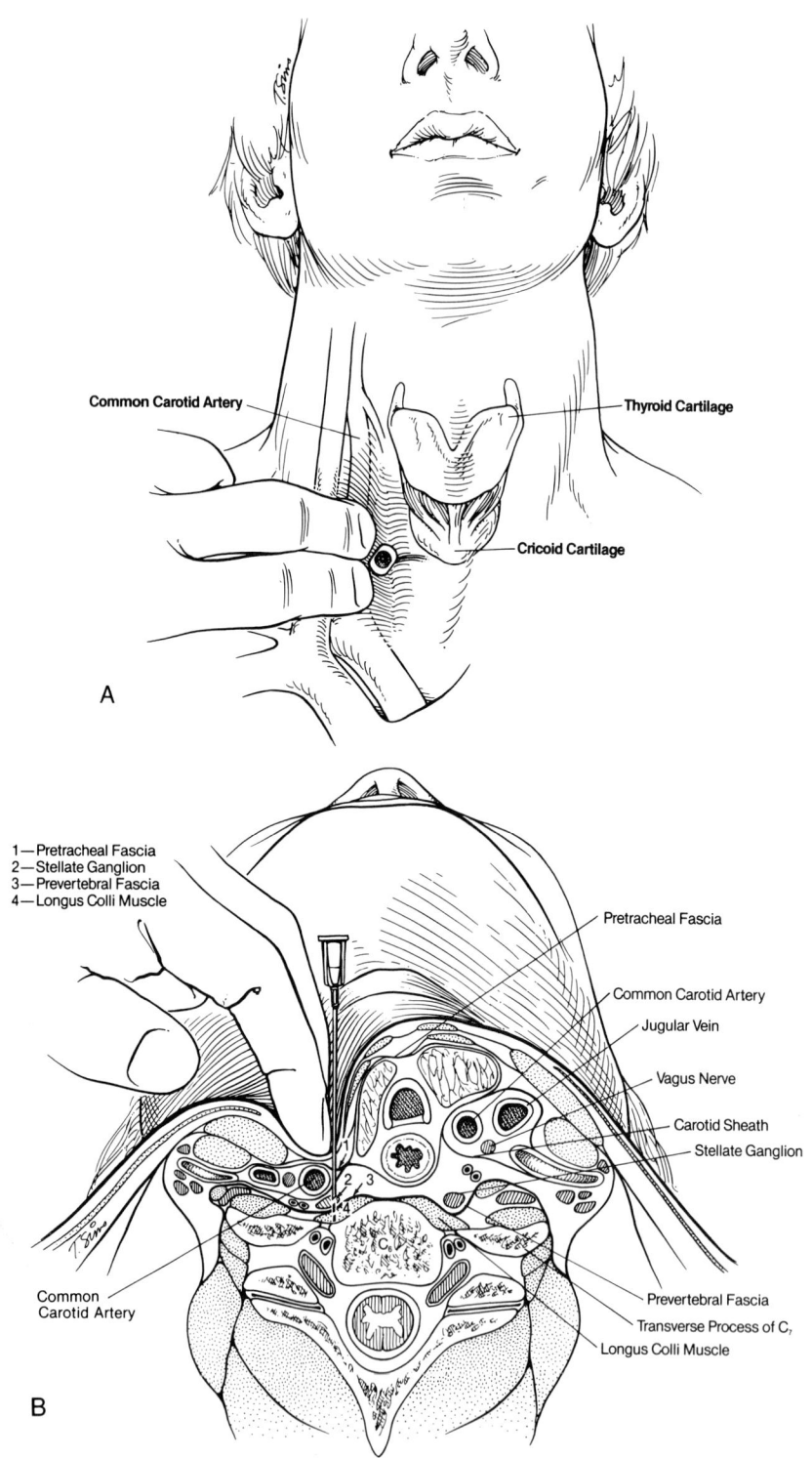

FIGURE 11-4 *See legend on opposite page*

distribution of the ophthalmic division of the fifth nerve. The pain is intense and sharp, lasting from seconds to minutes.[92] Bouts of pain can occur for weeks at a time. Pain is initiated by stimulating trigger zones. Causes include mechanical deformity of the nerve root entry zone and demyelinating diseases.

The mechanical deformity is due to pressure in the posterior fossa from a loop of the superior cerebellar artery. Pain caused by multiple sclerosis is usually suspected because of the typical fluctuating and changing neurologic symptoms. This condition must be distinguished from other causes of facial pain arising from the teeth, jaw, or sinuses. No sensory loss can be demonstrated with tic douloureux. Evaluation of the patient requires a history and physical examination including an oral and facial evaluation. It is necessary to obtain a CT scan to rule out space-occupying lesions.

Multiple therapeutic modalities have been used. Diphenylhydantoin (Dilantin) 300 to 600 mg per day is not used as often as it was in the past because it is associated with tachyphylaxis and incomplete control of pain.[93] Carbamazepine (Tegretol) 100 to 200 mg two to three times a day offers good pain relief in more than 60 per cent of patients.[94] Unfortunately, side effects include leukopenia, thrombocytopenia, and aplastic anemia and hepatocellular disease. Serial complete blood counts and liver function tests are mandatory when this drug is used. Baclofen, an antispasmotic, given in doses of 10 to 60 mg twice a day, has also been found to be effective.[95]

Block of the trigeminal ganglion using a local anesthetic or neurolytic agents has been shown to have short-lived results and has several side effects, including dysesthetic numbness, facial weakness, double vision, and anesthesia dolorosa, the pain of which can be severe and debilitating. Thermocoagulation of the trigeminal ganglion, radiofrequency percutaneous rhizotomy, and posterior fossa exploration have had varying success.[96]

Glossopharyngeal Neuralgia

The pain of glossopharyngeal neuralgia characteristically lasts 30 seconds and is followed by 2 to 5 minutes of a burning sensation in the posterior portion of the tongue, soft palate, and pharynx. It may radiate to the ear. It may be brought on by insidious movement of the mouth or tongue and is often followed by ipsilateral tearing and salivation.[97] There are no neurologic deficits. An idiopathic syndrome exists in which most of the symptoms subside after the fifth decade. The differential diagnosis includes

---

FIGURE 11–4. *A*, Stellate ganglion block. Surface landmarks and position of the needle for the stellate ganglion block. Note that the head is well extended. Fingers retract the carotid sheath laterally with the needle at C6 level in the paratracheal space. *B*, Stellate ganglion block, paratracheal approach. Transverse section at the level of C6, showing the needle medial to the finger retracting the carotid vessel laterally. (From Raj, P.P. Chronic pain. In Raj, P.P. (ed.). Handbook of Regional Anesthesia. New York, Churchill Livingstone, 1985. By permission.)

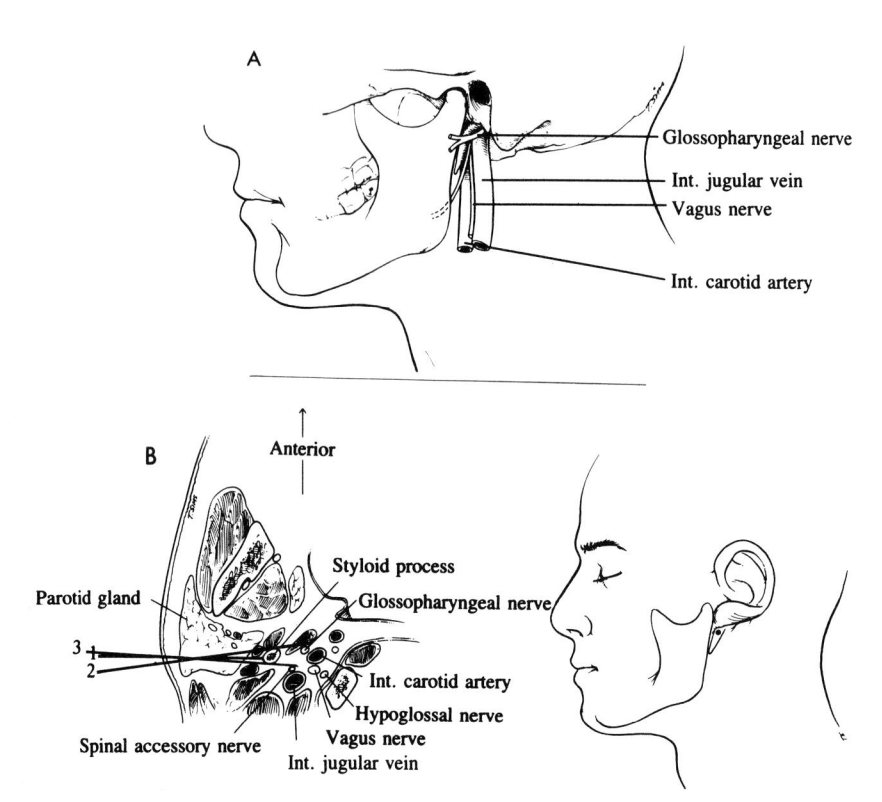

FIGURE 11–5. Glossopharyngeal nerve block. *A*, The 5-cm, 22-gauge needle is inserted halfway between the mastoid process and the angle of the mandible, seeking the styloid process. When this bony end point has been located, the needle is "walked" off the anterior aspect at the styloid process at the same depth (usually about 3 cm). A glossopharyngeal paresthesia should be obtained. A small bolus of 1–2 cc of either a local anesthetic or a neurolytic agent is sufficient for block at this site. Note the proximity of the underlying internal carotid artery and internal jugular vein, necessitating meticulous attention to aspiration testing. *B*, Point of entry of needle for glossopharyngeal and vagal nerve block. 1, The needle is inserted at the point of entry perpendicularly to the skin, until it touches the styloid process. 2, The needle tip is slipped anteriorly and seeks paresthesia of the glossopharyngeal nerve. 3, For vagal nerve block the needle tip is slipped posteriorly to the same depth (~ 3 cm). (From Murphy, T.M. Techniques of nerve blocks. In Raj, P.P. Practical Management of Pain. Chicago, Year Book Medical Publishers, 1986.)

anomalous arteries at the cerebellopontine angle, arachnoiditis, perineural fibrosis, elongation of the styloid process, and viral infections such as herpes zoster. Therapy is initiated with carbamazepine or phenytoin. If this is unsuccessful and symptoms persist, surgical division of the nerve near the medulla may be indicated.[98]

GLOSSOPHARYNGEAL NERVE BLOCK

Glossopharyngeal nerve block is occasionally performed for patients with idiopathic neuralgia. In chronic pain management, however, this block is indicated in patients with carcinoma invading the posterior third of the tongue or pharynx that has not responded to other therapies. It may be

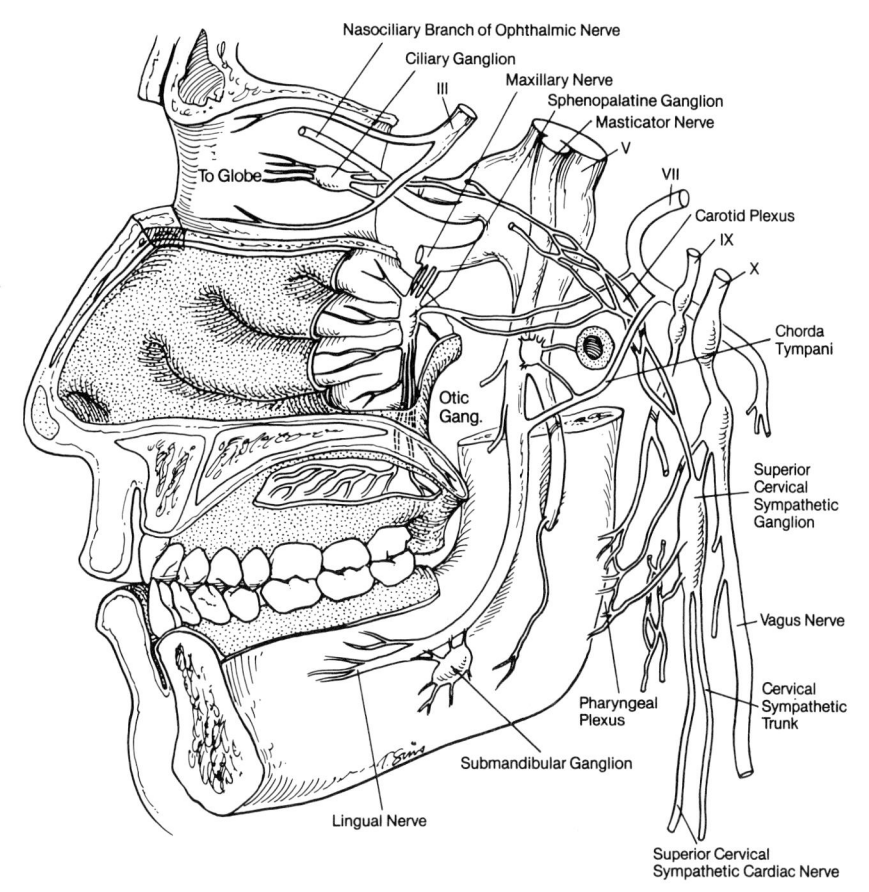

FIGURE 11–6. Autonomic nerves in the head. Sphenopalatine ganglion anatomy. (From Raj, P.P. (ed.). Handbook of Regional Anesthesia. New York, Churchill Livingstone, 1985.)

associated with significant complications. An extraoral block of the glossopharyngeal nerve can easily spread to the vagus and accessory nerves with resultant analgesia of the hemilarynx or trapezius or sternocleidomastoid paralysis. Because the internal carotid artery and internal jugular vein are near the site of injection, one must aspirate carefully to ensure that an intravascular injection does not occur. Abnormal swallowing with its associated risk of aspiration is a potential complication.[99]

The block is performed by inserting a 5-cm, 22-gauge needle midway between the mastoid process and the angle of the mandible until contact is made with the styloid process. The needle is walked off the styloid process posteriorly, at which point a paresthesia should be obtained. One to two ml of a local anesthetic or neurolytic agent is adequate to perform the block. The styloid process is easily palpable after a radical neck dissection, and this block is then easily performed (Fig. 11–5).

Block of the sphenopalatine ganglion has been useful for the management of several chronic pain syndromes, including musculoskeletal pain of the upper torso, head, and neck, neuralgia, vasospasm, reflex sympathetic dystrophy, low back pain, sciatica, and angina. The ganglion is covered by a 1- to 5-mm layer of connective tissue and mucous membrane and is located in the pterygopalatine fossa posterior to the middle turbinate. Topically applied local anesthetics can easily diffuse across the thin layer of tissue into the ganglion.

The ganglion has sensory effects through the trigeminal and facial nerves, visceral motor function through the parasympathetic activity of the superficial petrosal nerve, and sympathetic function through its connection to the cervical sympathetic chain via the great deep petrosal nerve. Studies have shown that 4 percent lidocaine and 10 percent cocaine offer equal improvement of pain secondary to several chronic pain states. It is thought that the effect of the sphenopalative ganglion is mediated by the autonomic nervous system.[88, 101–103] (Fig. 11–6).

Summary

The anesthesiologist is in a unique position to evaluate patients with chronic pain. Diagnostic and therapeutic nerve blocks are useful modalities in the care of patients with head and neck pain. Other, less invasive therapies such as biofeedback, hypnosis, and cryotherapy and pharmacotherapy complete the range of available therapies. Chronic pain syndromes of the head and neck include a large spectrum of disorders. A combined medical and psychological approach such as that used by modern pain clinics will provide the best clinical results.

References

1. Ng, L. K., et al. Pain Discomfort and Humanitarian Care. Amsterdam, Elsevier, 1980.
2. Taylor, H., et al. The Nuprin Pain Report. New York. Louis Harris and Associates, 1985, pp. 20 and 72.
3. Merskey, H. Classification of chronic pain, descriptions of chronic pain syndromes and definitions of pain terms. Pain (Suppl 3), 1986, p. S217.
4. Fordyce, W. E. Pain viewed as learned behavior. Adv Neurol 4:415–422, 1973.
5. Holzman, A., et al. Pain Management, A Handbook of Psychological Treatment Approaches. New York, Pergamon Press, 1986.
6. Pain Center Clinic Directory. Atlanta, American Society of Anesthesiologists, 1980.
7. Pain Clinic Organization and Administration. Manual of the Department of Anesthesiology. Charlottesville, Virginia, University of Virginia Medical Center, 1976.
8. Carpenter, M. B. Core Textbook of Neuroanatomy. Baltimore, Williams & Wilkins, 1985, pp. 74–81.
9. Gilman, S., et al. Essentials of Clinical Neuroanatomy and Neurophysiology. Philadelphia. F. A. Davis, 1982, pp. 33–40.

10. Guyton, A. C. Textbook of Medical Physiology. Philadelphia, W. B. Saunders Co., 1986, pp. 572–591.
11. Zimmerman, M. Somatovisceral sensibility: Processing in the central nervous system. In Schmidt, R. F., and Thews, G. Human Physiology. Berlin, Springer-Verlag, 1983, pp. 193–210.
12. Casey, K. L. Supraspinal mechanisms in pain: The reticular formation. In Kosterlitz, H. W., and Terenius, L. Y. (eds.). Pain and Society. Berlin, 1979, pp. 183–200.
13. Iggo, A. Segmental neurophysiology of pain control. In Kosterlitz, H. W., and Terenius, L. Y. (eds.). Pain and Society. Weinheim, Verlag Chemie, 1980, pp. 123–140.
14. Barchas, J. D., et al. Behavioral neurochemistry: Neuroregulators and behavioral states. Science 200:964–973, 1978.
15. Melzack, R., et al. Pain mechanisms: A new theory. Science 150:971–979, 1965.
16. Melzak, R., et al. The Challenge of Pain. New York, Basic Books, 1983.
17. Zimmerman, M. Recurrent persistent pain: Mechanisms and models. In Kosterlitz, H. W., and Terenius, L. Y. (eds.). Pain and Society. Weinheim, Verlag Chemie, 1980, pp. 367–382.
18. Abrams, S. E. Common pain syndromes and their therapy. In American Society of Anesthesiologists. Refresher Courses in Anesthesiology, Vol. 11. Philadelphia. JB Lippincott, 1986, pp. 11–12.
19. Warfield, C. A. The sympathetic dystrophies. Hosp Pract pp. 52C–52J, May 1984.
20. Abram, S. E. Sympathetic pain. In Raj, P. P. (ed.). Practical Management of Pain. Chicago, Year Book Medical Publishers, 1986, p. 209.
21. Mersky, H. Classification of chronic pain, descriptions of chronic pain syndromes and definitions of pain terms. Pain (Suppl. 3), 529, 1986.
22. Bonica, J. Causalgia and other reflex sympathetic dystrophies. In Bonica, J., et al. Advances in Pain Research and Therapy, Vol. 3. New York, Raven Press, 1979.
23. Gilman, A. G., et al. Analgesic-antipyretics and anti-inflammatory agents. In Gilman, A. G. (ed.). The Pharmacological Basis of Therapeutics. New York, Macmillan, 1985, pp. 674–689.
24. Moore, M. E. Use of drugs in the management of chronic pain. Anesthesiol Rev 14–18, August 1985.
25. Levy, G. Pharmacokinetics of salicylate in man. Drug Metab Rev 9(1)3–19, 1979.
26. Mehlisch, D. R. Review of the comparative analgesic efficacy of salicylates, acetaminophen and pyrazolones. Am J Med 47–52, November 1983.
27. Cooper, S. A. Comparative analgesic efficacies of aspirin and acetaminophen. Arch Intern Med 141:282–285, 1981.
28. Koch-Weser, J., et al. Nonsteroidal anti-inflammatory drugs, part 2. N Engl J Med 302:1237–1243, 1980.
29. Lanza, F. L. Endoscopic studies of gastric and duodenal injury after the use of ibuprofen, aspirin, and other nonsteroidal agents. Am J Med 19–24, July 1984.
30. Houde, R. W. Systemic analgesics and related drugs: Narcotic analgesics. In Bonica, J. J., et al. (eds.). Advances in Pain Research and Therapy. Vol. 2. New York, Raven Press, 1979, pp. 263–273.
31. Ramadhyani, U. Opioid and non-opioid analgesics. In Attia, R. R., Grogono,

A. W., and Domer, F. R. (eds.). Practical Anesthetic Pharmacology. Norwalk, Appleton-Century-Crofts, 1987, p. 129.
32. Snyder, S. Drug and neurotransmitter receptors in the brain. Science 224:22–30, 1984.
33. Stoelting, R. K., and Miller, R. D. Intravenous anesthetics. In Basics of Anesthesia. New York, Churchill Livingstone, 1984, p. 73.
34. Gilman, A. G., et al. Morphine and related opioids. In Gilman, A. G. (ed.). The Pharmacological Basis of Therapeutics. New York, Macmillan, 1985, pp. 495–513.
35. Gilman, A. G., et al. Tricyclic antidepressants. In Gilman, A. G. (ed.). The Pharmacological Basis of Therapeutics. New York, Macmillan, 1985, pp. 413–423.
36. Warfield, C. A. Psychotropic agents for pain control. Hosp Pract, May 15, 141–143, 1985.
37. Feinmann, C. Pain relief by antidepressants: Possible modes of action. Pain 23:1–8, 1985.
38. France, R. D., et al. Therapeutic effects of antidepressants in chronic pain. Gen Hosp Psychiat 6:55–63, 1984.
39. Fields, H. L. Pain. New York, McGraw Hill, 1987, pp. 285–306.
40. Ward, N. G. The effectiveness of tricyclic antidepressants in the treatment of coexisting pain and depression. Pain 7:331–341, 1979.
41. Rubin, E. H. Psychotropic therapy: Special concerns in the elderly. Hosp Pract, October 15, 95–105, 1986.
42. Johnson, K. S. Transcutaneous electrical nerve stimulation. In Raj, P. P. (ed.). Practical Management of Pain. Chicago, Year Book Medical Publishers, 1986, p. 793.
43. Pike, P. Transcutaneous electric stimulation. Anesthesia 33:165–171, 1978.
44. Nehme, A. E., et al: Cryoanalgesia: Freezing of peripheral nerves. Hosp Pract, January 15, 172–174, 1987.
45. Myers, R. R., et al. Biophysical and pathological effects of cryogenic nerve lesion. Ann Neurol 10(5):478–485, 1981.
46. Blumer, D., et al. Chronic pain as a variant of depressive disease, the pain-prone disorder. J Nerv Ment Dis 170:381–406, 1982.
47. Magni, G. On the relationship between chronic pain and depression when there is no organic lesion. Pain 31:1–21, 1987.
48. Gupta, M. A. Is chronic pain a variant of depressive illness? A critical review. Can J Psychiat 31:241–248, 1986.
49. Magni, G., et al. Chronic pain as a depressive equivalent. Postgrad Med 73:79–80, 1983.
50. Turk, D. C., et al. Chronic pain as a variant of depressive disease: A critical reappraisal. J Nerv Ment Dis 172(7):398–404, 1984.
51. American Psychiatric Association. Diagnostic and Statistical Manual of Mental Disorders, 3rd ed. Washington, D. C., American Psychiatric Association, 1980.
52. Katon, W., et al. The prevalence of somatization in primary care. Comprehensive Psychiat 25:208–215, 1984.
53. Dworkin, R. H., et al. Unraveling the effects of compensation, litigation and employment on treatment response in chronic pain. Pain 23:49–59, 1985.
54. Anderson, T. P., et al. Behavior modification of chronic pain: A treatment program by a multidisciplinary team. Clin Orthoped Rel Res 129:96–100, 1977.

55. Roberts, A. H., et al. The behavioral management of chronic pain: Long-term follow-up with comparison groups. Pain 8:151–162, 1980.
56. Krusen, E. M., et al. Compensation factor in low back injuries. JAMA 166:1128–1133, 1958.
57. Abrams, S. E., et al. Factors predicting short-term outcome of nerve blocks in the management of chronic pain. Pain 10:323–330, 1981.
58. Brena, S. F., et al. Conditioned responses to treatment in chronic pain patients: Effects of compensation for work-related accidents. Bull Los Angeles Neurolog Soc 44:48–52, 1980.
59. Taylor, S. E. Health Psychology. New York, Random House, 1986.
60. Beecher, H. K. Measurement of Subjective Responses. New York, Oxford University Press, 1959.
61. Shapiro, A. K. Factors contributing to the placebo effect. Their implications for psychotherapy. Am J Psychother 18:73–88, 1964.
62. Lebovits, A. H., et al. Chronic pain and Crohn's disease: Treatment difficulties. Clin J Pain 3:31–38, 1987.
63. Cox, G. B., et al. The MMPI and chronic pain. The diagnosis of psychogenic pain. J Behav Med 1:437–444, 1978.
64. Dahlstrom, W. G., et al. An MMPI Handbook. Vol. 1. Clinical Interpretation. Minneapolis, University of Minnesota Press, 1972.
65. Bond, M. R. Pain: Its Nature, Analysis, and Treatment. Edinburgh, Churchill Livingstone, 1979.
66. Bradley, L. Relationships between the MMPI and the McGill Pain Questionnaire. In Melzack, R. (ed.). Pain Measurement and Assessment. New York, Raven Press, 1983.
67. Holzman, A. D., et al. The cognitive-behavioral approach to the management of chronic pain. In Holzman, A. D., and Turk, D. C. (eds.). Pain Management. A Handbook of Psychological Treatment Approaches. New York, Pergamon Press, 1986.
68. Maruta, T., et al. Chronic pain: Which patients may a pain management program help? Pain 7:321–329, 1979.
69. Fordyce, W. E., et al. Operant conditioning in the treatment of chronic pain. Arch Phys Med Rehab 54:399–408, 1973.
70. Gentry, W. D., et al. Pain groups. In Holzman, A. D., and Turk, D. C. (eds.). Pain Management. A Handbook of Psychological Treatment Approaches. New York, Pergamon Press, 1986.
71. Mersky, W. Traditional individual psychotherapy and psychopharmacotherapy. In Holzman, A. D., and Turk, D. C. (eds.). Pain Management. A Handbook of Psychological Treatment Approaches. New York, Pergamon Press, 1986.
72. Lefkowitz, M., et al. Management of chronic pain syndrome in a quadriplegic patient. A case report. Clin J Pain 3:119–122, 1987.
73. Phero, J. C., et al. Common headaches. In Raj, P. P. (ed.). Practical Management of Pain. Chicago, Year Book Medical Publishers, 1986, p. 374.
74. Murphy, T. M., et al. Techniques of nerve block—Spinal nerves. In Raj, P. P. (ed.). Practical Management of Pain. Chicago, Year Book Medical Publishers, 1986, pp. 600–601.
75. Murphy, T. M., et al. Techniques of nerve blocks—spinal nerves. Medical Publishers, pp. 600–601, 1986.
76. Carron, H. Control of pain in the head and neck. Otolaryngol Clin North Am 14(3):631–652, August 1981.

77. Berges, P. U. Myofascial pain syndromes. Postgrad Med 53:(6), 1973.
78. Raj, P. P. Myofascial trigger point injection. In Raj, P. P. (ed.). Practical Management of Pain. Chicago, Year Book Medical Publishers, 1986, pp. 569–572.
79. Travell, J. Myofascial pain and dysfunction. In The Trigger Point Manual. Baltimore, Williams & Wilkins, 1983, Chaps. 2 and 3.
80. Berkow, R., et al. Herpes zoster. In Windholz, M. (ed.). The Merck Index, 10th ed. Rahway, NJ, Merck & Co., 1983, p. 187.
81. Whitley, R. J. Varicella-zoster virus infections. In Braunwald, E. et al. Harrison's Principles of Internal Medicine. New York, McGraw Hill, 1987, pp. 689–692.
82. Ibid., p. 1123.
83. Sandrock, N. J. G., et al. Managing the pain of herpes zoster. Hosp Pract November 30, 81–93, 1986.
84. Epstein, E. Triamcinolone-procaine in the treatment of zoster and post-zoster neuralgia. Calif Med 115(2):6–10, 1971.
85. Mayne, G. E., et al. Pain of herpes zoster and post-herpetic neuralgia. In Raj, P. P. (ed.). Practical Management of Pain. Chicago, Year Book Medical Publishers, 1986, pp. 358–359.
86. Lilley, J. P., et al. Sensory and sympathetic nerve blocks for postherpetic neuralgia. Regional Anesth 11:165–167, 1986.
87. Abram, S. E., et al. Pain syndromes and rationale for management. In Raj, P. P. (ed.). Practical Management of Pain. Chicago, Year Book Medical Publishers, 1986, pp. 184–189.
88. Raj, P. P. Handbook of Regional Anesthesia. New York, Churchill Livingstone, 1985, p. 114.
89. Stanton-Hicks, M., et al. Sympathetic blocks. In Raj, P. P. (ed.). Practical Management of Pain. Chicago, Year Book Medical Publishers, 1986, p. 663.
90. Anatomy of the stellate ganglion. Reproduced with permission from Stanton-Hicks, M., et al. Sympathetic Blocks in Raj, P. P. Practical Management of Pain. Chicago. Yearbook Medical Publishers. 1986, pp. 662.
91. Victor, M., et al. Diseases of the cranial nerves. In Braunwald E., et al. Harrison's Principles of Internal Medicine. New York, McGraw-Hill, 1987, pp. 2035–2040.
92. Jannetta, P. J. Trigeminal neuralgia and hemifacial spasm—etiology and definitive treatment. Trans Am Neurol Assoc 100:89–91, 1975.
93. Berkow, R., et al. Trigeminal neuralgia. In Windholz, M. (ed.). The Merck Index, 10th ed. Rahway, NJ, Merck & Co., 1983, p. 1376.
94. From, G., et al. Baclofen in trigeminal neuralgia. Effect on the spinal trigeminal nucleus: A pilot study. Arch Neurol 37:768–771, 1980.
95. Steiner, J. Trigeminal neuralgia. In Raj, P. P. (ed.). Practical Management of Pain. Chicago, Year Book Medical Publishers, 1986, pp. 379–388.
96. Phero, J. C., et al. Less common syndromes causing pain. In Raj, P. P. (ed.). Practical Management of Pain. Chicago, Year Book Medical Publishers, 1986, p. 403.
97. Victor, M., et al. Diseases of the cranial nerves. In Braunwald, E., et al. Harrison's Principles of Internal Medicine. New York, McGraw-Hill, 1987, p. 2039.
98. Murphy, T. M. Techniques of nerve blocks—cranial nerves. In Raj, P. P. (ed.). Practical Management of Pain. Chicago, Year Book Medical Publishers, 1986, pp. 594–595.

99. Ibid., p. 594.
100. Murphy, T. M. Techniques of nerve blocks—cranial nerves. In Raj, P. P. (ed.). Practical Management of Pain. Chicago, Year Book Medical Publishers, 1986, p. 594.
101. Berger, J., et al. Does topical anesthesia of the sphenopalatine ganglion with cocaine or lidocaine relieve low back pain? Anesth Analg 65:700–702, 1986.
102. Reder, M. A., et al. Sphenopalatine ganglion block in treatment of acute and chronic pain. In Hendler, N. H., Long, D. M., and Wise, T. N. (eds.) Diagnosis and Treatment of Chronic Pain. Boston, John Wright, 1982, p. 104.
103. Ruskin, A. P. Sphenopalatine (nasal) ganglion: Remote effects including "psychosomatic" symptoms, rage reaction, pain, and spasm. Arch Phys Med Rehabil 60:353–359, 1979.

Index

Note: Page numbers in *italics* refer to illustrations. Page numbers followed by the letter (t) refer to tables.

A-alpha fibers, TENS therapy and, 310
Abducens nerve, functional evaluation of, 14
Aberrant reference, 10
Abutments, for tooth restoration, 122
Acetazolamide, for corneal disease, 93
Acids, ingestion of, 142
Acquired immunodeficiency syndrome (AIDS), cobblestoned esophagus with, 143, *144*
　fungal pharyngitis with, 137
　inflammatory nasal lesions with, 102, *102*
　postherpetic neuralgia and, 318
Actinomycosis, neck pain with, 148, *149*
Action potentials in electromyography, 276
Acupuncture, for myofascial pain syndrome, 318
Acupuncture-like TENS, 283
Acute angle closure glaucoma, 92–93
Acute necrotizing ulcerative gingivitis (ANUG), 124
Addiction, drug therapy for pain and, 17, 306
A-delta fibers, in afferent pain pathways, 8
　gate control theory and, 303
　neurophysiology of pain, 9
　pain transmission with, 302
　TENS therapy and, 310
Adenocarcinomas, in nasal region, 106–107
Adenoid cystic carcinoma, oropharyngeal pain and, 141
Adenoid obstruction, middle ear otalgia and, 64
Adenovirus, pharyngitis caused by, 136
Adjuvant analgesics, for chronic pain, 308, 310
　role in pain therapy, 17
Affective disorders, 291
Afferent pain pathways, 8
Age, as factor in trigeminal neuralgia, 28
　mandibular posture and, 159
　optics and, 81
Agonist-antagonist drugs, role in pain therapy, 17
AIDS. See *Acquired immunodeficiency syndrome.*
Air travel, middle ear otalgia and, 65

Alcmaeon, 4
Alcohol ingestion, sphenopalatine neuralgia and, 40–41
Alkalis, ingestion of, 142
Allergic rhinitis, nasal inflammation with, 103
　treatment of, 113
Amblyopia, 86
Amitriptyline (Elavil), 17
　for depression-related facial pain, 46
　for pain syndrome, 297
　for postherpetic neuralgia, 39
　for Raeder's syndrome, 44
Ancient civilizations, pain theories in, 2–3
Angiography, cerebral, 15
　for otalgia, 58
Anisometropic asthenopia, 83
Antianxiety agents, for pain syndrome, 296
Anticonvulsants, for chronic pain, 310
　G-32883, for trigeminal neuralgia, 31
Antidepressants, for pain syndrome, 296–297
Antipsychotic agents, for pain syndrome, 295–297
Arachnoid membrane, 257
Arnold-Chiari malformations, occipital neuralgia and, 41
Arthrography, temporomandibular joint dysfunction, 192–194, *194*
Articular disk, disorders of, 206
Articular eminence, 154
Articulation, atlantoaxial, 268–269, 269(t)
Aspirin, acetaminophen and, 307
　for chronic pain, 306–308, 307(t), *309*
Asthenopia, 81–87
　accommodative, 81–84, 84–85
　　hyperopia, 81–82, *82*
　　paresis of, 84
　　presbyopia, 82–83
　anisometropic, 83
　astigmatic, 83

331

Asthenopia *(Continued)*
  corneal degeneration and, 92
  diagnosis of, 86, *87*
  muscular, 85–87
  myopia, 83, *84*
  psychological factors in, 84
Astigmatic asthenopia, 83
Atarax, for pain syndrome, 296
Ativan, for pain syndrome, 296
Atlantoaxial articulation, 268–269, 269(t)
Atlas vertebra, anatomy of, 255
Atrophic rhinitis, 109
  treatment of, 114
Audiometry, middle ear otalgia and, 63–64
Auditory-vestibular nerve, functional evaluation of, 14
Autoimmune disease, benign mucous membrane pemphigoid as, 140
  otalgia and, 74–75
Autonomic nervous system, anatomy of, *323*, 323–324
  nose structure and, 100
Avicenna, 6
Axis vertebra, anatomy of, 255

Babinski's sign, testing for in spinal cord lesions, 271
Baclofen, for geniculate neuralgia, 38
  for trigeminal neuralgia, 32, 321
  for vagoglossopharyngeal neuralgia, 37
Bacterial culture, for oral cavity disease, 126
Barotrauma, middle ear otalgia and, 64–65
Bed rest, for neck and arm pain, 277
Behavior therapy, 294
Bell, C., 7
Bell's palsy, Ramsay-Hunt syndrome and, 69
Benign mucous membrane pemphigoid, oropharyngeal pain with, 139–140
Benign tumors, in nasal region, 106
Benzodiazepines, for chronic pain, 310
  for pain syndrome, 296
Bernard, Claude, 7
Beta-endorphin, endogenous analgesia and, 11
Bioelectric measurement, of mandibular function, 180–188
Biofeedback, for pain syndrome, 295
Biting, tooth sensitivity localization with, 120–121. See also *Bruxism*.
Blepharitis, 89, *90*
BNS-40 instrument, 214
Borderline personality disorder, 291
Bruxism, in craniomandibular disorders, 167, 175
  in myofacial pain dysfunction, 205–206
  oral pain and, 118–119
  temporomandibular joint trauma from, 210
Bulb of Krause, afferent pain pathways in, 8
Bullous myringitis, 63
Bupivacaine, for myofascial pain syndrome, 317
Burns, on external ear, 59

C1–C2 arthrosis, occipital neuralgia and, 41, 42(t)
C fibers, afferent pain pathways and, 8
  gate control theory and, 303
  neurophysiology of pain and, 9
  pain transmission with, 302
  TENS therapy and, 310
Candida, fungal pharyngitis and, 137
Canker sores, pharyngitis with, 138, *138*
Carbamazepine, for geniculate neuralgia, 38
  for trigeminal neuralgia, 31–32, 321
  for vagoglossopharyngeal neuralgia, 37
Carotidynia, neck pain with, 151
  otalgia and, 75
Causalgia, pain transmission and, 303–304
  reflex sympathetic dystrophy and, 44
  skin tenderness and, 270
Caustic ingestion, hypopharyngeal pain and, 142
Cell theory, pain theory and, 7
Celsus, 5
Cerebral angiography, 15
Cerebral circulation, analysis of, 15–16
Cerebrospinal fluid (CSF), 15
Cervical disk degeneration, 263
Cervical muscles, in craniomandibular disorders, palpation and examination of, *169*, 170
Cervical myelopathy, spinal cord compression with, 260–261
Cervical myeloradiculopathy, 261
  lower extremity weakness and paralysis in, 267
  rheumatoid arthritis and, 269
Cervical orthoses, 277, 277–278
Cervical radiculopathy, pain with, 261–266, *264–265*
Cervical spine, anatomy of, 255–258
  facet joints and, 256
  intervertebral disk and, 256
  joints of Luschka and, 256
  ligaments and, 257
  nerve roots and, 258
  periosteum and, 257
  spinal cord and, 257
  vertebrae and, 255–256, *256*
  vertebral artery and, 258
  physical examination of, 267–272
    compression-extension maneuver in, 269
    distraction-flexion maneuver in, 269
    functional state in, 272
    inspection of muscle in, 270
    joints in, 269
    loss of lordosis in, 268
    muscle strength in, 271
    muscle tone in, 270–271
    neurologic examination and, 269–270
    passive range of motion in, 268–269, 269(t)
    posture in, 267–268
    reflex testing in, 271–272
    sensory examination and, 271
    torticollis in, 268
Cervical spine lesions, clinical symptoms of, 258–267
  pain as, 258–266, 259(t)

Index 333

Cervical spine lesions *(Continued)*
  diagnostic studies of, 272–276
    electrodiagnostic testing in, 273–276
    electromyography in, 275–276
    motor nerve conduction studies in, 274
    radiologic studies in, 272–273
    sensory nerve conduction studies in, *264–265*, 274–275
    somatosensory evoked potentials in, 276
  lower extremity weakness and, 267
  management of, 276–285
    anti-inflammatory drugs in, 278
    conditioning exercises in, 284
    cryotherapy in, 281
    electrical stimulation in, 282–284
    heat treatments in, 280
    high-voltage galvanic stimulation in, 283–284
    immobilization in, 277, *277–278*
    iontophoresis in, 284
    muscle relaxants in, 278–279
    nerve blocks in, 279
    occupational therapy in, 284–285
    physical therapy in, 279–280
    range of motion exercises in, 284
    rest in, 277
    return to work and, 285
    specialist referrals in, 279
    traction in, 281–282
    transcutaneous electrical nerve stimulation in, 282–283
    vocational counseling in, 285
  posterior paravertebral muscle spasms with, 278–279
  upper extremity weakness and, 266–267
Cervical spondylosis, lower extremity weakness and paralysis in, 267
  pain with, 260–261, *261–263*
Character disorders, 291–292
Cheeks, physical examination of, 125
Chest x-rays, nasal pain diagnosis and, 111
China, pain theory in, 3–4
Chlamydia, conjunctivitis and, 91
Cholesteatomas, middle ear otalgia and, 65–66, *66*
Chronic pain, classification of, 16–17
  defined, 300–301
  economic impact of, 299–300, 300(t)
  head and neck syndromes and, 314–324
    glossopharyngeal neuralgia as, 321–324
    myofascial pain syndrome as, 315–318
    occipital headache as, 315
    postherpetic neuralgia as, 318–319
    trigeminal neuralgia as, 319, 321
  personality factors in, 313–314
  psychological aspects of, 312–313
  treatment modalities for, 305–312
    cryoanalgesia as, 311–312
    nerve blocks as, 305
    pharmacotherapy as, 306–310
    transcutaneous electrical nerve stimulation as, 310–311
Ciliary dysmotility syndromes, 107

Circulation, cerebral, analysis of, 15–16
Clenching, EMG recording of, 225, *227*. See also *Bruxism.*
Clicking, in temporomandibular joint disorders, 167–168
  reciprocal clicking, 167–168
Clonazepam, for trigeminal neuralgia, 32
  for vagoglossopharyngeal neuralgia, 37
Cluster headaches, onset and duration of, 12
  signs and symptoms of, 25
  sphenopalatine neuralgia and, 40–41
Cocaine test, for Raeder's syndrome, 43
  for vagoglossopharyngeal neuralgia, 37
Code of Hammurabi, 2–3
Cognitive therapy, 294
Collagen disease, otalgia and, 74–75
Compensation neurosis, pain in, 20
Compression-decompression surgery, for trigeminal neuralgia, 33–34
Compression-extension maneuver, with spinal examination, 269
Compulsive personality disorder, 291
Computed tomography (CT), cine, 195
  for laryngeal trauma, 144–145
  nasal pain diagnosis with, 110–111
  of cervical spine, *262*, 273
  oral cavity disease and, 126
  otalgia and, 57–58
  role in diagnosis, 15
  temporomandibular joint dysfunction and, 195, *195–196*
  three-dimensional, 195
Conditioning exercises, for neck pain, 284
Condyle, anatomy and physiology of, 154–158
  displacement of, diagnosis of, 189, *189–190*, 191–192
Confrontation fields examination, 78–79
Congenital cysts, neck pain with, 148–149
Congenital disorders, in nasal region, 107
Conjunctiva, 90–91, *91*
  examination of, 79
Contact dermatitis, on external ear, 59
Convergence, hyperopia and, 82
  insufficiency, 87–88
Convulsions, with vagoglossopharyngeal neuralgia, 36–37
Cornea, diseases of, 91–92
  examination of, 79
Coronoplasty, 225–228, *227*
Corynebacterium diphtheriae, 136
Crackling, in temporomandibular joint disorders, 168
Cranial nerves, evaluation for pain diagnosis, 132
  role in head and neck pain, 14
Craniomandibular disorders, anatomy and physiology of system, 154–162
  mandibular elevators and depressors in, 159–162, *160*
  musculoskeletal system and, 158, *158–162*
  temporomandibular joint and, 154–158, *155–156*

Craniomandibular disorders *(Continued)*
  clinical presentation of, 163
  defined, 153
  dental problems and, 115–116
  diagnostic evaluation of, 178–198
    bioelectronic measurement techniques in, 180–188
    imaging modalities in, 188–198
    mandibular function measurements in, 179–180
  extracapsular disorders, 153–154
    myofacial pain dysfunction syndrome, 198–206, 199(t)–200(t), 202(t), *205*
  interdisciplinary approach to, team diagnostic approach, 241–242
    treatment and referral coordination in, 242
  intracapsular disorders, 154, 206–210
    articular disk disorders in, 206
    inflammatory joint disease in, 208–209
    joint capsule disorders in, 207–208
    retrodiskal fiber disorders in, 206–207
    temporomandibular joint neoplasms in, 209–210
  patient history in, 162
  physical examination and, 163–178
    intraoral examination in, *171*, 171–176
    mandibular excursive movement in, 165–166, *166*
    muscle palpation in, 168–171, *169–170*
    observation of head in, 163, *164*
    occlusion instability in, *174–175*, 174–175
    opening and closing movements in, 163–165, *165*
    oral breathing in, 172–173, *173*
    summary of, 176–178, 177(t)–178(t), 179(t)
    temporomandibular joint examination in, *164*, 166–167
    temporomandibular joint sounds in, *164*, 167–168
  prognosis for, 240–241
  therapy for, 210–240
    evaluation of results and, 240
    musculoskeletal dysfunction and, 210–211
    neuromuscular approach in, 213–239
    repositioning appliances and, 211–213
    sequential approach to, 210
    variations in terminology and, 198
Crepitus, in temporomandibular joint disorders, 168
Cricoarytenoid joint arthritis, laryngeal inflammation and, 146–147
Cricopharyngeal spasm, 141
  hypopharyngeal pain and, 141
Crowns (dental), occlusion modification with, 235, *237*. See also *Coronoplasty*.
Cryotherapy, for chronic pain, 311–312
  for neck pain, 281
Conjunctival hyperemia, 79
Cystic lesions, in nasal region, 107, 113
  in oral cavity, 126

Da Vinci, Leonardo, 6–7
Dark Ages, pain theory in, 6–7
De Re Medicina, 5
Deep pain, in visceral organs, 9–10
Degenerative joint disease, temporomandibular joint and, 208
Denervation potentials, 276
Denial of illness, prevalent in head and neck pain, 19
Dental caries, as cause of pain, 116–117
  defective restorations of, 122
  treatment for, 122
Dental problems, atypical facial pain and, 45
  causes of, 116–118
  diagnostic procedures for, 120–121
  electronic tracking of, 188
  intraoral pain and, 115–116
  otalgia during, 74
  patient history and, 118–119
  physical examination and, 119–120
  prognosis for, 123–124
  symptoms of, 116
  treatment for, 121–123
Dental radiography, 120
  in oral cavity disease, 125–126
Dentists, psychiatrists and, 291
Dentures, healthy muscle function with, 235, *238*
Depression, atypical facial pain and, 45–46
  pain syndrome and, 20, 291
  with chronic pain, 311
    as precipitating or sequential factor, 312
Dermatomal sensory nerve innervation, *264–265*, 275
Dermatome chart, *264*, *265*
Developmental cysts, in nasal region, 107
Diabetes mellitus, external otitis and, 60–61
Digastric muscle, 161
Digital subtraction angiography, 15
Dilantin, for trigeminal neuralgia, 30, 321
  for vagoglossopharyngeal neuralgia, 37
Diphtheria, causes and treatment of, 136
Diplopia, hyperopia and, 82
Disk displacement and perforation, with arthrography, 193, *194*
  magnetic resonance imaging of, 196, *197*
Dissection, 3
Distraction-flexion maneuver, with spinal examination, 269
Dorsal horn, gate control theory and, 303–304
  pain transmission and, 302
Dorsal roots, function of, 258
Drug abuse, chronic pain therapy and, 17, 306
Drug therapy, for chronic pain, 306–310
  for pain, 16–17
  for trigeminal neuralgia, 30–32, 31t
  prescription, avoidance of, 23
Dura mater, 257
"Dural pain," with spinal cord injury, 261
Dyadic therapy (one-on-one), 294

Index

Eagle's syndrome, 71, 72
Ear, sensory innervation of, 53–54
  temporomandibular joint and, 171–172
Ear canal, otalgia and, 58–62
Ear, nose and throat (ENT) evaluation, 46
Ear pain. See *Otalgia*.
Economic impact of pain, 17–18
  chronic pain and, 299–300, 300(t)
  headaches and, 1
Ectropion, 89–90, *90*
Edwin Smith papyrus, 3
Egypt, pain theory in ancient times, 3
Elavil. See *Amitriptyline*.
Electric shock therapy, for pain syndrome, 295
Electrical stimulation, for neck pain, 282–284
Electrodes, used in electromyography, 183–184, *184*
Electrodiagnostic testing, of cervical spine, 273–276
Electroencephalograms (EEG), 15
Electromyography (EMG), clenching muscle action and, 225, *226*
  function testing with, 235, *238–239*
  mandibular function and, 182–186
    electrode placement in, 183, *184*
    muscle clenching activity in, 184, 185(t)
    position determination in, 220, *223*
    resting activity in, 184, 185(t)
  monitoring orthotic appliances with, *233*
  of cervical spine, 275–276
  role in TENS treatment, 214(t), 215–217, *217*
  temporalis and masseter muscle function and, 220, *221*
Electronystagmogram (ENG), mandibular function and, 186, *187*
Emotional factors in pain, 19–20
Endocrine alterations, nasal inflammations with, 103
Endodonture (root canal therapy), for periapical disease, 126
  for traumatized teeth, 121–122
Endogenous analgesia system, discovery of, 10–11
Endorphins, depletion of, and atypical facial pain, 46
  endogenous analgesia and, 10–11
Enkephalin, as endogenous analgesia, 11
Entropion, 89–90, *90*
Enzyme-linked immunosorbent assays (ELISA), 135
Epidemics (Hippocrates), 4–5
Epstein-Barr virus (EBV), 137
Equilibration, 225–228, *227*
Erasistratus of Cheor, 5
Erythema multiforme, 140
Esophageal candidiasis, hypopharyngeal pain with, 141, 143
Esophagus, cobblestoned appearance of, 143, *144*
Esotropia, 85, 85–86, *86*
Ethmoid pain, defined, 100
Ethmoid sinusitis, signs of, 109–110, *110*

Ethyl chloride, for myofascial pain syndrome, 317–318
  for postherpetic neuralgia, 39
Etidocaine, for myofascial pain syndrome, 317
Eustachian tube dysfunction, middle ear otalgia and, 65
Exophthalmos, 79
External ear, otalgia and, 58–62
External otitis (furunculosis), 60
  treatment of, 60–61
Extracapsular craniomandibular disorders, 198–206
  defined, 153–154
Eye examination, lid margins in, 78
  missing lashes in, 78
  optical system in, *80*, 80–81
Eye pain, background to, 77
  corneal foreign bodies and, 92
  nonocular conditions with, 96–97
  physical examination for, 77–80
Eyelids, 89–90, *90*

Face pain, classification of, 23–24, 24t
  rhinologic causes of, 99–114
Facet joint, anatomy of, 256
  arthropathy of, 266
Facial nerve, functional evaluation of, 14
Facial pain, atypical, 29, 44–46, 45t
  myofacial pain dysfunction and, 199, 199(t)
Family history, importance of, 2
Farsightedness (hyperopia), 81–82, *82*
Fiberoptic endoscopy, laryngeal trauma and, 144
"Five-joint complex," 260
Flexion-hyperextension injury. See *Whiplash injury*.
Fluoride, dental caries and, 116–117
Focal entrapment neuropathy, muscle atrophy and, 270
Foreign bodies, external ear and, 59–60
  hypopharyngeal pain and, 141–142, *142*
  in alveolar bone, 123
  in cornea, 92–93
  in tongue or tonsils, 140
  nasal inflammation from, 103, *104*
Fractured teeth, restoration of, 122
Free nerve endings, afferent pain pathways and, 8
Frontal sinusitis, treatment of, 112, *112*
Frostbite, on external ear, 59
Functional state testing, with spinal injury, 272
Fungal pharyngitis, 137
Furunculosis, 60
  treatment of, 60–61
Fusional reserve, muscular asthenopia and, 85

Galen, pain theories of, 5–6
Gallium-labeled metabolites, temporomandibular joint dysfunction and, 192

Gastrointestinal pain, cause of, 9
Gate control theory of pain, 9, 303–304
  TENS therapy and, 213
Geniculate neuralgia, 38
Geniohyoid muscle, 161
Germ theory of disease, 7
Glaucoma, 92–93
Glenoid fossa, 154
Glossopharyngeal nerve, oropharyngeal pain and, 132, 134, *134*
Glossopharyngeal nerve block, *322*, 322–323
Glossopharyngeal neuralgia. See *Vagoglossopharyngeal neuralgia.*
Glycerol instillation, for trigeminal neuralgia, 33–34
Goldscheider's pain theory, 8
Gradenigo's syndrome, 70–71
Gram-positive bacteria, middle ear otalgia and, 64
Greco-Roman pain theories, 4–6
Grisel's syndrome, neck pain with, 150

Habitual centric occlusion (HCO), in craniomandibular disorders, 165–166, *166*
  with myofacial pain dysfunction, 201–202
Halo devices, 277
Handedness, unilateral trigeminal neuralgia and, 29
Harvey, William, 7
Head pain. See also *Headache.*
  chronic pain syndromes of, 314–324
  ocular conditions with ocular findings and, 88–96
  ocular conditions without ocular findings and, 80–88
Head position, and craniomandibular disorders, 163, *164*
Headache. See also types of headaches, e.g., *Vascular headaches.*
  classification of, 23–24, 24t
  economic impact of, 1
  frequency, duration and severity of, 2
  location of, 2
  myofacial pain dysfunction and, 199, 199(t)
  occipital, 315
  onset and duration of, 12
  otogenic brain abscess and, 70
  pain-sensitive head structures and, 24–25
  patient history as diagnostic aid to, 12
  physical and psychological impact of, 1
Hearing loss, diagnostic tests for, 57
  middle ear otalgia and, 63–64
Heat therapy, contraindications for, 280
  for neck pain, 280
Hematoma, in external ear, 58
Hemophilus influenzae, inflammatory nasal lesions and, 102
  middle ear otalgia and, 64
Herophilus, 5
Herpangina, 137
Herpes simplex, association with trigeminal neuralgia, 28
  corneal lesions and, 92, *92*

Herpes zoster infection, in ocular region, 88–89, *89*
  postherpetic neuralgia and, 39–40, 318
Herpes zoster oticus, 39, 68–69
Herpetic esophagitis, 143
Herpetic gingivostomatitis, 136–137
Herpetic infection, laryngeal inflammation and, 146
Heterophoria, 85
  diagnosis of, 86, *87*
Heterotropia, 85
  diagnosis of, 86, *87*
High-voltage galvanic stimulation, for neck pain, 283–284
Hippocrates' pain theory, 4
History. See *Family history; Patient history.*
Hoarseness, laryngeal neoplasms and, 73, *74*
Hodgkin's lymphomas, oropharyngeal pain and, 141
Horner's syndrome, confusion with cluster headache, 25
  Raeder's syndrome and, 42–44
  vertebral artery compromise and, 266
Household bleach, ingestion of, 142
Humors, theory of, 4–5
Hyperalgesia, defined, 10
Hyperopia (farsightedness), 81–82, *82*
Hyperpathia, defined, 10
Hyperesthesia, defined, 10
Hypertension, Raeder's syndrome and, 42
Hypopharyngeal diverticula, 141
Hypopharyngeal pain, 141–144
  infectious causes of, 143, *144*
Hypothyroidism, nasal inflammation with, 103
Hysteria, chronic pain and, 20
Hysterical conversion syndrome, atypical facial pain and, 45
Hysterical personality disorder, 291

Idiopathic nasal lesions, 109
Imhotep, 3
Immobilization for neck and arm pain, 277, 277–278
Immunoglobulin E, allergic rhinitis and, 103
Impacted teeth, 118
  signs of, 119
  treatment for, 122–123
Impedance audiometry, 57
India, pain theory in, 3
Infectious arthritis, temporomandibular joint and, 208
Infectious mononucleosis, pharyngitis with, 137
Inflammation, of external ear, 60
Inflammatory lesions, nasal pain from, *102*, 102–105
Innervation, of larynx, 144
Interchange therapies, 294
Intercuspal position (ICP), in craniomandibular disorders, 165–166, *166*
  with myofacial pain dysfunction, 201–202
Interspinous ligaments, 257
Intervertebral disk, anatomy of, 256
  herniation of, 260

Index

Intracapsular temporomandibular joint disorders, 206–210
   articular disk disorders and, 206
   defined, 154
   inflammatory joint disease and, 208–209
   joint capsule disorders and, 207–208
   retrodiskal fiber disorders and, 206–207
Intracranial lesions, headaches from, 25
Intranasal defects, sphenopalatine neuralgia and, 40–41, 73
Intraoral examination, in craniomandibular disorders, *171*, 171–176
   summary of, 176–178, 177(t)-179(t)
Iontophoresis, for neck pain, 284

Jawlash, tooth trauma and, 118
   with retrodiskal fiber disorders, 206–207
Joint capsule disorders, 207–208
Joints, physical examination of, 269
Joints of Luschka, 256

Kartagener's syndrome, 107
Klebsiella ozaenae, nasal lesions from, 109

Laminae, pain transmission with, 302
Laryngeal carcinoma, vagoglossopharyngeal neuralgia and, 35
Laryngeal pain, 144–147
   carcinomas as cause of, 147
   inflammation and, 145–147
   innervation and, 144
   neuralgia and, 145
   trauma and, 144, *145*
Laryngeal tuberculosis, 145–146
Laryngitis, 145
Laryngocele, laryngeal inflammation and, 147
Larynx, neoplastic lesions in, 73, *74*
Latency, in cervical spine, 274, *275*
Leprosy, laryngeal inflammation and, 146
Librium, for depression-related facial pain, 45–46
   for pain syndrome, 296
Lifestyle habits, role in pain diagnosis, 12
Ligamenta flava, 257
Ligaments, anatomy of, 257
   lesions of, 259
Light sensitivity, in migraine, 96
Lithium carbonate, for chronic pain syndrome, 296
Long-term therapy, for craniomandibular disorders, 234–240
Longitudinal fracture, temporal bone, 68
Longitudinal ligaments, anterior and posterior, 257
Lordosis, loss of, 268
Lower extremity weakness, with spinal cord lesions, 267
Lumbar puncture, 15
Lymphadenitis, 148
Lymphangioma, 149, *149*
Lymphatic system, role in TENS therapy, 213–214

Madison scale of pain evaluation, 19–20
Magendie, E., 7
Magnetic resonance imaging (MRI), mandibular muscle physiology and, 162
   nasal pain diagnosis and, 111
   of cervical spine, 262, 273
   oral cavity disease and, 126
   otalgia and, 57–58
   role in diagnosis, 15
   temporomandibular joint dysfunction and, 196–198, *197*
Malignant external otitis, 61, *61*
Malignant intranasal neoplasms, 106–107
Malocclusion, role in myofacial pain dysfunction, 203–204
Mandible, palpation and examination of, *170*, 171
   rest position with myofacial pain dysfunction, 202, 202(t)
   structure and function of, 156–157
Mandibular elevators and depressors, 159–162, *160*
Mandibular excursive movements, in craniomandibular disorders, 165–166, *166*
Mandibular function, bioelectric measurement techniques of, 180–188
   electromyography and, 182–186, *184*, 185(t)
   mandibular tracking and, 180–182, *181*, *183*
   significance of electronic testing in, 186–188, *187*
   mechanical measurement of, 179–180
Mandibular kinesiograph (MKG), 180–182, *181*
   for craniomandibular disorders, 165, *165*
   mandibular rest position determination and, 220, *223*
   mandibular tracking for long-term therapy and, 235, *237*
   schematic representation of, *182–183*
   TENS therapy and, 215, 217, *217*
   and neuromuscular occlusion, 218–220, *219*
   rest position in, 215, *217*, 222–224
Mandibular-malleolar ligament, 75
Mandibular posture, 158–159
Mandibular repositioning, orthotic appliances for, 211–213
   sequential therapy with, 210
Mandibular tracking, 180–182, *181*
   for long-term therapy, 235, *237*
Marcus-Gunn phenomenon, optic nerve inflammation and, 94
   pupil dilatation and, 78
Masochistic personality disorder, 291–292
Masseter muscle, anatomy and physiology of, 159–160
   electromyographic measurement of, 184
   function at rest, 220, *222*
   function in clenching, 220, *221*
   palpation in craniomandibular disorder examination, 168, *169*
   relationship to temporalis muscle, 220, *224*
Masticatory muscles, *158*, 158–163, *160*
Mastoid cavity infections, 61–62
Mastoidectomy, canal down "radical," 61–62

Mastoiditis, *69*, 69–70
  chronic, 65–66
  temporal bone neoplasms and, *70*, 70–71
Maxillary sinusitis, 100–101
  oral pain as sign of, 119
Mechanical measurement, of mandibular function, 179–180
Mechanical traction devices, 281
Meissner's and pacinian corpuscles, afferent pain pathways and, 8
Mellaril, for chronic pain syndrome, 295–296
Mephensin carbamate, 31
Microvascular decompression, for trigeminal neuralgia, 34–35
Microwave diathermy, 280
Middle ear, examination of, 56
  otalgia in, 63–67
Migraine headaches, causes of, 9
  hereditary heritage of, 2
  ocular symptoms and, 96
  onset and duration of, 12
  ophthalmoplegic, 96
Miltown, for pain syndrome, 296
Minnesota Multiphasic Personality Inventory (MMPI), 314
Mixed dentition, in craniomandibular disorders, 173–174, *174*
Monoamine oxidase inhibitors, for pain syndrome, 296–297
Mononeuritis, muscle atrophy and, 270
Motor nerve conduction studies, in cervical spine, 274
Motorized traction devices, 281
Mouth breathing, in craniomandibular disorders, 172–173, *173*
Mouth opening, lateral deviations in, *164*, 164
Mucosal disorders, nasal inflammation with, 104–105
Mucous membrane, evaluation of, 132
  of frontal sinus, 100
Multidisciplinary approach to pain, importance of, in head and neck pain, 12
  pain clinics and, 301–302
Multiple sclerosis, optic nerve inflammation and, 94
  trigeminal neuralgia and, 28–29
Muscle atrophy, in cervical spine lesions, 270
Muscle contraction headache, signs and symptoms of, 25
Muscle palpation, in craniomandibular disorder examination, 168–171, *169–170*
Muscle relaxants, for neck pain, 278–279
Muscle splinting, for joint capsule disorders, 208
  for myofacial pain dysfunction, 204, *205*
Muscle strength testing, in spinal cord lesions, 271
Muscles of mastication, *158*, 158–163, *160*
Muscular asthenopia, *85*, 85–87, *86*
Muscular kinesiography, monitoring orthotic appliances with, *232*–233
  of vertical freeway space, *231*
Musculoskeletal dysfunction, electromyography and, 183, *184*

Musculoskeletal dysfunction *(Continued)*
  prognosis for, 240, 241(t)
  therapy for, 210–211
Musculoskeletal system, anatomy and physiology of, *158*, 158–162
Mycotic infections, laryngeal inflammation and, 146
Myeloradiculopathy. See *Cervical myeloradiculopathy.*
Mylohyoid muscle, 161
  palpation of, in craniomandibular disorder examination, 168, *169*
Myo-monitor, 214
  TENS function-clench test and, natural occlusion in, 220, *221*
  neuromuscular occlusion in, 220, *221*
Myofacial pain dysfunction, 198–206
  chronic pain with, 315–318
  coordination of therapy and referral in, 242
  defined, 154
  diagnosis of, 172
    criteria for, 316
  electronic tracking of, 186, *187*
  etiology of, 201–206
    dental occlusal position in, 201–202
    mandible resting position in, 202, 202(t)
    nasal obstruction in, 202–203
    perpetuating factors in, 204–206
    precipitating factors in, 204
    predispositions for, 203–204
  long-term therapy for, 234–240
  muscle tenderness in, 270
  otalgia and, 75
  sequential therapy for, 210
  symptoms of, 199–201, 199(t)–200(t)
    dysfunctional symptoms as, 199–201
    painful symptoms as, 199
    self-destructing dentition and, 201
  trigger areas for, 316–317
    treatment at, 317–318
Myopia, 83, *84*
Myringotomy, middle ear otalgia and, 64

Naloxone, endogenous analgesia reversal and, 10
  placebo effect and, 11
Narcissistic disorders, 291
Narcotic analgesics, 308, 310(t)–311(t). See also *Addiction.*
  role in pain therapy, 17
  synthetic analgesics, 17
Nardil, for depression-related facial pain, 45
Nasal cysts, 113
Nasal discharge culture, nasal pain diagnosis and, 111–112
Nasal obstruction, with myofacial pain dysfunction, 202–203
Nasal pain, etiology of, 101–109
  congenital and developmental lesions in, 107, *107*
  idiopathic lesions in, 109
  inflammatory lesions in, 102–105

Index 339

Nasal pain *(Continued)*
  etiology of, neoplasms in, 105–107, *106*
    neurologic lesions in, 108–109
    trauma and, 107–108, *108*
  neuroanatomy and, 99–101
  patient evaluation for, 109–112, *110–111*
  treatment of, *112*, 112–114
Nasopharyngoscope, cavity examination with, 132
Natural dentition, TENS function-clench test and, 226
Neck pain, 148–151. See also *Cervical spine lesions.*
  chronic pain syndromes of, 314–324
  in cervical radiculopathy, 262–266, *264–265*
  in facet joint arthropathy, 266
  in spinal cord injury, 261–262
  in vertebral artery compromise, 266
  management of, anti-inflammatory drugs in, 278
    conditioning exercises in, 284
    cryotherapy in, 281
    electrical stimulation in, 282–284
    heat in, 280
    immobilization in, 277, 277–278
    muscle relaxants in, 278–279
    nerve blocks in, 279
    occupational therapy in, 284–285
    physical therapy in, 279–280
    range of motion exercises in, 284
    return to work and, 285
    specialist referrals in, 279
    traction in, 281–282
    vocational counseling in, 285
    with rest, 277
  physical and psychological impact of, 1
  with cervical spine lesions, 258–259, 259(t)
  with cervical spondylosis, 260–261, *261–263*
Necrotizing sialometaplasia, 105
Neoplasms, ear examination and, 57
  hypopharyngeal pain and, 142–143, *143*
  in middle ear, 66, *67*
  in oral cavity, 126–127
  incidence of trigeminal neuralgia and, 29
  laryngeal, 147
  of nasal region, 105–107, *106*
    diagnosis and, 110, *110–111*
    treatment of, 113
  oropharyngeal pain and, 140–141
  Raeder's syndrome and, 42
  temporal bone, *70*, 70–71
  temporomandibular joint, 209
Nerve blocks, for chronic pain, 305
  for postherpetic neuralgia, 318
  for trigeminal neuralgia, 321
  glossopharyngeal, *322*, 322–323
  occipital, 315, *316*
  sphenopalatine ganglion, *323*, 323–324
Nerve root, anatomy of, 258
  compression of, 260
Nervous system, autonomic, anatomy of, *323*, 323–324
  nose structure and, 100
Nervus intermedius neuralgia, 38

Network therapy, 294
Neuralgias, classification of, 26–44
  nervus intermedius (geniculate neuralgia) in, 38
  occipital neuralgia in, 41, 42t
  postherpetic neuralgia in, 38–40
  Raeder's paratrigeminal syndrome in, 41–44, 43t
  reflex sympathetic dystrophy (causalgia) in, 44
  sphenopalatine neuralgia in, 40–41
  trigeminal neuralgia in, 26–35
  vagoglossopharyngeal neuralgia in, 35–38
  laryngeal pain and, 145
Neuroanatomy, nose structure and, 99–101
Neurodermatitis, 59
Neuroendocrinology, 10–11
Neurogenic tumors, in nasal region, 106
Neurologic examination, of cranial nerve function, 14
  with cervical spine lesions, 269–270
Neurologic lesions, nasal pain and, 108–109
Neurologic perspective on pain, 7–11
Neuromuscular occlusion, establishment of, 225–229
  coronoplasty and, 225–228, *227*
  long-term modification of, 234–240
Neuromuscular pain, in neck, 150
Neuromuscular therapy, for craniomandibular disorders, 213–239
  coronoplasty as, 225–228
  neuromuscular occlusion as, *217*, 218–229
  orthotic appliances as, 228–229, *230–233*
  transcutaneous electrical neural stimulation (TENS) as, 213–218
Neuromuscular trajectory of movement, TENS therapy and, 215, *217*
Neurotransmitters, pain transmission and, 303
Nickel exposure, nasal neoplasms from, 106–107
Nociception, pain transmission and, 302
  gate control theory and, 303
Nonbenzodiazepine, for pain syndrome, 296
Noninfectious pharyngitis, 137–138
Nonpurulent middle ear effusion, otalgia and, 64
Nonsteroidal anti-inflammatory agents (NSAIDs), for chronic pain, 306–308, 307(t), *309*
  for craniomandibular disorders, 211
  for neck pain, 278
  gastrointestinal bleeding with, 307
  role in pain therapy, 17
Norpramin, for pain syndrome, 297
Nuprin Pain Report, 299–300, 300(t)
Nystagmus, middle ear otalgia and, 66

Occipital headache, 315
Occipital nerve block, 315, *316*
Occipital neuralgia, 41, 42t
Occipitoatlantal articulation, 268–269, 269(t)
Occlusion, habitual centric (HCO), 165–166, *166*
  in craniomandibular disorders, examination of, *171*, 171–176, *173*
  instability of, 174–175, *175*

Occlusion *(Continued)*
  electromyographic measurement of, 184
  long-term modification of, 234–240
  neuromuscular, coronoplasty and, 226–228, *227*
  normal, 215, *217*
  otalgia and, 75
  position changes with MPD, 201–202
  reduced vertical dimension of, 171
  role in myofacial pain dysfunction, 203–204
Occupational therapy, for cervical spine lesion patients, 284–285
Ocular pain. See *Eye pain.*
Oculomotor nerve, functional evaluation of, 14
Olfactory nerve, testing of, 14
Opening and closing movements, craniomandibular disorders and, 163–165, *165*
Ophthalmoplegic migraine, 96
Ophthalmoscopy, for eye pain, 79–80
Opiate receptors, pain transmission and, 303
Opioids, effects of, 308, 310
  endogenous, analgesic effects of, 10–11
    released with TENS therapy, 310–311
Opium, alkaloids and derivatives of, 17
  for chronic pain relief, 308
Optic nerve, functional evaluation of, 14
  inflammation of, 94
Optics, *80,* 80–81
Oral cavity, examination of, in pain diagnosis, 132, *133*
  soft and hard tissue disease in, 124–127
Oral pain, 112–127
  dental problems and, 116–124
    causes of, 116–117
    diagnostic measures for, 120–121
    patient history in, 118–119
    physical examination and, 119–120
    prognosis for, 123–124
    symptoms of, 116
    treatment methods for, 121–123
  oropharyngeal pain and, 132–141
  soft and hard tissue disease and, 124–127
    causes of, 124
    diagnostic measures and, 125–126
    patient history in, 124–125
    physical examination and, 125
    prognosis for, 127
    symptoms of, 124
    treatment for, 126–127
Orbital cellulitis, ethmoid sinusitis and, *110*
Orbital disease, 95, 95–96
Orbital examination, nasal pain diagnosis and, 109–110
Oropharyngeal gonorrhea, 136
Oropharyngeal pain, 132–141
  neoplastic causes of, 140–141
Orthotic appliances, mandibular repositioning with, 211–213
  monitoring effectiveness of, 229, 231(t)–232(t), 232–233
  neuromuscular occlusion and, 228–229, *230–233*
Osteomas, in nasal region, 106
Osteophytes, in cervical spondylosis, 260, *261–262*

Otalgia, causes of, 53–55, 54t
  diagnosis of, 53–54
  tests for, 57–58
  disease as cause of, 55
  in craniomandibular disorders, 166–167
  myofacial pain dysfunction and, 199, 199(t)
  nonotogenic causes of, 71–76
  otogenic causes of, 58–71
    external ear and ear canal in, 58–62
    middle ear in, 63–67
    temporal bone (mastoid and inner ear) in, 68–71
    tympanic membrane in, 62–63
  psychogenic causes of, 75–76
  tube patency and function in, 57
Otitis, external, 60
  treatment of, 60–61
Otitis media, chronic, 65–66
  middle ear and, 63
Otoscopy, 62
  chronic ear disease and, 66

Pacinian corpuscles, afferent pain pathways and, 8
Pain. See also specific types of pain, e.g., *Neck pain.*
  acute vs. chronic, 300–301
  as psychobiologic phenomenon, 131–132
  associated with trigeminal neuralgia, 30
  chronic. See *Chronic pain.*
  clinical perspective on, 11–16
  clinical types of, 9–10
  defined, 299
  economic impact of, 17–18
    chronic pain and, 299–300, 300(t)
  gate control theory of, 303–304
  historical perspectives on, 2–7
  neurologic perspectives on, 7–11
  neurophysiology of, 9
  pharmocologic management of, 16–17
  psychiatric aspects of, 18–20, 287–297
  transmission of, anatomy and physiology of, 302–303
Pain clinic, development of, 301(t), 301–302
  referrals to, 279
Pain syndrome, defined, 300–301
  psychiatric consultation and, 287–291
  secondary effects of, 292–293
  treatment modalities for, 293–297
Palate, physical examination of, 125
Panoramic dental x-rays, temporomandibular joint function and, 189, *191*
Papillomas, in nasal region, 106
Paralysis, flaccid, 270–271
  with spinal cord lesions, 267
Paranoid schizophrenics, 290
Parapharyngeal space infection, 138
Paré, Ambrose, 7
Paredrine, for Raeder's syndrome, 43
Paresis of accommodation, 84
Parkinsonlike syndrome, 295

Passive range of motion, 268–269, 269(t)
Patient history, craniomandibular disorders and, 162
　eye pain and, 77–78
　for dental problem diagnosis, 118–119
　for otalgia, 55
　importance of, 2
　nasal pain diagnosis and, 109–112
　oral cavity disease (soft and hard tissue) and, 124–125
　physical appearance of patient and, 14
　psychiatric consultation for, 287–291
　role in pain diagnosis, 12, 131–132
Pemphigoid, 91
Pemphigus, nasal inflammation with, 104–105
　oropharyngeal pain with, 139–140
　treatment of, 126–127
Penicillin G, for streptococcal pharyngitis, 135
Perception of pain, 1
Percussion, of sensitive teeth, 120
Percutaneous stereotaxic rhizotomy, for trigeminal neuralgia, 34–35
Periapical disease, root canal therapy for, 126
Perichondritis, 59
Periodontal pain, causes of, 117
　treatment for, 123
Periodontal surgery, 126. See also *Endodonture.*
Periosteum, anatomy of, 257
Peripheral polyneuropathy, muscle atrophy and, 270
Peritonsillar space infection, 138–139
Personality factors. See also *Affective disorders; Character disorders; Narcissistic disorders.*
　in chronic pain, 313–314
Phantom pain, defined, 10
　with spinal cord injury, 261
Pharmacotherapy. See *Drug therapy.*
Pharyngitis, 135–139
　bacterial, 135–136
　fungal, 137
　noninfectious, 137–138
　viral, 136–137
Phenothiazine, for chronic pain, 310
　for pain syndrome, 295
　for postherpetic neuralgia, 39
Philadelphia collar, 278
Physical examination, craniomandibular disorders and, 163–178
　　intraoral examination in, *171*, 171–176, *173*
　　mandibular excursive movements in, 165–166, *166*
　　muscle palpation in, 168–171, *169–170*
　　observation of head in, 163, *164*
　　opening and closing movements in, 163–165, *165*
　　summary of, 176–178, 177(t)-179(t)
　　temporomandibular joint examination in, *164*, 166–167
　　temporomandibular joint sounds in, *164*, 167–168
　eye pain and, 77–80
　for dental problems, 119–120

Physical examination *(Continued)*
　for otalgia, 74–75
　importance of, 2–3
　nasal pain diagnosis, 109–112
　of cervical spine, 267–272
　of ear, 55–57
　oral cavity disease (soft and hard tissue), 125
　role in pain diagnosis, 131–132
　with trigeminal neuralgia, 30
Physical therapy, for neck pain, 279–280
Physician's attitude toward pain, 18–19
Pia mater, 257
Pinto's ligament, 157
Placebo effect, 11
Plain skull films, importance of, 15
Plato, 5
Pneumatic otoscopy, 56, *56*
Positron emission tomography, 16
Postherpetic neuralgia, 38–40
　chronic pain with, 318–319
　cryoanalgesia for, 310–311
　oropharyngeal pain with, 135
Posture, craniomandibular disorders and, 163, *164*
　examination of, during spine injury, 267–268
　mandibular, 158–159
　role in myofacial pain dysfunction, 204–206
Pregnancy, nasal inflammation with, 103
Presbyopia, 82–83
Primary pain, defined, 70
Procaine block, for postherpetic neuralgia, 39
Prognostic blocks, for chronic pain, 305
Prostaglandins, aspirin synthesis and, 306
Provider-patient interactions, chronic pain and, 313
Pseudomonas, external otitis and, 60–61
Psychiatric aspects of pain, 287–297
　goals of consultation in, 289–292
　historical perspective on, 287–288
　referrals and, 288–289
　treatment recommendations and implementation in, 293–297
　　antipsychotic agents as, 295–297
　　psychosocial treatments as, 293–295
　　somatic therapies as, 295
Psychobiological perspectives on pain, 18–20
Psychodynamic-psychoanalytic therapy, 294
Psychological factors in pain, 1–2
　in asthenopia, 84
　in atypical facial pain, 45
　in chronic pain, 312–314
　in craniomandibular disorders, 162
　of otalgia, 75–76
　role in myofacial pain dysfunction, 204
　with trigeminal neuralgia, 30
Psychological pain, 19–20. See also *Phantom pain.*
Psychosocial treatment for pain syndrome, 293–295
Psychotherapy, time limits on, 294–295
Psychotropic drugs, for postherpetic neuralgia, 39
Pterygoid muscles, dysfunction in, 166
　lateral, 161
　　not measured by electromyography, 183
　　palpation of, in craniomandibular disorder examination, 168, *169*

Pterygoid muscles *(Continued)*
  medial, 160–161
    palpation of, in craniomandibular disorder examination, 168, *169*
Ptosis, 79
Pulp vitality, electrical testing for, 120
Pulpal hyperemia, dental treatment as cause of, 117–118
Pulpal necrosis, in tooth fractures, 117
Punishment, perception of pain as, 18
Pupil size and contractility, eye pain and, 78
Pythagoras, 4

Radiofrequency heating, for trigeminal neuralgia, 33–34
Radiographic imaging, dental, 120, 125–126
  in nasal pain diagnosis, 110
  of cervical spine, 272–273
  otalgia and, 57–58
  temporomandibular joint disorders and, 188
Radionuclide scanning, temporomandibular joint function and, 192, *193*
Raeder's paratrigeminal neuralgia, 41–44, 43t
  confusion of, with cluster headache, 25
  etiology of, 42
  Horner's syndrome and, 42–44
  trigeminal nerve involvement in, 43
Ramsay-Hunt syndrome, 39
  etiology of, 68–69
Range of motion exercises, for neck pain, 284
  passive, 268–269, 269(t)
Reciprocal clicking, temporomandibular joint disorders and, 167–168
Referrals. See also *Multidisciplinary approach to pain.*
  for neck pain relief, 279
  psychiatric, 288–289
Referred pain, defined, 70
Reflex esophagitis, 137
Reflex sympathetic dystrophy, 44
  pain associated with, 304–305
  skin tenderness and, 270
Reflex testing, in spinal cord lesions, 271–272
Remodeling, of temporomandibular joint, 157–158
Renaissance, pain theory in, 6–7
Rest, for dental problems, 121
  for neck and arm pain, 277
Retinitis, 93–94, *94*
Retrodiskal fiber disorders, 206–207
  pseudodisk creation with, 212
Retropharyngeal space infections, 138
Returning to work, after spinal injury, 285
Rheumatoid arthritis, joint examination for, 269
  laryngeal inflammation and, 147
  temporomandibular joint, 208–209
Rhinitis, allergic, 103
  treatment of, 113
  atrophic, 109
    treatment of, 114
  vasomotor, nasal lesions from, 109

Rhinitis medicamentosa, 103
  treatment of, 113
Rhinoscleroma, 102–103, *103*
  laryngeal inflammation and, 146, *146*
Rinne tests, middle ear otalgia and, 65
Root canal therapy. See *Endodenture.*
Ruffini end-organs, afferent pain pathways and, 8

Saddle nose deformity, 104, *105*
Salivary gland pain, 150
Salivary gland tumors, oropharyngeal pain and, 141
Sarcoidosis, nasal inflammation with, 104
  treatment of, 113
Schizophrenic disorders, pain syndromes in, 290
Sclera, inflammation of, 95
Secondary gain, from chronic pain, 313
Self-destructing dentition, myofacial pain dysfunction and, 201
Sensor array, mandibular function measurement and, 180, *181*
Sensory examination, in spinal cord lesions, 271
Sensory innervation, nose pain and, 100
Sensory nerve conduction studies, in cervical spine, 264–265, 274–275
Sequential therapy, for craniomandibular disorders, 210
Serial tomography. See also *Computed tomography.*
  temporomandibular joint function and, 190–191, *192*
Serognathograph, 180
Serotonin-agonists, pain control and, 11
Sex ratios, incidence of trigeminal neuralgia and, 28–29
Shortwave diathermy, 280
Single plane radiography, temporomandibular joint function, 189–190
Sinus of Morgagni syndrome, 73–74
Sinus pain, etiology of, 101–109
  frontal pain and, 100–101
  post-surgical, 108
Sinusitis, ethmoid, signs of, 109–110, *110*
  maxillary, 100–101
    oral pain as sign of, 119
Sjögren's syndrome, nasal inflammation with, 104
  treatment of, 113
Skeletal pain, ischemic cause of, 9
Skin, in ocular region, 88–89
  pain in, 9
Sluder's neuralgia. See *Sphenopalatine neuralgia.*
Sodium valproate, for trigeminal neuralgia, 32
Soft collar, 278
Soft tissue examination, with arthrography, 193, *194*
  with computed tomography, 195
Soft tissue shadow, pharyngeal, 138, *139*
Somatic therapy, for pain syndrome, 295
Somatization disorder, with chronic pain, 312–313
Somatosensory evoked potentials, in cervical spine, 276
  spinal cord lesions and, 267

Index

SOMI (Sterno-Occipital-Mandibular-Immobilizer), 277–278
Sore, canker, pharyngitis with, 138, *138*
Sore throat. See *Pharyngitis.*
Space infection, lymphangioma as, 149, *149*
  oropharyngeal pain with, 138–139
Spasticity, with spinal cord lesions, 270–271
Sphenoid pain, defined, 100
Sphenopalatine ganglion, nerve block of, *323,* 323–324
Sphenopalatine neuralgia, 40–41
  nasal lesions and, 108–109
  nasal pain with, 113–114
  otalgia in, 71, 73
Spinal cord, anatomy of, 257
  compression of, in cervical spondylosis, 260, *261–262*
  injury to, pain with, 261
Spinal reflex, sympathetic pain and, *304,* 304–305
"Spinal shock phase" of spine injury, 270
Squamous cell carcinomas, hypopharyngeal pain and, 142–143, *143*
  oropharyngeal pain and, 140–141
Staphylococcus aureus, 60, 102
Stelazine, for pain syndrome, 295
Stellate ganglion block, for postherpetic neuralgia, 319, *320*
  for reflex sympathetic dystrophy, 305
Sternocleidomastoid muscle, in craniomandibular disorders, *170,* 170
Steroids, eye damage from, 94
  for chronic pain, 310
  for postherpetic neuralgia, 39, 319
Stevens-Johnson syndrome, 91, 104–105
Stilbamine, trigeminal neuralgia therapy with, 30–31
Streptococcal pharyngitis, 135–136
Streptococcus pneumoniae, 102
Stress, analgesia and hyperalgesia, 11
Stylohyoid muscle, 161
  in craniomandibular disorders, *170,* 171
Styloid process pain, in glossopharyngeal neuralgia, 70
  oropharyngeal pain and, 140
Subarachnoid space, in spinal cord, 257
Subdural space, in spinal cord, 257
Substantia gelatinosa, pain transmission and, 303
Supine or sitting traction, 282
Suprahyoid muscles, 161
Surgical therapy, for dental problems, 123
  for postherpetic neuralgia, 39–40
  for temporomandibular joint disorders, 212–213
  for trigeminal neuralgia, 33(t), 33–35
  for vagoglossopharyngeal neuralgia, 37–38
Sweetness sensitivity, in teeth, 119
Swinging light test, 78
Sympathetic nerve blocks, for postherpetic neuralgia, 318–319
  for reflex sympathetic dystrophy, 305
Sympathetic pain, spinal reflexes and, *304,* 304–305
Syncope, with vagoglossopharyngeal neuralgia, 36–37

Synovial joints, structure and function of, 154–156
Syphilis, laryngeal inflammation and, 146
  pupil size and, 78

Talking therapies, 293–294
Tardive dyskinesia, 295
Team approach, to craniomandibular disorders, 241–242
Tear film abnormalities, 89–90
Technetium-labeled metabolites, temporomandibular joint dysfunction and, 192
Teeth. See also *Dental problems.*
  destruction of, with myofacial pain dysfunction, 201
  exfoliating primary, 118
  fractured, therapy for, 121–122
  impacted, 118
  in craniomandibular disorders, 172–173, *173*
    crowded, spread, or loose teeth in, 175–176
    missing posterior teeth in, 172–173, *174*
    occlusion instability and, 174–175, *175*
  sensitive, percussion of, 120
Temperature sensitivity, in teeth, as sign of dental problems, 116
  pulpal vitality and, 119
Temporal arteritis, otalgia and, 74–75
Temporal bone (mastoid and inner ear) fracture, 68–71
  otalgia in, 68–71
Temporalis muscle, anatomy and physiology of, 159
  dominance over masseter, 220, *224*
  electromyographic measurement of, 184–186
  function at rest, 220, *222*
  function in clenching, 220, *221*
  in craniomandibular disorders, 169–170
Temporomandibular joint, anatomy and physiology of, 154–158, *155–156*
  arthrography of, 192–194
  computed tomography of, *195,* 195–196
  development of, 157–158
  dysfunction of, tooth trauma and, 118
  ear and, 171–172
  imaging modalities for, 188–198
    transcranial radiographs and, 188–192, *189–190*
  inflammatory diseases of, 208–209
  magnetic resonance imaging of, 196–198, *197*
  otalgia and, 75
  pain presentation in, 163
  physical examination of, *164,* 166–167
  prognosis for, 240–241
  radionuclide scanning of, 192, *193*
  sounds of, *164,* 167–168
Tendon reflexes, deep, in spinal cord lesions, 271
Tenon's capsule, 94
TENS. See *Transcutaneous electrical nerve stimulation.*
Tensor tympani muscle, 157
Tensor veli palatini muscle, 157
Thalamic pain levels, 8
Thalamus, pain transmission from, 302

Therapeutic nerve blocks, 305
Thoracic outlet syndrome, 151
Thorazine, for pain syndrome, 295
Thyroglossal duct cysts, 149–150
Thyroid disease, orbital disease and, 95, 95–96
Thyroiditis, neck pain with, 150
Tic doulourex, 27. See also *Trigeminal neuralgia.*
Timolol, for corneal disease, 93
"Tincture of time," as treatment for otalgia, 62–63
Tizanidine, for trigeminal neuralgia, 32
Tocainide, for trigeminal neuralgia, 32
Tofranil, for pain syndrome, 297
Tolerance of pain, 19
Tongue, condition of, in craniomandibular disorders, 172–173, *173*
　mobility of, as diagnostic aid, 132, *133*
　physical examination of, 125
　positioning of, for MPD alleviation, 205
Tonsillectomy, middle ear otalgia and, 64
　vagoglossopharyngeal neuralgia associated with, 35
Tooth fractures, as cause of pain, 117
Torticollis, 268
　neck pain with, 150
Tract of Lissauer, afferent pain pathways and, 8
Traction, contraindications for, 281–282
　for cervical spine, 281–282
Transcranial radiography, 188–192, *189–190*
　cephalometric tracings, 235, *236*
Transcutaneous electrical nerve stimulation (TENS)
　contraindications for, 283
　electrode placement during, 214, *216*
　electromyographic measurements and, 214(t)
　for chronic pain, 310–311
　for craniomandibular disorders, 213–218
　for myofacial pain syndrome, 318
　for neck pain, 282–283
　for postherpetic neuralgia, 39
　neuromuscular occlusion and, *217–218*, 218–225
　mandibular function diagnosis and, 186
　　before and after results, *187*
　modes of, commonly used, 282–283
　sequential therapy with, 210
　spectral analysis, 214, *215*
Transillumination, for dental problems, 120
Transverse fracture, of temporal bone, 68
Trapezius muscle, in craniomandibular disorders, *170*, 170–171
Trauma, cervical spine injuries and, 267
　in oral cavity, 124
　nasal and facial pain from, 107–108, *108*
　　treatment of, 113
　oropharyngeal pain with, 140
　Raeder's syndrome and, 42
　specialist referrals for, 279
　temporomandibular joint and, 209–210
　to larynx, 144–145, *145*
　to teeth, 117, 118–119
Traumatic arthritis, in temporomandibular joint, 208
"Trench mouth." See *Vincent's angina.*
Triadic (couples) therapy, 294

Tricyclic antidepressants (TCAs), for chronic pain, 308, 310
　for depression-related facial pain, 46
　for pain syndrome, 296–297
　for postherpetic neuralgia, 319
Trigeminal nerve, functional evaluation of, 14
　involvement in Raeder's syndrome, 43
　maxillary division of, 100, *101*
　nasociliary branch of, 100
　role in TENS therapy, 214, *216*
Trigeminal neuralgia, age and sex factors for, 28–29
　atypical. See *Sphenopalatine neuralgia.*
　chronic pain syndrome with, 319, 321
　classification of, 26–35
　herpes simplex virus associated with, 28
　historical background on, 26–27
　incidence of, 29
　medical therapy for, 30–33, 31(t)
　otalgia during, 73–74
　pathology of, 27(t), 27–28
　psychodynamic factors in, 30
　risk factors for, 28–29
　signs and symptoms of, 30
　surgical therapy for, 32–35, 33t
　tumor incidence and, 29
　unilaterality of, 29
Trochlear nerve, functional evaluation of, 14
Trotter's syndrome, otalgia during, 73–74
Tuberculosis, laryngeal, 145–146
Tumors. See *Neoplasms.*
Tuning forks, middle ear otalgia and, 64
Tympanic membrane, 62–63
　physical examination of, 56
Tympanometry, 57
　middle ear otalgia and, 63–64

Ultrasound heat therapy, 280
Upper extremity weakness, with spinal cord lesions, 266–267
Uveitis, 93–94, *94*

Vagoglossopharyngeal neuralgia, background on, 35
　characteristics of, 35, 36(t)
　chronic pain syndrome with, 321–324
　cocaine test for diagnosis of, 37
　idiopathic nature of, 35
　incidence and age of onset of, 35–36
　left-sided preponderance of, 36
　medical therapy for, 37
　oropharyngeal pain with, 132, 134, *134*
　otalgia and, 70
　signs and symptoms of, 36–37
　surgical therapy for, 37–38
Valium, for pain syndrome, 296
Valsalva maneuver, female preponderance of, 25
　tympanic membrane motion and, 56
　vascular headaches and, 25
Vascular headaches, onset and duration of, 12
　pulsatile quality of, 25
　signs and symptoms of, 24–25

Index

Vasomotor rhinitis, nasal lesions from, 109
Ventral roots, function of, 258
Ventralis posterolateralis (VPL), 8
Vertebrae, anatomy of, 255–256, *256*
Vertebral artery, anatomy of, 258
    compression of, 260, *263*
        bulbar signs with, 267
        reflex testing for, 272
    pain with compromise of, 266
Vertical freeway space, muscular kinesiography of, *231*
    neuromuscular occlusion and, 225–228
    orthotic appliances and, 228–229, *230–233*
Vertigo, middle ear otalgia and, 66
Vidian neuralgia, otalgia and, 73
Vincent's angina, 124, 136
Viral pharyngitis, 136–137
Visual acuity testing for eye pain, 78
Vocal cord nodules, laryngeal inflammation and, 147
Vocational counseling, after spinal injury, 285
Von Frey pain theory, 8

Wallenberg's syndrome, pain with artery compromise in, 266

Weber test, middle ear otalgia and, 65
Wegener's granulomatosis, 103–104, *105*
    treatment of, 113
Whiplash injury, pain associated with, *259*, 259–260
    tooth trauma and, 118
    with retrodiskal fiber disorders, 206–207
Wisdom teeth, 118

Xanax, for pain syndrome, 296
X-ray, chest, nasal pain diagnosis and, 111
    panoramic dental, temporomandibular joint function and, 189, *191*

Yale cervicothoracic orthosis, 277
Yin and yang, pain theory and, 3–4

Zenker's diverticula, 141
Ziehl-Neelsen stain, nasal culture and, 111–112